Evidence Based
Physical Therapy

Evidence Based Physical Therapy

Linda Fetters, PhD, PT, FAPTA
Professor
Skyes Family Chair in Pediatric Physical Therapy,
Health & Development
Division of Biokinesiology & Physical Therapy
Department of Pediatrics, Keck School of Medicine
University of Southern California
Los Angeles, California

Julie Tilson, PT, DPT, MS, NCS
Associate Professor of Clinical Physical Therapy
Division of Biokinesiology and Physical Therapy
University of Southern California
Los Angeles, California

F.A. Davis Company • Philadelphia

1915 Arch Street
Philadelphia, PA 19103
www.fadavis.com

Printed in the United States of America

Last digit indicates print number: 10 9 8 7 6 5 4 3

Acquisitions Editor: Margaret M. Biblis
Manager of Content Development: George W. Lang
Developmental Editor: Peg Waltner
Manager of Art and Design: Carolyn O'Brien

Cover Image: Avian/Shutterstock.com

As new scientific information becomes available through basic and clinical research, recommended treatments and drug therapies undergo changes. The author(s) and publisher have done everything possible to make this book accurate, up to date, and in accord with accepted standards at the time of publication. The author(s), editors, and publisher are not responsible for errors or omissions or for consequences from application of the book, and make no warranty, expressed or implied, in regard to the contents of the book. Any practice described in this book should be applied by the reader in accordance with professional standards of care used in regard to the unique circumstances that may apply in each situation. The reader is advised always to check product information (package inserts) for changes and new information regarding dose and contraindications before administering any drug. Caution is especially urged when using new or infrequently ordered drugs.

Library of Congress Cataloging-in-Publication Data

Fetters, Linda, 1948-
  Evidence-based physical therapy / Linda Fetters, Julie Tilson.
      p. ; cm.
  Includes bibliographical references and index.
  ISBN 978-0-8036-1716-2 (pbk. : alk. paper)
  I. Tilson, Julie. II. Title.
  [DNLM: 1. Physical Therapy Modalities. 2. Evidence-Based Medicine. WB 460]
615.8'2—dc23

                                        2012002237

Teaching and learning is a constant dynamic. My dedication is to the world's most dynamic teacher both in the classroom and in life, my husband Mike Fetters; to all the students and colleagues who continue to give me feedback about best teaching, including my co-author Julie Tilson, and to my sons Seth and Zachary, who taught me how to learn.
LF

Life is neither in the wick, nor in the wax, but in the burning. My dedication is to those who light my way in life: my parents, Mike and Jennifer, who taught me to believe in myself; the many students and colleagues who inspire me, particularly my co-author Linda Fetters, who generously invited me on this journey; and most important, my ever supportive and loving husband Donovan Steutel, truly the light of my life.
JT

Foreword

As someone interested in action, I rarely read forewords. So I will keep this one short and cut to the chase. The last few decades have seen a revolution in medical care, particularly in physiotherapy. Research is shedding light on many old and new practices. Harnessing this research for the benefits of patients means that modern practitioners will need new skills—evidence based practice (EBP)—that are complementary to the clinical skills and patient orientation needed for good care. Good clinical practice now requires the three pillars shown in Chapter 1, Figure 1.1, of this book: (1) clinical expertise (gained by good training plus years of experience with feedback), (2) understanding of patient values (requiring good history-taking skills and shared decision-making skills), and (3) skills in locating and appraising research literature: all three the subjects of this book.

The ideas behind EBP—the empirical testing of theories about treatment and diagnosis by careful study in groups of patients—date back many centuries to at least the 10th century and Al Rhazi in Persia (for those interested in learning more about Al Rhazi, Lind, Bradford-Hill, and the whole history of clinical trials, an excellent resource is www.jameslindlibrary.org). The 20th century saw a rapid development in the methods for both clinical research and connecting this research directly to clinical practice. A pivotal moment in this long development was the coining of the term "evidence-based medicine" for a series of articles — the "user guides" — published in the Journal of the American Medical Association (JAMA) in the 1990s. The new term and the JAMA series helped spark worldwide interest of clinicians across countries and disciplines. Professional curricula have been slowly catching up with this revolution. Whereas some educational programs still debate the need to include EBP, for many others it has become the norm. The three pillars of EBP are seen as essential skills in the lifelong learning now needed in the fast-moving world of clinical care.

Physiotherapy has undergone its own revolution in the past few decades, emerging from its apprenticeship craft to become a more scientifically focused discipline. The growth in research has been astonishing. The Physiotherapy Evidence Database (PEDro) (www.pedro.org.au) now contains over 19,000 randomized trials, systematic reviews, and clinical practice guidelines in physiotherapy, and it continues to grow rapidly. Currently, the number of randomized trials in physiotherapy doubles about every 7 years (see Chapter 7, Figure 7.2). That implies that the last 7 years has seen as many trials as in all the previous history of physiotherapy. Whereas some trials merely confirm current practice as correct, some will overturn ideas, and others will introduce new methods and practices. This growth and change is potentially a great blessing for patients. However, for that blessing to reach the bedside, clinicians must be highly skilled in accessing, interpreting, and applying this wealth of research evidence.

The goal of this book is to support the learning of those skills. However, EBP must be adapted to be adopted. Although the fundamental principles are the same, the needs and contents of each health-care discipline require the principles of EBP to be framed and applied in ways that suit its special issues and research base. EBP looks somewhat different in medicine, psychiatry, nursing, and physiotherapy. This book, then, is an essential bridge to assist the application of EBP to physiotherapy.

Dr. Fetters and Dr. Tilson have done an excellent job in describing the fundamentals of EBP and expertly adapting them to the needs of physiotherapists using everyday clinical examples to illustrate the processes. Using this book will help in learning these vital skills for 21st century practice. But that is not enough. The methods of EBP must also be practiced and integrated into your professional life and clinical care for the real benefits to patients to be seen. I wish you well with that vital task.

Paul Glasziou
Professor, Centre for Research in Evidence-Based Practice
Bond University

Preface

We created this book as a learning tool for physical therapy students and clinicians who want to become evidence based practitioners. It can also serve as a tool for more experienced physical therapists who want to continue to improve their knowledge and skills as evidence based therapists. With this book you can develop skills to search the literature for the best and most applicable research for your patients and critically appraise this literature for quality and clinical application. We have included chapters on the use of current technology and forms of communication in order to support realistic practice in the busy clinical workplace.

This book is the product of our years of teaching evidence based practice (EBP) to physical therapy students, physical therapists, and faculty. Our teaching has taken many forms including online, classroom, laboratory, and through institutes organized specifically for faculty who teach EBP to physical therapists. Throughout our teaching years, we searched for a book that was targeted to physical therapists and supported the dynamic learner. When our search failed, we decided to write our own book! During this process, we asked and received feedback from many students and colleagues. This feedback was critical to our final product; the book has been greatly improved as a result. We owe thanks to the anonymous reviewers who were solicited by F.A. Davis. Their thoughtful and thorough reviews were valuable to our process. Finally, a special thanks to Weslie Holland, whose enthusiastic, prompt, and expert assistance was greatly appreciated.

Writing a book is a lot of work over an extensive period. One sure way to complete a book is to be passionate about the subject and, more important, to be passionate about not just teaching the subject, but learning the subject. We are both. In addition, it helps to have a sense of humor. In fact, a sense of humor helps everything in life, particularly those aspects that are a lot of work over an extensive period. Our passion for teaching and learning has always been complemented by our humor, enjoyment of the content and process, and respect and enjoyment of each other. We wish you a successful journey toward becoming an evidence based physical therapist.

Linda Fetters
Julie Tilson

Reviewers

Peter Altenburger, MS, PT
Assistant Professor
University of Nevada
Henderson, Nevada

Sherrilene Classen, PhD, MPH, OTR
University of Florida
Gainesville, Florida

Deanna C. Dye, PT, PhD
Assistant Professor
Idaho State University
Pocatello, Idaho

Marie Earl, PhD, PT
Assistant Professor
Dalhousie University
Halifax, Nova Scotia, Canada

Steven Z. George, PT, MS, PhD
Assistant Professor
University of Florida
Gainesville, Florida

Shelley Goodgold, PT, ScD
Professor
Simmons College
Boston, Massachusetts

Brenda L. Greene, PT, PhD
Assistant Professor
Emory University
Atlanta, Georgia

Penelope J. Klein, PT, EdD
Professor
D'Youville College
Buffalo, New York

Barbara J. Norton, PT, PhD
Associate Professor and Associate Director
Washington University
St. Louis, Missouri

Jena B. Ogston, PhD, PT
Associate Professor
College of St. Scholastica
Duluth, Minnesota

Christopher Powers, PhD, PT
Associate Professor
University of Southern California
Los Angeles, California

Kelly Sass, PT, MPT
Assistant Academic Coordinator and Associate Faculty
University of Iowa
Iowa City, Iowa

Joseph Schreiber, PT, MS, PCS
Assistant Professor
Chatham College
Pittsburgh, Pennsylvania

Contents

How to Use This Book

Goals and Audience

This book was created for the physical therapy student and clinician who want to practice evidence based physical therapy. Our goal is to provide sufficient information to guide the development of the necessary skills to become an independent evidence based practitioner. We recognize that, just like any other skill, practice is essential to effective and efficient learning. We assume the reader is at the beginning of the learning process and, therefore, the content of the book includes the necessary information to become an entry-level evidence based physical therapist.

Content

The book is divided into three sections, but chapters can be used independently.

Section I: Finding and Appraising Evidence to Improve Patient Care

Section II: Appraising Other Types of Studies: Beyond the Randomized Clinical Trial

Section III: Communication and Technology for Evidence Based Practice

Each chapter in our book was designed to "stand alone," such that each chapter can be assigned in any order and does not necessarily proceed from Chapter 1 through Chapter 12. The organization of the content of this book does, however, reflect our teaching process. More important, it reflects the learning process that our students have taught us. Over our years of teaching both separately and together, we have organized our evidence based practice (EBP) course using various sequences of the topics included in this book. Our students have commented on each sequence, and we have reflected on the students' knowledge and skills achieved through the use of each sequence. Although there is no one sequence that is "best" to teach EBP, we suggest that the novice to EBP benefits from reading *Section I: Finding and Appraising Evidence to Improve Patient Care*, Chapters 1–4, first and in this order. These chapters provide the basics of identifying clinical questions that can be searched effectively in the literature and the necessary search skills to find the best available research evidence (Chapters 1 and 2). Basic appraisal skills for intervention research that can be combined effectively with clinical expertise and patient goals and values are the topics of Chapters 3 and 4. Many of the basic skills that are developed in Chapters 1–4 can then be applied to specific topic areas found in *Section II: Appraising Other Types of Studies: Beyond the Randomized Clinical Trial* (Chapters 5–8). Section II includes, for example, appraisal skills for the diagnostic literature (Chapter 5) and the prognostic literature (Chapter 6). But teachers and learners combine in unique ways, and this book is designed to be used effectively for a variety of teaching and learning styles.

Most chapters include "Digging Deeper" sections. These sections include material that offers depth in a topic and may be considered either optional or required learning material. We designed these for the learner who wants more information on a topic, but with the view that the material presented in these sections may be beyond entry level. We also include "Self-Tests" in most chapters. These should be used as opportunities for learners to reflect on their knowledge and skills in EBP and determine if additional study of a topic is warranted.

The text is abundantly supported with visual information to support EBP concepts. Teachers and learners may find it helpful to concentrate first on the illustrations of a concept and later on the text supporting the concept.

We believe that this book can be used to support the learning of effective and efficient skills to become evidence based physical therapists.

1 The Evidence Based Practice Model

PRE-TEST

1. Can you explain to someone else what evidence based practice (EBP) is and why it is important?

2. Can you describe the three primary sources of evidence for EBP?

3. What are the five steps of EBP?

4. What is known about EBP in the real world?

CHAPTER-AT-A-GLANCE

This chapter will help you understand the following:

- Definition and purpose of EBP

- Three principal sources of evidence for EBP: research, patient perspective, clinical expertise

- The five steps of EBP: identify a question, search, appraise, integrate, evaluate

- The challenges of and solutions for EBP in the real world

■ Introduction

What is EBP and Why is it Important?

Evidence based practice (EBP) is a method of clinical decision making and practice that integrates the best available scientific research evidence with clinical expertise and a patient's unique values and circumstances.[1,2] For the evidence based therapist, these three sources of evidence (scientific research, clinical expertise, and patient values and circumstances) form a foundation on which you and your patients will work together to determine the best course of physical therapy care in any given circumstance (Fig. 1.1). The goal of evidence based therapists is to ensure that the best available evidence informs patient care to optimize the benefit that patients gain from therapy.

As an evidence based therapist, you will provide care that is grounded in scientific research, guided by clinical expertise, and ultimately directed by your patients' individual values and circumstances. Third-party payers, patients, and the general health-care community have a steadily increasing expectation that physical therapists will be evidence based. The effort that you put into EBP will not only fulfill the expectations of others, it will also enhance the quality and credibility of your services. This will lead to enhanced confidence and ability to assist patients in choosing their best options for physical therapy care. EBP moves the physical therapy profession away from practice based on habit and toward a careful, systematic assessment of the best available evidence to inform patient care. By carefully appraising what is known from multiple reference points, you will be better prepared to provide your patients with the best care that physical therapy has to offer.

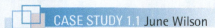

CASE STUDY 1.1 June Wilson

Consider June Wilson, a 17-year-old swimmer referred to your outpatient clinic for neck pain 3 days before the state high school swimming championships in which she is scheduled to compete. June and her parents will expect you, the movement expert, to be able to answer their questions. June might ask you:

"Why does my neck hurt?"
"What are the chances that I will be able to swim without pain in 3 days?"
"What will you be able to do to help me get better?"

As an evidence based therapist, you will be able to give June and her family answers based on the best available evidence from scientific research, clinical expertise, and June's personal values and circumstances. This is likely to enhance the quality of your care and increase your credibility with June and her parents. In addition, your EBP skills can make you more effective when working with medical care providers, third-party payers, and legislators.

June and her family maintain ultimate control over all of her medical decisions. As a therapist, you make recommendations about how June should proceed in physical therapy. As an evidence based therapist you will be able to provide patients with the information and education they need to work with you to make a shared-informed decision. A shared-informed decision is defined as a choice that is generated through a partnership between the therapist and patient and that is informed by the best evidence.[3] **This case is followed from Chapters 1 through 4.**

EBP provides a structured method for thinking about and collecting the different types of evidence used to make clinical decisions. As described above and in Figure 1.1, evidence can be thought of as coming from three different sources:

1. Scientific research
2. Clinical expertise
3. Patient values and circumstances

 ### DIGGING DEEPER 1.1

What do you expect when you are the patient?

Think back to the last time that you or a close friend or family member saw a health-care provider for a medical problem. Did you expect that the diagnosis, treatment plan, and prognosis to be based on current research, the medical professionals' experience, and consideration for you or your loved one? Would you have been satisfied if those decisions had been based on knowledge that was out of date, the most recent market fad, or information that the physician learned in school 20 years ago?

Picture yourself sitting in an orthopedic surgeon's office receiving a diagnosis of rotator cuff tear. The surgeon would need to decide whether to recommend that you have surgery.

■ List three things the surgeon would need to know about you to guide the decision making.

■ Name the key decision makers who would help you decide whether to have surgery.
■ What questions would you need to ask the surgeon to ensure that the right decision was made about your care?
■ What sources of information would you expect the surgeon to use to answer your questions?

Patients expect, even demand, that medical care be based on the best available evidence. Patients and the public expect this of you as a physical therapist.

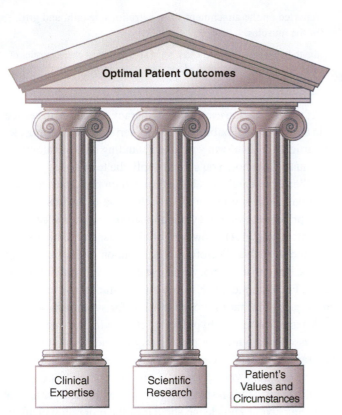

FIGURE 1.1 The three pillars of evidence that support optimal outcomes for patients. The patient and the therapist contribute evidence to the decision-making process. As the evidence is collected, the therapist and the patient engage in a dynamic process using evidence to make a shared-informed decision.

Figure 1.2 illustrates how the patient and therapist use the three sources of evidence to identify a shared-informed decision that is likely to lead to the best possible outcomes.

■ Understanding the EBP Model

What are the Sources of Evidence?

Continuing with the case, June Wilson and her parents will expect your answers to their questions and recommendations for June's care to be based on high-quality evidence. As an evidence based therapist it is important to consider all three sources of evidence—together the three sources are stronger than any one source on its own. In this section the three sources of evidence are presented in detail.

Scientific Research

Scientific research evidence is empirical evidence acquired through systematic testing of a hypothesis. Therapists access two general types of scientific research, clinical research and basic science research. **Clinical research** involves human subjects and answers questions about diagnosis, intervention, prevention, and prognosis in relation to disease or injury.

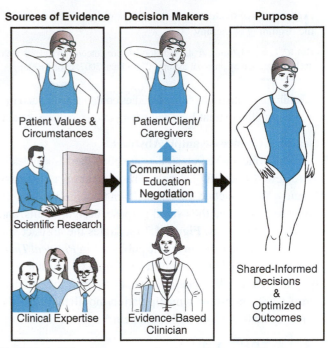

FIGURE 1.2 The three sources of evidence that are used by the patient-clinician team to achieve a shared-informed decision.

For example:

A *diagnostic* study by Wainner et al[3] showed that several tests conducted together (Upper Limb Tension Test A, cervical rotation <60°, cervical distraction test, and Spurling A) are more effective for identifying cervical radiculopathy than is any individual test.

Wainner RS, Fritz JM, Irrgang JJ, et al. Reliability and diagnostic accuracy of the clinical examination and patient self-report measures for cervical radiculopathy. *Spine.* 2003;28:52-62.

An *intervention* study conducted by Cleland et al[4] determined that for people with neck pain, thrust mobilization/manipulation of the thoracic spine results in significantly greater short-term reductions in pain and disability compared with non-thrust mobilization/manipulation of the thoracic spine.

Cleland JA, Glynn P, Whitman JM, et al. Short-term effects of thrust versus nonthrust mobilization/manipulation directed at the thoracic spine in patients with neck pain: A randomized clinical trial. *Phys Ther.* 2007;87(4):431-440.

A *prevention* study conducted by Linton and Andersson[5] found that cognitive behavior group intervention can lower the risk of developing long-term disability among patients with spinal pain who perceived that they were at risk of developing chronic pain.

Linton SJ, Andersson T. Can chronic disability be prevented? A randomized trial of a cognitive-behavior intervention and two forms of information for patients with spinal pain. *Spine.* 2000;25:2825-2831.

A *prognostic* study conducted by Hill et al[6] found that the amount of recovery from neck pain that can be expected 6 weeks after physical therapy is influenced by patients' social class, expectations of treatment success, and severity of neck pain at the beginning of therapy.

Hill JC, Lewis M, Sim J, et al. Predictors of poor outcome in patients with neck pain treated by physical therapy. Clin J Pain. 2007;23:683-690.

Familiarity with each of these studies could influence and improve your ability to treat June and other patients with neck pain.

Research Evidence—Sample Abstract

Results of clinical research studies are published as articles in peer-reviewed scientific journals. The **abstract** is a summary of a study. With practice, therapists learn to quickly review an abstract to understand the overall purpose, design, results, and conclusions of a study. Figure 1.3 illustrates the abstract and author information from an article published in *Physical Therapy* (www.ptjournal.org), the official journal of the American Physical Therapy Association, that compared the efficacy of thrust with non-thrust manipulation/mobilization to the thoracic spine in persons with neck pain.[4]

■ SELF-TEST 1.1

Read the abstract in Figure 1.3, then close the book and write down as many facts about the study as you can remember. As you gain skills as an evidence based therapist you will find that key facts from the abstract help you to quickly understand the fundamental aspects of a research study.

When there is insufficient clinical research on a particular topic, therapists can look to research in similar fields (e.g., studies on healthy participants) and basic science research. From these studies you can extrapolate, with caution, how patients will respond in a clinical situation. Studies of healthy individuals help therapists understand what is normal and can lead to hypotheses about how best to care for persons with an injury or disease condition.

For example:

A study by Kluemper et al[7] involving swimmers without pain or injury found that a shoulder stretching and strengthening program reduced forward shoulder posture after 6 weeks.

Kluemper M, Uhl T, Hazelrigg H. Effect of stretching and strengthening shoulder muscles on forward shoulder posture in competitive swimmers. *J Sport Rehab.* 2006;15:58-70.

If, based on your knowledge of anatomy and biomechanics, you believe that June's pain is associated with forward shoulder posture, this study could affect your prescription of shoulder stretching and strengthening exercises.

Basic science research often involves non-human research and is fundamental to evidence based physical therapy.

For example:

A study by Smith et al[8] involved a series of 13 dissections of serratus anterior muscles in human cadavers. The study reported on the attachment sites, serrations, length, and girth of the muscles.

Smith R, Nyquist-Battie C, Clark M, et al. Anatomical characteristics of the upper serratus anterior: Cadaver dissection. *J Ortho Sports Phys Ther.* 2003;33:449-454.

If you decided to use a manual therapy technique to reduce pain and increase flexibility of June's serratus anterior muscle, this article could inform your understanding of the anatomy of this muscle and how you should apply the technique.

Clinical research should be founded on principles learned from basic science research with the goal of understanding those principles when they are applied in the patient care environment (Fig. 1.4). However, clinical research is time- and resource-intensive. Therefore, it is common to find intriguing basic science that has not been investigated in a patient population. For example, the Kluemper et al[7] study reported an exercise program that improved posture for swimmers without neck pain. You might hypothesize that swimmers *with* neck pain associated with poor posture might benefit from the same program. A clinical research study involving patients with neck pain would help you to know if your hypothesis is correct. Until the program is tested on swimmers with shoulder and/or neck injury, your knowledge about how the program will affect patients is limited. In this case, however, if the Kluemper et al[7] study is judged to be of sufficient quality, you might tell swimmers such as June that this particular stretching and strengthening program might improve forward shoulder posture. Naturally, when you educate a patient about research evidence, it is important to use layperson terms and to confirm that the patient understands by asking follow-up questions.

Therapists have the primary responsibility to identify, evaluate, and summarize research evidence concerning a patient's care. Sometimes, however, a patient will acquire research evidence relevant to his or her condition. In this case, the clinician can assist the patient to ensure accurate evaluation and interpretation of the evidence. Methods for effectively and efficiently appraising research evidence are presented in Chapters 3 through 10.

Clinical Expertise

Clinical expertise refers to implicit and explicit knowledge about physical therapy diagnosis, treatment, prevention, and prognosis gained from cumulative years of caring for patients with disease and injury and working to improve and refine that care. Therapists share a collective professional wisdom acquired through decades of providing patient care. Much of that wisdom has yet to be tested, and some cannot be tested, by scientific inquiry. Professional clinical expertise is passed from clinician to clinician in the formal academic setting, post-professional education (e.g., continuing education courses, residencies), formal mentorship, and informally between colleagues. As a new therapist you will discover that identifying an expert mentor who readily shares his or her clinical

Research Report

Short-Term Effects of Thrust Versus Nonthrust Mobilization/Manipulation Directed at the Thoracic Spine in Patients With Neck Pain: A Randomized Clinical Trial

Joshua A Cleland, Paul Glynn, Julie M Whitman, Sarah L Eberhart, Cameron MacDonald, John D Childs

Background and Purpose

Evidence supports the use of manual physical therapy interventions directed at the thoracic spine in patients with neck pain. The purpose of this study was to compare the effectiveness of thoracic spine thrust mobilization/manipulation with that of nonthrust mobilization/manipulation in patients with a primary complaint of mechanical neck pain. The authors also sought to compare the frequencies, durations, and types of side effects between the groups.

Subjects

The subjects in this study were 60 patients who were 18 to 60 years of age and had a primary complaint of neck pain.

Methods

For all subjects, a standardized history and a physical examination were obtained. Self-report outcome measures included the Neck Disability Index (NDI), a pain diagram, the Numeric Pain Rating Scale (NPRS), and the Fear-Avoidance Beliefs Questionnaire. After the baseline evaluation, the subjects were randomly assigned to receive either thoracic spine thrust or nonthrust mobilization/manipulation. The subjects were reexamined 2 to 4 days after the initial examination, and they again completed the NDI and the NPRS, as well as the Global Rating of Change (GROC) Scale. The primary aim was examined with a 2-way repeated-measures analysis of variance (ANOVA), with intervention group (thrust versus nonthrust mobilization/manipulation) as the between-subjects variable and time (baseline and 48 hours) as the within-subject variable. Separate ANOVAs were performed for each dependent variable: disability (NDI) and pain (NPRS). For each ANOVA, the hypothesis of interest was the 2-way group X time interaction.

Results

Sixty patients with a mean age of 43.3 years (SD=12.7) (55% female) satisfied the eligibility criteria and agreed to participate in the study. Subjects who received thrust mobilization/ manipulation experienced greater reductions in disability, with a between-group difference of 10% (95% confidence interval [CI] =5.3–14.7), and in pain, with a between-group difference of 2.0 (95% CI=1.4 –2.7). Subjects in the thrust mobilization/manipulation group exhibited significantly higher scores on the GROC Scale at the time of follow-up. No differences in the frequencies, durations, and types of side effects existed between the groups.

Discussion and Conclusion

The results suggest that thoracic spine thrust mobilization/manipulation results in significantly greater short-term reductions in pain and disability than does thoracic nonthrust mobilization/manipulation in people with neck pain.

JA Cleland, PT, DPT, PhD, OCS, FAAOMPT, is Assistant Professor, Department of Physical Therapy, Franklin Pierce College, 5 Chenell Dr, Concord, NH 03301 (USA); Research Coordinator, Rehabilitation Services, Concord Hospital, Concord, NH; and Faculty, Manual Physical Therapy Fellowship Program, Regis University, Denver, Colo. Address all correspondence to Dr Cleland at: joshcleland@comcast.net.

P Glynn, PT, DPT, OCS, FAAOMPT, is Physical Therapy Clinical Specialist, Newton-Wellesley Hospital, Newton, Mass, and Fellow, Manual Physical Therapy Fellowship Program, Regis University.

JM Whitman, PT, DSc, OCS, FAAOMPT, is Assistant Faculty, Department of Physical Therapy, and Faculty, Manual Physical Therapy Fellowship Program, Regis University.

SL Eberhart, PT, MPT, is Physical Therapist and Clinical II, Rehabilitation Services, Concord Hospital.

C MacDonald, PT, DPT, GCS, OCS, FAAOMPT, is Physical Therapist, Centennial Physical Therapy, Colorado Sport and Spine Centers, Colorado Springs, Colo.

JD Childs, PT, PhD, MBA, OCS, FAAOMPT, is Assistant Professor and Director of Research, Doctoral Program in Physical Therapy, US Army–Baylor University, San Antonio, Tex.

[Cleland JA, Glynn P, Whitman JM, et al. Short-term effects of thrust versus nonthrust mobilization/manipulation directed at the thoracic spine in patients with neck pain: a randomized clinical trial. *Phys Ther.* 2007;87:431–440.]

 For The Bottom Line: www.ptjournal.org

FIGURE 1.3 Abstract from Cleland JA, Glynn P, Whitman JM, Eberhart SL, MacDonald C, Childs JD. Short-term effects of thrust versus nonthrust mobilization/manipulation directed at the thoracic spine in patients with neck pain: A randomized clinical trial. *Phys Ther.* 2007;87:431-440.

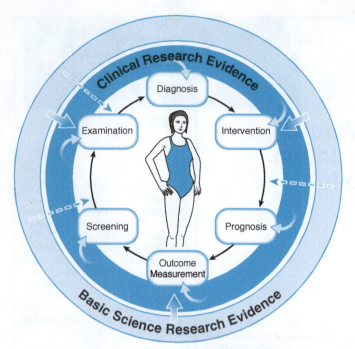

FIGURE 1.4 How different types of research contribute to evidence based patient care. Basic science research evidence informs clinical research evidence, which informs how we provide care in all aspects of patient management (screening, examination, diagnosis, intervention, prognosis, and outcome measurement). The dashed line arrows indicate that basic science research evidence informs patient management when clinical research evidence is not sufficient.

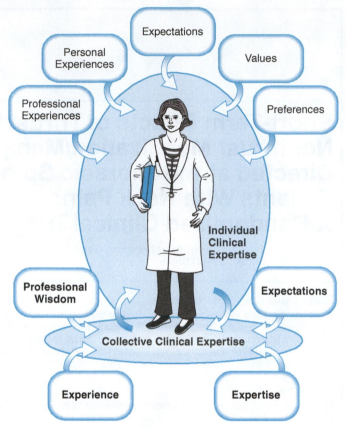

FIGURE 1.5 The interplay between components of collective and individual clinical expertise.

expertise with you is a critical component to becoming an evidence based therapist. As does research evidence, clinical expertise needs to be appraised for quality.

In addition to gaining evidence from experts in the profession, each individual therapist develops his or her own clinical expertise (Fig. 1.5). Reflective therapists develop clinical knowledge by explicitly thinking about their clinical encounters with patients.[9] As a reflective therapist, you will use experience from previous patients to generate expectations for future patients. Those expectations play an important role in the shared decision-making process with patients. Finally, as an individual, each therapist uses his or her own values and preferences as evidence. Our values and preferences are important, but they naturally lead to biases in decision making. It is important to evaluate and recognize your biases so that they do not overpower other sources of evidence.

Let's explore clinical expertise as a source of evidence with respect to caring for June Wilson (Case Study 1.1). Although there are numerous studies that have examined what tests and measures should be used to diagnose June's condition and which interventions are most likely to reduce her pain and improve her function, there will never be research evidence that describes the effectiveness of every element of your interaction with June. For example, suppose June has a significant forward head-and-shoulders posture. Studies that report the value of educating a 17-year-old swimmer with neck pain about the

impact of body mechanics during swimming may not exist. However, based on anatomical evidence, physical therapists have hypothesized that forward head-and-shoulders posture can put increased strain on the soft-tissue structures of the neck, causing pain. As June's therapist, you would need to use clinical expertise and your observations of her movement to inform the degree to which postural education should constitute June's physical therapy treatment.

Patient Values and Circumstances

The patient and his or her caregivers create the most important pillar of evidence to the decision-making process. Figure 1.6 illustrates that evidence from the patient can be divided into two categories: values and circumstances. Patient values include the beliefs, preferences, expectations, and cultural identification that the patient brings to the therapy environment.[1] Fundamentally, values are the core principles that guide a person's life and life choices. Therapists will encounter patients with diverse values that affect their physical therapy care. For example, patients may weigh the value of family involvement and independence differently. Consider June; she may feel strongly that her parents should be directly involved in all therapy decisions. Conversely, she may have a strong desire for personal independence, wishing to have autonomous control

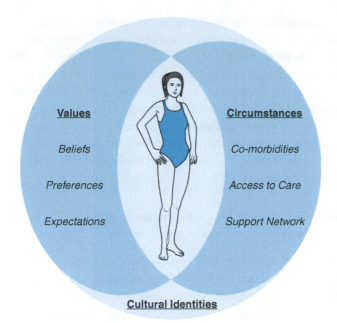

Values

Beliefs

Preferences

Expectations

Circumstances

Co-morbidities

Access to Care

Support Network

Cultural Identities

FIGURE 1.6 Components of patient values and circumstances that contribute to patient perspective as evidence.

over as many decisions as possible. Either scenario, if recognized by the therapist, can be leveraged to help June benefit optimally from therapy. Values are generated from personal and spiritual beliefs and must be respected and accommodated even when they do not match yours.

Patient preferences serve as important evidence for guiding treatment decisions. For example, some patients excel at completing a therapy exercise program consistently on a daily basis. They can readily incorporate a prescribed home exercise program into their lifestyle and monitor their progress independently. Other patients prefer to avoid therapeutic exercise to the fullest extent possible. If the latter represents June's preference, she may need to see a direct benefit before she will engage in any exercise program to address her neck pain. When patients are resistant to sharing preferences, consider whether they lack sufficient understanding of the situation to develop a preference, lack confidence to make or share a preference, or feel uncomfortable or embarrassed about their preference. Considering the situation from the patient's perspective can significantly enhance communication.

Patient expectations may also affect their responses to physical therapy. If June's father had previous physical therapy for an anterior cruciate ligament (ACL) repair, the family might conclude that physical therapy for June's neck injury will be painful (often the case for ACL repair rehabilitation programs but rarely for neck pain). In addition, because June is slated to swim in her state championships in 3 days, she is likely to have high expectations for a rapid solution to her pain. Conversely, she and/or her parents might have unusually high or low expectations for June's recovery depending on previous life experiences.

Patient circumstances encompasses information about the patient's medical history (e.g., co-morbidities), access to medical services (e.g., rural versus urban or insured versus uninsured), and family environment (e.g., lives with parents versus lives in foster home). For example, if June has a history of juvenile rheumatoid arthritis, the use of thrust and non-thrust manipulation of the thoracic spine for reduction of neck pain may not be appropriate.

All patient values and circumstances can be influenced by the culture(s) with which a patient identifies. Some cultural identifications are easy to recognize, whereas others are more subtle. The therapist who learns about the cultural norms of unique patient populations and remembers that individuals may or may not follow those norms will be well served. For example, if June and her family are recent immigrants from Iraq, the therapist might expect that the family will have significant concerns about June exposing her torso to a male therapist.[10] That said, if the male therapist did not discuss this with the family but rather referred June to a female therapist without explanation, June might interpret this action as unwarranted rejection.

The ability to integrate what you, as an evidence based therapist, learn from scientific research, from clinical expertise, and from patient values and circumstances is essential to providing the best possible physical therapy care. Integration of the three evidence pillars into daily patient interactions takes practice. Patients benefit when you judiciously share the clinical bottom-line message from quality research articles. You can share clinical experience and expectations with your patients, using phrases such as, "I have found that" or "You may respond best to." By conducting a skilled interview, you learn about patient values and circumstances. Figure 1.7 illustrates an example of the contributions that different components of evidence can make for both you and the patient.

■ The EBP Process: What Does the Evidence Based Therapist Actually Do?

EBP can be thought of as having five fundamental steps (Fig. 1.8) that facilitate successful evidence collection, appraisal, and integration.[11] This section summarizes each of the steps and indicates where they are addressed in this book.

Five Steps in the EBP Process

STEP 1: Identify the need for information and develop a focused and searchable clinical question

The first step of EBP involves collecting information from the patient and identifying a need for additional information for

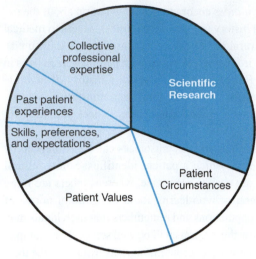

Example of a possible distribution of sources of evidence for a **therapist**

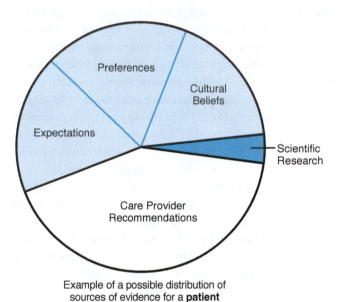

Example of a possible distribution of sources of evidence for a **patient**

FIGURE 1.7 An example of the diverse sources of information that contribute to patient and therapist evidence when making a decision about best health care.

clinical decision making. Once you identify that you need information, you will develop a specific question called a **searchable clinical question.** In Chapter 2 we will explore the different types of searchable clinical questions, and you will have a chance to practice writing your own. A well-developed searchable clinical question has a specific structure that makes it easier to search databases for the best available research evidence. A question that is too narrow may not lead to any applicable articles. A question that is too broad could result in an overwhelming set of possible articles.

STEP 2: Conduct a search to find the best possible research evidence to answer your question

The second step of the EBP process involves using electronic databases to search for specific research evidence to answer your clinical question. Chapter 2 describes how to search for and retrieve the best available research to inform your question from step 1. First, you need to know what type of research evidence will assist you in making clinical decisions. The Evidence Pyramid (Fig. 1.9) illustrates a hierarchy that can be used as an initial filter for identifying high-quality research evidence. Systematic Reviews (SRs), studies that combine other studies, are at the top of the pyramid and represent the highest level of research evidence. Below SRs are individual studies including randomized clinical trials (RCTs) and cohort studies. Evidence based clinical practice guidelines (CPGs) are illustrated separately from the pyramid but slightly above SRs. CPGs are not research studies but rather a comprehensive summary of research studies developed by experts in the field. CPGs include direct recommendations for practice that combine best clinical research and clinical expertise.

The most efficient way to search for the best research evidence is to start by searching for CPGs and then, if necessary

Step 1	Identify the need for information and develop a focused and searchable **clinical question**.
Step 2	Conduct a **search** to find the best possible research evidence to answer your question.
Step 3	Critically **appraise** the research evidence for applicability and quality.
Step 4	**Integrate** the critically appraised research evidence with clinical expertise and the patient's values and circumstances.
Step 5	**Evaluate** the effectiveness and efficacy of your efforts in Steps 1–4 and identify ways to improve them in the future.

FIGURE 1.8 The five-step EBP process. This figure is used throughout this book to orient you to the step being addressed.

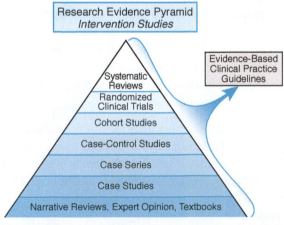

FIGURE 1.9 The Evidence Pyramid illustrates a hierarchy of best sources of evidence for searchable clinical questions. Categories of research evidence are ordered from top to bottom; higher levels on the pyramid represent the most likely sources of high-quality research evidence. This pyramid is specific to studies about treatment intervention.

(as is frequently the case), proceed down the levels of the pyramid. Learning to search in research databases, such as PubMed, to find the best research evidence takes practice and persistence.

STEP 3: *Critically appraise the research evidence for applicability and quality*

After identifying potentially useful research evidence, you will begin the appraisal process. Study **appraisal** is the process of determining whether an article is applicable to your question and if it is of sufficient quality to help you make a decision. Chapters 3 through 10 are dedicated to helping you learn to appraise different types of studies on the Evidence Pyramid. Figure 1.10 illustrates the rating of research evidence on two scales—applicability and quality. It is unusual for an article to have perfect applicability and perfect quality. Rather, articles fall along a continuum on each scale, and it is up to you to determine if an article is or is not valuable for answering your clinical question. When you are appraising an article, it is important to balance skepticism with open-mindedness. Every study has some deficits—you will learn to read studies critically while avoiding the temptation to dismiss imperfect studies that have value to clinical practice.

STEP 4: *Integrate the critically appraised research evidence with clinical expertise and the patient's values and circumstances*

Having identified and appraised relevant and quality research to inform your searchable clinical question, the fourth step is to integrate the three pillars of EBP. Chapter 11 addresses the art of integrating and communicating the best available evidence to colleagues and patients. As discussed above, research evidence does not provide answers about how to rehabilitate patients. Rather, it informs and provides a framework for practice. Integration of research evidence, clinical expertise, and patient values and circumstances is completed in partnership with the patient and/or his or her family and caregivers. Each case example throughout the book will explore the process of integrating clinical expertise and patient values and circumstances with appraised research evidence to inform your clinical practice.

STEP 5: *Evaluate the effectiveness and efficacy of your efforts in Steps 1 Through 4 and identify ways to improve them in the future*

In step 5 the evidence based therapist reflects on the EBP process and looks for ways to improve. You can do this at the level of the individual patient and at the level of overall practice habits and skills. Chapters 11 and 12 explore methods that you can use to reflect on and continually improve your skills as an evidence based therapist. For example, by using standardized outcome measures consistent with those used in physical therapy research, you will be able to compare your patients' progress with results in the literature. In addition, by learning to use technologies developed to support the evidence based therapist, you can improve your efficiency and effectiveness. By reflecting on your overall habits and skills as a clinician, you will identify knowledge gaps that, when addressed, can lead to a more effective and rewarding quality of life as a practitioner.

To help you picture the five steps in action, Figure 1.11 provides an example of how the EBP process might look for the care of June Wilson.

■ EBP in the Context of Real-Time Clinical Practice: Can EBP Work in the Real World?

You may be wondering if EBP is a realistic expectation for physical therapists working under the pressure of the modern health-care system. In fact, although physical therapists as a group report high value for the importance of EBP they also identify barriers that must be addressed.[12,13] In this book we address these barriers directly to provide you with the tools you need to overcome them. Table 1.1 summarizes these barriers and describes suggestions for how to overcome them.

In 2000, the American Physical Therapy Association established Vision 2020. The vision states that "physical therapists and physical therapist assistants will render evidence based services throughout the continuum of care."[14] With a commitment to lifelong learning, all physical therapists can contribute to the achievement of this goal. Chapters 11 and 12 address mechanisms that you can use to develop lifelong EBP habits and ultimately become a leader in the effort for physical therapy to be an evidence based profession.

Two Independent Scales for Research Evidence Appraisal:

1) **Applicability** to your question:

Low ————————————→ High

■ Study 1
■ Study 2
□ Study 3

2) **Quality** of the study:

Low ————————————→ High

One study can have very different rankings on the two scales.

FIGURE 1.10 Research studies are ranked on two distinct scales: applicability and quality. Study 1 has low applicability to the therapist's case and high quality. Study 2 has moderate applicability and quality. Study 3 has high applicability and low quality. Weighing strengths and weaknesses of each of these studies, the clinician may glean value from all three for guiding practice. The appraisal process allows clinicians to determine the extent to which individual studies should influence their practice.

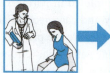

The EBP process starts with a patient interaction, in this case, your initial evaluation of June Wilson.

Step 1:   Clinical Question

In June's case you ask: "For a 17 year old female swimmer, is manual therapy combined with therapeutic exercise more effective than therapeutic exercise alone for rapid reduction of pain and return to swimming?"

Step 2:   Search

You search in PubMed for Randomized Controlled Trials or Systematic Reviews that investigate the merits of manual therapy and therapeutic exercise compared with therapeutic exercise alone.

Step 3:   Appraise

You find a randomized controlled trial by Walker et al published in the journal *Spine* in 2008. You determine that the study is of high quality and has acceptable applicability to your question. You learn that a program of manual therapy and exercise was more effective than a minimal exercise and education program for adults with a primary complaint of neck pain.

Step 4:   Integrate

You talk again with June and her parents and learn that June's mother has high anxiety about the use of 'cracking' treatments of the spine. You know from your knowledge of skeletal development that June's age is not a contraindication for mobilization. You also feel strongly that movement patterns could be contributing to June's pain based on anatomical principles. With June and her parents, you develop a program that includes non-thrust mobilization, daily home exercise, and postural reeducation. You will monitor June's progress with standardized outcome measures to assess her progress.

Step 5:   Evaluate

After June's first treatment she is feeling 50% better. You are pleased with this progress. You wonder if you had looked for a Systematic Review or Clinical Practice Guideline you would have found evidence from more than one study to inform June's care. Next time you might try that first and see how it goes.

FIGURE 1.11 The EBP model contains five steps that start with the patient. Each step is described in the context of Case Study 1.1 concerning June Wilson.

TABLE 1.1   Breaking Down Barriers to EBP

BARRIER	BARRIER BUSTER
Time	Time is the most common barrier to using EBP. Faster searches and study appraisal are keys to success and we will teach you how to optimize speed while maintaining quality in these processes.
Lack of generalizability of research	Therapists treat individual patients but research evidence generally addresses groups of patients. In the chapters on appraisal you will learn how to determine if a study can be applied to a particular patient even if the study sample is not a perfect fit with your patient. You will see that critical thinking skills are an important component to informing care for individual patients with research evidence.
Lack of research skills	Chances are that you did not decide to become a physical therapist so that you could do research. This is the beauty of EBP. As an evidence based therapist you only need to learn to be a *consumer* of research, not a *doer* of research. This book focuses on the skills you need to be a consumer of research.
Lack of understanding of statistics	Statistics are an integral part of most research studies and they can be intimidating. This book will help you to understand and interpret the most common statistical concepts encountered in clinical physical therapy literature.
Lack of search and appraisal skills	Searching for research evidence and appraising it for quality and applicability take practice. Just like completing a subjective history—you won't be very good at it at first. But with practice, you can learn to become very skilled. The examples and exercises in this book will guide your skill development in these key areas.

TABLE I.I   **Breaking Down Barriers to EBP—cont'd**

BARRIER	BARRIER BUSTER
Lack of Information Resources	Dissemination of information is a business. Many therapists encounter barriers when trying to search for and retrieve research evidence. In this book we focus on *free* resources to ensure that any therapist with an Internet connection can find the best available evidence without breaking the bank.
Inconsistent Culture of EBP in Physical Therapy	Physical therapists have vastly different EBP skills and knowledge. In addition, although most studies show that the majority of therapists value EBP, there are certainly therapists who do not. As a new learner of EBP you may be challenged to justify your efforts to integrate all three sources of evidence into patient care. In this book we illustrate this type of conflict through patient cases and study questions to help you develop your leadership skills as an evidence based therapist.

SUMMARY

Evidence based practice (EBP) is defined as the integration of the best available research evidence with clinical expertise and patients' unique values and circumstances. The purpose of EBP is to use the best available evidence from all sources to optimize our patients' benefit from physical therapy. There are three principal sources of evidence for EBP:

1. Research evidence
2. Clinical expertise
3. Patient values and circumstances

The five steps of EBP are designed to facilitate a structured approach to EBP. By making a habit of following the five steps, you will find it easier to succeed as an evidence based therapist. They are:

Step 1: Identify a need for information and construct a focused and searchable clinical question.
Step 2: Conduct a search to find the best possible research evidence to answer your question.

Step 3: Critically appraise the research evidence for validity and applicability.
Step 4: Integrate the critically appraised research evidence with clinical expertise and patient values and circumstances.
Step 5: Evaluate the effectiveness and efficacy of your efforts in Steps 1 through 4 and identify ways to improve them in the future.

Your efforts to become an evidence based therapist will be heavily influenced by the clinical environment in which you practice. Key challenges to EBP reported by therapists are insufficient time, inability to generalize research, lack of knowledge about statistics and research, lack of search and appraisal skills, and the presence of a culture that does not consistently support EBP. This book is designed to help you overcome each of these barriers and become an agent of change as the physical therapy profession earns the reputation of being an evidence based profession.

REVIEW QUESTIONS

1. Define and describe the purpose of EBP. What health-care professions are or are not evidence based? How does being evidence based (or not) influence a profession's reputation? Do you think outsiders would consider physical therapy to be evidence based? How could EBP strengthen the quality of care that you and other therapists provide?

2. Think back to a person whom you know (yourself, a family member, a patient) with a medical condition who received medical or therapy care.

   ■ Describe what you know about the patient's perspective in this situation (consider the person's values, preferences,

   expectations, and circumstances). Did the patient's perspective influence the care that he or she received?
   ■ Describe any clinical expertise (your own or others) that influenced the care that the person received.
   ■ What do you know about the research evidence that influenced the person's care?
   ■ What questions do you have about the diagnostic process, intervention plan, or prognosis associated with this person's health condition?
   ■ Can you describe how the five steps of EBP would guide you to answer one of those questions?

Continued

REVIEW QUESTIONS —cont'd

3. Can you think of an instance when you have observed EBP in action? Describe the situation. Can you identify evidence that came from each of the three sources of evidence in EBP?

4. You might want to know if ultrasound therapy would be effective for reducing the neck pain experienced by patient June Wilson in Case Study 1-1. Complete the following steps to focus your learning efforts in future chapters:

Step 1. Identify a gap in your knowledge about ultrasound therapy for neck pain and try writing a searchable clinical question.

Step 2. List sources you might use to find research evidence to answer this question. Can you name some of the benefits and drawbacks of those sources? Do you know what type of research evidence you might look for to answer your question?

Step 3. When you find research evidence, how will you decide if the research is applicable to your question? How will you decide if the research has sufficient quality to influence your practice? How will you decide if the results of the research are of sufficient magnitude to change your practice?

Step 4. What questions would you ask June and her parents to ensure that you understood the patient and family's values and circumstances? How would you balance that information with your own and others' clinical expertise and the patient perspective that you have gathered?

Step 5. What questions will you ask yourself to ensure that you reflect on this process to facilitate your growth in the future?

REFERENCES

1. Straus S, Richardson S, Glasziou P, et al, eds. *Evidence-Based Medicine: How to Practice and Teach EBM.* 3rd ed. Endinburgh, UK, Elsevier Churchill Livingstone; 2005.
2. Towle A, Godolphin W. Framework for teaching and learning informed shared decision making. *BMJ.* 1999;319:766-771.
3. Wainner RS, Fritz JM, Irrgang JJ, et al. Reliability and diagnostic accuracy of the clinical examination and patient self-report measures for cervical radiculopathy. *Spine.* 2003;28:52-62.
4. Cleland JA, Glynn P, Whitman JM, et al. Short-term effects of thrust versus nonthrust mobilization/manipulation directed at the thoracic spine in patients with neck pain: a randomized clinical trial. *Phys Ther.* 2007;87(4):431-440.
5. Linton SJ, Andersson T. Can chronic disability be prevented? A randomized trial of a cognitive-behavior intervention and two forms of information for patients with spinal pain. *Spine.* 2000;25:2825-2831.
6. Hill JC, Lewis M, Sim J, et al. Predictors of poor outcome in patients with neck pain treated by physical therapy. *Clin J Pain.* 2007;23: 683-690.
7. Kluemper M, Uhl T, Hazelrigg H. Effect of stretching and strengthening shoulder muscles on forward shoulder posture in competitive swimmers. *J Sport Rehab.* 2006;15:58-70.
8. Smith R, Nyquist-Battie C, Clark M, et al. Anatomical characteristics of the upper serratus anterior: cadaver dissection. *J Orthop Sports Phys Ther.* 2003;33:449-454.
9. Jensen GM, Gwyer J, Shepard KF, et al. Expert practice in physical therapy. *Phys Ther.* 2000;80:28-43.
10. Milne D. Culture, religion frame care for Muslim patients. *Psychiatr News.* 2005;40:13-58.
11. Dawes M, Summerskill W, Glasziou P, et al. Sicily statement on evidence based practice. *BMC Med Educ.* 2005;5:1.
12. Salbach NM, Jaglal SB, Korner-Bitensky N, et al. Practitioner and organizational barriers to evidence-based practice of physical therapists for people with stroke. *Phys Ther.* 2007;87:1284-1303.
13. Jette DU, Bacon K, Batty C, et al. Evidence-based practice: beliefs, attitudes, knowledge, and behaviors of physical therapists. *Phys Ther.* 2003;83:786-805.
14. American Physical Therapy Association. www.apta.org Accessed April 1, 2008.

2 Asking a Clinical Question and Searching for Research Evidence

PRE-TEST

1. Why is it important to construct a searchable clinical question?

2. Can you give an example of a background question and a foreground question?

3. What is the difference between a database and a search engine?

4. Name a search engine that anyone can access for free on the Internet. What are this tool's strengths and weaknesses for helping therapists find research evidence?

5. Name three important techniques for narrowing a search in the PubMed search engine. Do the same for expanding a search.

6. Where could you locate a repository of full-text articles mandated by the U.S. Congress?

CHAPTER-AT-A-GLANCE

This chapter will help you understand the following:

- Searchable clinical questions

- Searching for research evidence

- Accessing full text of research articles

■ Introduction

This chapter develops your knowledge and skills in the first two steps of evidence based practice (EBP) (Fig. 2.1):

- **Step 1:** Identify a need for information, and develop a focused and searchable **clinical question.**
- **Step 2:** Conduct a **search** to find the best possible research evidence to answer your question.

These steps take you through the process of obtaining research evidence. Most therapists find that research evidence is the most difficult type of evidence to obtain. This chapter will help you learn to obtain research evidence quickly and efficiently.

STEP 1: Identify the Need for Information and Develop a Focused and Searchable Clinical Question

How Do I Know if I Need Information?

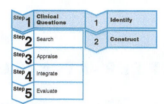

Step 1 can be divided into two parts—identifying a need for information and then constructing a focused, searchable clinical question. How do you identify a need for information? During your physical therapy education, you are flooded with information about how to care for patients. As an evidence based therapist and lifelong learner, you will be constantly adding to your knowledge. Every patient is different, and many will present in ways that push you to find new information to optimize their care. Also, scientific evidence rapidly changes. There are now over 2000 new clinical trials published every year related to physical therapy (Fig. 2.2). You cannot know the answer to every clinical question that will arise. The key is to identify important knowledge gaps and know how to fill them with the best available evidence.

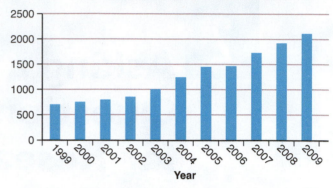

Number of Physical Therapy Clinical Trials Published Each Year from 1999 to 2009*

*Search conducted in PubMed, limited to 'clinical trials' and using the terms: physical rehabilitation or "physical therapy" treatment or physiotherapy.

FIGURE 2.2 The growing number of physical therapy–related clinical trials published each year.

Identification of your needs for information may occur before you see a patient and throughout a patient's course of care. The American Physical Therapy Association defines *patient management* as having six components: examination, evaluation, diagnosis, prognosis, intervention, and outcomes measurement (Fig. 2.3).[1]

We describe the use of EBP for each of these components throughout this book. This chapter addresses clinical questions related to diagnosis, prognosis, and intervention. The information that the evidence based therapist needs during day-to-day patient care usually falls into these three categories.

Let's revisit our patient from Chapter 1, June Wilson (Case Study 1.1). Figure 2.4 illustrates some basic information about June.

From this information, you might have questions about several areas of patient care:

- What special tests should be done to determine the cause of her pain? (Diagnosis)
- What treatments will be most effective for reducing her pain quickly? (Intervention)
- How likely is neck pain to recur? (Prognosis)

These are examples of background questions. **Background questions** ask about general information and are not specific to an individual patient. When you are less familiar with a particular condition, you ask more background questions. As your knowledge about a condition increases, the frequency of your background questions diminishes, and your need increases for foreground clinical questions.

Answers to background questions are usually best found in a general resource (e.g., textbook, reliable Web page) rather than in a specific research study. In contrast, **foreground questions** are specific to a particular patient, condition, and

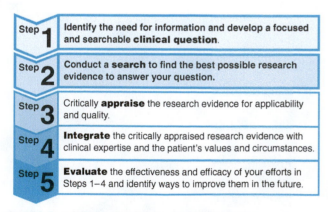

Step 1	Identify the need for information and develop a focused and searchable **clinical question**.
Step 2	Conduct a **search** to find the best possible research evidence to answer your question.
Step 3	Critically **appraise** the research evidence for applicability and quality.
Step 4	**Integrate** the critically appraised research evidence with clinical expertise and the patient's values and circumstances.
Step 5	**Evaluate** the effectiveness and efficacy of your efforts in Steps 1–4 and identify ways to improve them in the future.

FIGURE 2.1 EBP steps 1 and 2 discussed in this chapter.

The Elements of Patient/Client Management Leading to Optimal Outcomes

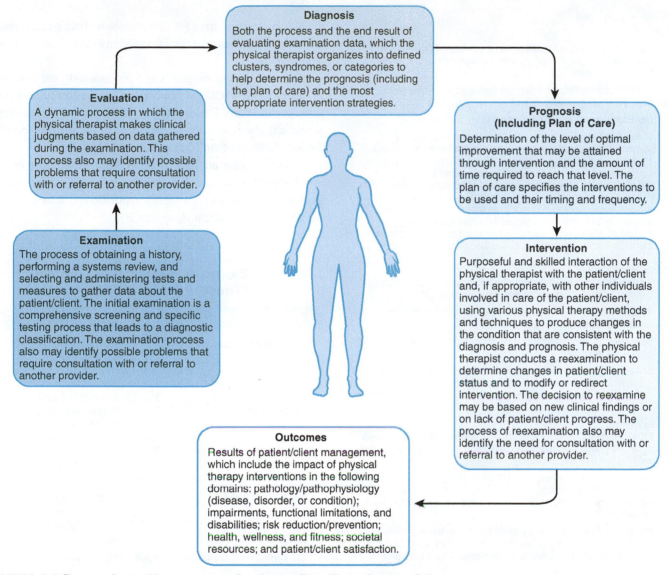

Diagnosis
Both the process and the end result of evaluating examination data, which the physical therapist organizes into defined clusters, syndromes, or categories to help determine the prognosis (including the plan of care) and the most appropriate intervention strategies.

Evaluation
A dynamic process in which the physical therapist makes clinical judgments based on data gathered during the examination. This process also may identify possible problems that require consultation with or referral to another provider.

Prognosis (Including Plan of Care)
Determination of the level of optimal improvement that may be attained through intervention and the amount of time required to reach that level. The plan of care specifies the interventions to be used and their timing and frequency.

Examination
The process of obtaining a history, performing a systems review, and selecting and administering tests and measures to gather data about the patient/client. The initial examination is a comprehensive screening and specific testing process that leads to a diagnostic classification. The examination process also may identify possible problems that require consultation with or referral to another provider.

Intervention
Purposeful and skilled interaction of the physical therapist with the patient/client and, if appropriate, with other individuals involved in care of the patient/client, using various physical therapy methods and techniques to produce changes in the condition that are consistent with the diagnosis and prognosis. The physical therapist conducts a reexamination to determine changes in patient/client status and to modify or redirect intervention. The decision to reexamine may be based on new clinical findings or on lack of patient/client progress. The process of reexamination also may identify the need for consultation with or referral to another provider.

Outcomes
Results of patient/client management, which include the impact of physical therapy interventions in the following domains: pathology/pathophysiology (disease, disorder, or condition); impairments, functional limitations, and disabilities; risk reduction/prevention; health, wellness, and fitness; societal resources; and patient/client satisfaction.

FIGURE 2.3 Elements of patient/client management. *From: American Physical Therapy Association: Guide to Physical Therapist Practice, ed 2. Author, Alexandria, VA, 2001; with permission.*

clinical outcome of interest. Foreground questions are typically answered using a research study or evidence based clinical practice guideline. Electronic databases house thousands to millions of articles and guidelines. To conduct an efficient and effective search, you must first develop a focused, searchable clinical question.

What Is a Searchable Clinical Question?

Searchable clinical questions are foreground questions about a patient that are structured to help you find the necessary research evidence as efficiently as possible. Many hours of frustration can be avoided by following a formula to focus your

search. Focused, searchable, clinical questions contain three elements:

1. *Patient characteristics:* Include the most important patient characteristics that relate to a patient's health condition.
2. *Patient management* (e.g., intervention, diagnosis, prognosis): Define the component of interest for patient management. Study designs differ for questions about interventions, diagnostic tests, and prognosis. By specifying the component of patient management, you focus your question on a particular type of research.
3. *Outcome of interest:* Determine your patient's goals, and identify an appropriate outcome. This is often difficult for

Patient Information Summary

Name: Wilson, June
Age: 17

Current Condition: Ms. Wilson is a 17-year-old female who presents to physical therapy with worsening neck pain over the past 2 weeks.

Past Medical History: Previous episodes of similar neck pain with high intensity swim training.

Medications: Ibuprofen 400 mg 3x/day for 1 week

Disability/Social History: Ms. Wilson is a high school student and member of her school's swim team. She swims 10,000+ yards 5 days per week. She has excelled in the current competition season and is scheduled to compete in the state high school championships (100 yard free-style, 100 yard individual medley) in three days. She has had progressively worsening neck pain that is exacerbated by swimming and prolonged sitting. Her sleep is slightly disturbed. Ms. Wilson lives with her parents who are present at the examination and supportive of her swimming activities.

Functional Status
Sitting Tolerance: 30 minutes before onset of pain—affects comfort in classroom and doing homework.

Sleep: Difficulty falling asleep due to pain, "difficult to find a comfortable position."

Self-care: Slow in the AM due to "morning stiffness" but otherwise unlimited.

Swimming: Able to complete full 10,000 yard workouts but with pain. Pain is worst with free-style and butterfly strokes. Swim speed has been only mildly affected by the injury (< 5%).

Impairments
ROM: Limited cervical ROM for right rotation (45°), side bend right (15°), and extension (30°)—all with pain. Shoulders—full, pain-free range bilaterally.

Strength: Bilateral shoulders 5/5 strength for all major muscle groups. Isometric testing of neck musculature reproduces pain for extension and right sidebend. No overt cervical muscle weakness.

Pain: Neck pain average 4/10; radiates into her right arm to the elbow, interrupts her sleep (<1 hour/night) and during swim practice it increases to 7/10. Better with ice, ibuprofen.

FIGURE 2.4 Information regarding patient June Wilson. *Format from: Quinn & Gordon, Functional Outcomes Documentation for Rehabilitation, 2003.*

new learners. Digging Deeper 2.1 will help you develop this skill more thoroughly.

PICO (Patient, Intervention, Comparison, Outcome)

PICO is an acronym that comprises the key components of a searchable clinical question about interventions. The letters stand for the following:

- Patient (or Population) and clinical characteristics
- Intervention
- Comparison (referring to an alternative intervention)
- Outcome

It is common to have PICO questions without a *C* (comparison). Table 2.1 illustrates two intervention PICO questions about June Wilson.

Questions about diagnosis and prognosis do not conform as easily to the PICO framework but can be formulated into three general parts. Diagnostic questions can include the diagnostic test characteristcs (Question A) or the possible results for a particular patient (Question B) (Table 2.2).

Questions may address a patient population rather than a specific patient. Table 2.3 illustrates searchable clinical questions about prognosis for a patient population (Question A) and for an individual patient (Question B).

TABLE 2.1 Example Searchable Clinical Questions About Interventions

	QUESTION ELEMENT	PICO	QUESTION
1	Patient characteristics	P	For a 17-year-old female swimmer with neck pain . . .
2	Patient management: **Intervention**	I C	is manual therapy or . . . therapeutic exercise more effective . . .
3	Outcome of interest	O	for improving function and sport performance?

Searchable Clinical Question:

For a 17-year-old female swimmer with neck pain, is manual therapy or therapeutic exercise more effective for improving function and sport performance?

1	Patient characteristics	P	For a 17-year-old female swimmer with neck pain . . .
2	Patient management: **Intervention**	I	are manual therapy techniques effective . . .
3	Outcome of Interest	O	for short-term pain reduction?

Searchable Clinical Question:

For a 17-year-old female swimmer with neck pain, are manual therapy techniques effective for short-term pain reduction?

■ SELF-TEST 2.1 Writing Clinical Questions

 CASE STUDY 2.1 Mr. Jose Lopez

Let's consider another patient, Jose Lopez. Figure 2.5 illustrates some basic information about him. Mr. Lopez is a 52-year-old grandfather. He works on a peach farm and has had increasing knee pain for the past 4 months. He is not aware of a specific mechanism of injury. His pain has become so severe that he is unable to pick peaches or carry his 5-year-old grandson.

Reflect on the information provided about Mr. Lopez.

1. Write your questions about his care.

2. Determine if each question is a background or a foreground question.

3. Determine the component of patient management for each question (diagnosis, intervention, or prognosis).

4. For the questions that you believe are foreground questions, underline the three key components: patient characteristics, patient management (diagnosis, intervention, or prognosis), and outcome. If the question does not have all of those parts, try rewriting.

 DIGGING DEEPER 2.1

International Classification of Functioning, Disability and Health

The outcome(s) component of clinical questions refers to the particular outcome of interest to the patient and/or clinician. When considering the outcome, the International Classification of Function, Disability and Health (ICF) model (Fig. 2.6) may help you to frame and focus your question.[2]

The World Health Organization is encouraging health professionals to use a common language to communicate issues of health and wellness. ICF terms include body functions and structures, activity, and participation. Impairments describe problems at the level of body functions and structures. Activity describes actions such as walking, climbing stairs, or getting out of bed. Problems with activity are referred to as activity limitations. Participation includes work, school, and community involvement; participation restrictions describes problems at this level.

An outcome is defined at the level of body structures and function (e.g., pain, strength), at the activity level (e.g., prolonged sitting, swimming), or at the participation level (e.g., attend high school, participate on a sports team).

■ SELF-TEST 2.2 Practice Using the ICF Model

 CASE STUDY 2.2 Mr. Ed Dean

You are working with a 55-year-old truck driver, Ed Dean, who has developed low back pain associated with prolonged periods of sitting. When not working, Mr. Dean enjoys working on antique tractors and doing odd jobs around the house. He is married and has eight grandchildren.

List five outcome measures at the body structure and function, activity, and participation levels that pertain to Mr. Dean.

Use the outcome measures you have listed above under the three ICF categories to complete the following foreground questions:

■ For a 55-year-old truck driver with low back pain, is physical therapy care or chiropractic care more effective for

_____?

■ For a 55-year-old male with low back pain, are stabilization exercises or strength-training exercises more effective for

_____?

■ For a 55-year-old male with low back pain, is bedrest or a walking program more likely to improve

_____?

Body Structure and Function	Activity	Participation
Example: Lumbar spine range of motion	Example: Prolonged sitting	Example: Occupation— truck driver
1.	1.	1.
2.	2.	2.
3.	3.	3.
4.	4.	4.
5.	5.	5.

TABLE 2.2 **Example Searchable Clinical Questions About Diagnosis**

QUESTION ELEMENT	QUESTION
1 Patient characteristics	For a 17-year-old female with radiating neck pain . . .
2 Patient management: **Diagnosis (test characteristics)**	how sensitive and specific is the Spurling's test for . . .
3 Outcome of interest	detecting cervical nerve root impingement?

(A) Searchable Clinical Question:

For a 17-year-old female with radiating neck pain, how sensitive and specific is the Spurling's test for detecting cervical nerve root impingement?

1 Patient characteristics	For an athlete with neck pain and a positive Spurling's test . . .
2 Patient management: **Diagnosis (test result)**	what is the likelihood that . . .
3 Outcome of interest	the person has cervical nerve root impingement?

(B) Searchable Clinical Question:

For an athlete with neck pain and a positive Spurling's test, what is the likelihood that the person has cervical nerve root impingement?

TABLE 2.3 **Example Searchable Clinical Questions About Prognosis**

QUESTION ELEMENT	QUESTION
1 Patient characteristics	For a competitive swimmer with recurrent neck pain . . .
2 Patient management: **Prognosis**	what is the likelihood that the athlete will develop . . .
3 Outcome of interest	chronic neck pain?

(A) Searchable Clinical Question:

For a competitive swimmer with recurrent neck pain, what is the likelihood that the athlete will develop chronic neck pain?

1 Popoulation characteristics	Among competitive high school swimmers . . .
2 Patient management: **Prognosis**	what risk factors are associated with onset of . . .
3 Outcome of interest	cervical disk herniation?

(B) Searchable Clinical Question:

Among competitive high school swimmers, what risk factors are associated with onset of cervical disk herniation?

STEP 2: Conduct a search to find the best possible research evidence to answer your question

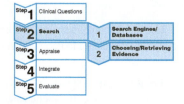

The second step in EBP involves searching for the best available research evidence to answer your clinical question. Most often, you will accomplish this by searching a database. In the context of EBP, a **database** is a compilation of research evidence resources, primarily lists of peer-reviewed journal articles, designed to organize the large amount of research published every year. Before choosing the best database to search, you will need to decide which type of research evidence you want to find.

Which Types of Studies are You Looking for?

The Evidence Pyramid (Fig. 2.7) illustrates a hierarchy that can serve as an *initial* filter for identifying high-quality

evidence. Study designs at the top of the pyramid are least likely to produce biased results. **Bias** occurs when a study's results are affected by unknown or unacknowledged errors resulting from the study's design or protocols. Your ability to recognize different study types will improve as you proceed through the chapters of this book.

When searching for research evidence about *interventions,* first search for evidence based clinical practice guidelines, followed by systematic reviews, randomized controlled trials, and so on down the pyramid. Randomized controlled trials are often not an appropriate design for studies on diagnosis or prognosis. For those categories, first search for systematic reviews, and then search for cohort studies. Subsequent chapters support your increased ability to identify these different study designs.

Using Search Engines to Find Research Evidence

A **search engine** is the user interface that allows specific articles to be identified in a database. Sometimes several search

Patient Information Summary

Name: Lopez, Jose
Age: 52

Current Condition: Mr. Lopez presents to physical therapy with worsening right knee pain over the past 4 months.

Past Medical History: Hypertension

Medications: Diuril (Chlorothiazide)

Disability/Social History: Mr. Lopez works as a crop manager and peach picker at a peach farm. He is on his feet 6-8 hours per day, often climbing on and off ladders and tractors. He lives with his wife, daughter and son-in-law and their two children (2 and 5 years). He has had progressively worsening right knee pain that is exacerbated by prolonged standing.

Functional Status

Standing Tolerance: 3 hours before onset of pain—affects work and home activities, requiring standing.

Sleep: Generally uninterrupted by knee pain.

Self-care: Unlimited.

Climbing Ladders: Knee feels unstable as if it might give out. This limits Mr. Lopez's efficiency and confidence working on the farm.

Tractor Driving: Knee becomes painful/stiff after long hours of driving tractor due to constant use of foot pedals.

Impairments

		R Knee	L Knee	R Hip	L Hip	R Ankle	L Ankle
Passive ROM	Extension/PF	5°	0°	0°	0°	50°	50°
	Flexion/DF	100°	120°	120°	120°	5°	5°
Active ROM	Extension/PF	5°	0°	0°	0°	50°	50°
	Flexion/DF	90°	110°	120°	120°	5°	10°
Strength	Extension/PF	3+/5	5/5	5/5	5/5	5/5	5/5
	Flexion/DF	3+/5	5/5	5/5	5/5	5/5	5/5

Pain: 6/10 pain with end range ROM and maximal contraction effort. Worst in past week = 7/10, best 1/10, average 4/10. Better with rest (sitting and gentle ROM), ace wrap.

FIGURE 2.5 Information regarding patient Jose Lopez. *Format from: Quinn & Gordon, Functional Outcomes Documentation for Rehabilitation, 2003.*

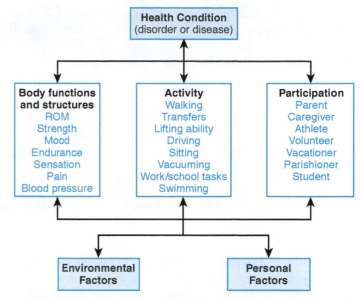

FIGURE 2.6 Different types of outcome measures organized by categories established in the International Classification of Function, Disability and Health model. *Modified from: International Classification of Functioning, Disability and Health: ICF.: World Health Organization, Geneva, Switzerland, 2001, with permission of the World Health Organization.*

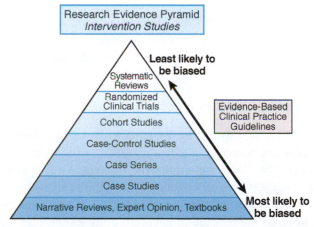

FIGURE 2.7 Consider the evidence pyramid when searching in databases for research evidence. *Adapted from: http://library.upstate.edu/evidence/ pyramid/#critically, Evidence-Based Practice (EBP) Resources, 2011.*

engines can be used to search the same database. For example, Medline,[3] one of the most comprehensive databases of medical research articles, can be searched using numerous search engines (e.g., PubMed,[4] Ovid Medline, and ProQuest). One search engine may also allow you to search numerous databases. For example, the Translating Research into Practice (TRIP)[5] search engine searches over 21 databases at once. This chapter focuses on freely available and effective search engines and databases. Figure 2.8 illustrates search engines and important databases for evidence based physical therapists, including the following:

National Guidelines Clearinghouse

National Guidelines Clearinghouse[6] (www.guidelines.gov) is a database of clinical practice guidelines (CPGs) developed by the

Agency for Healthcare Research and Quality (AHRQ). The clearinghouse allows authors of CPGs to post their guidelines for public reference. The site has its own search engine, which has limited functionality but allows searching for broad terms. This database contains numerous CPGs that are not indexed in MEDLINE.

Physiotherapy Evidence Database (PEDro)

The Physiotherapy Evidence Database (PEDro)[7] (www.pedro. org.au) is a freely available database and search engine of abstracts for physical therapy–specific literature. The database

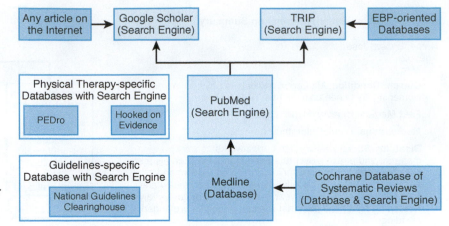

FIGURE 2.8 The relationships between common databases and search engines that are either available for free or available to members of the American Physical Therapy Association.

covers only intervention-related literature but does include clinical practice guidelines, systematic reviews, and other clinical studies. PEDro developers have created a well-documented rating system for determining the quality of clinical trials called the PEDro scale.[8,9] The scale ranges from 0 to 10; studies rated as 10/10 are considered to have the least risk for bias.

Hooked on Evidence

Hooked on Evidence[10] (www.hookedonevidence.com) is a physical therapy–specific database developed by the American Physical Therapy Association (APTA). This database is only available to APTA members.

The Cochrane Library of Systematic Reviews

The Cochrane Library of Systematic Reviews[11] (www.cochrane.org/reviews) is a database of systematic reviews conducted by Cochrane-approved reviewers. All Cochrane Systematic Reviews are conducted using the same methods, which are considered the gold standard. Cochrane Systematic Reviews are indexed in PubMed; using a supplemental search engine is not necessary to find these articles. A separate Cochrane search engine is, however, available as well.

MEDLINE Database

MEDLINE Database[3] indexes over 5200 journals published from around the world and across numerous medical and related disciplines. The journals indexed in MEDLINE are reviewed for quality by the U.S. National Library of Medicine. MEDLINE includes over 19 million research articles.

PubMed

PubMed[4] (www.pubmed.gov) is a freely available search engine developed by the U.S. National Library of Medicine and National Center for Biotechnology Information. Almost all of the articles that PubMed searches are contained in the MEDLINE database.

Google Scholar

Google Scholar (www.google.com/scholar) is a search engine developed by the company Google. The search engine is designed to search the Internet for journal articles. The Google Scholar search engine also links to the full text of articles (both free and paid). Google Scholar searches all entries included in PubMed and National Guidelines Clearinghouse.

Translating Research Into Practice (TRIP)

Translating Research Into Practice (TRIP)[5] (http://www.tripdatabase.com) is a powerful search engine designed to assist medical practitioners in searching numerous databases to find the best available evidence. TRIP searches PubMed/MEDLINE, National Guidelines Clearinghouse, and more than 20 other prescreened databases and databases focused on EBP.

Searching in PubMed

This chapter highlights the PubMed search engine (Fig. 2.9). PubMed is the most comprehensive and powerful freely available search engine for finding EBP research evidence. Learning the skills to use PubMed efficiently is important to EBP. Most powerful search engines will have tools similar to those of PubMed but with a different user interface. The choice to use one search engine over another is a matter of purpose and personal preference. You should find a search engine that is user-friendly and efficient for initial searches. Backup search engines can be used when necessary. The outcome of the search is more important than the tool used. Beyond this text, practice and working with a therapist or librarian skilled in medical literature searches can be helpful for developing your skills. Screenshots are included in this book to guide your learning. Although the look of screenshots will change over

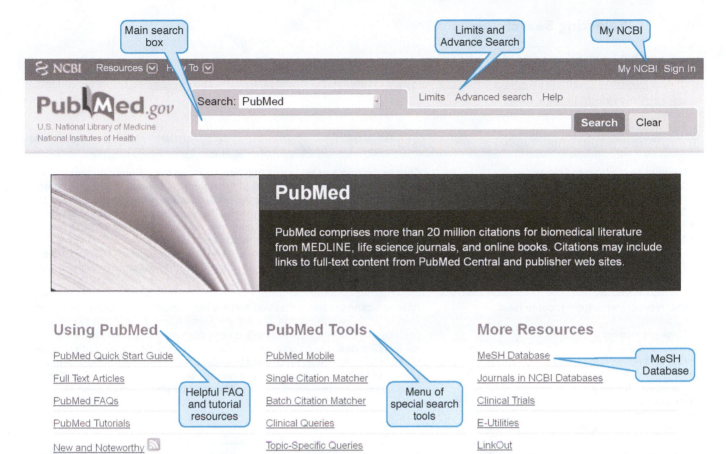

FIGURE 2.9 Screenshot from the PubMed homepage. The main search box includes areas in which **terms** are entered to search. The Limits and Advanced Search links provide access to tools for refined searches. MyNCBI allows the user to customize and save information at PubMed (see Digging Deeper 2.2 and Chapter 11). The MeSH database is a helpful resource for identifying appropriate search terms. Special tools are available for specific types of searches; several of these are addressed in Digging Deeper, "Additional Tools for Searching in PubMed." Several frequently asked questions (FAQs) and tutorials about PubMed are helpful for new users.

time, the general concepts of how to use the various online services will remain relatively constant.

Students familiar with Web browsers have experience using search engines for general Web searches. Research article databases, however, do not function exactly like all-purpose Internet search engines. Developing refined, efficient search skills takes practice. To use research article databases, you will need to learn the most appropriate terms to enter; how to combine terms; how to limit search results; and how to search by different categories such as author, year, journal, or keyword.

Following is a searchable clinical question about the patient June Wilson (Case Study 1.1) to illustrate several key skills for searching in PubMed:

Searchable Clinical Question:

For a 17-year-old swimmer with neck pain, is a combination of manual therapy and exercise effective for reducing pain and improving function?

Identify Your Search Terms

The first step in searching PubMed is to identify your search terms. When you enter a term into the PubMed search box, PubMed searches for articles using that term in the title and abstract. **Key words** are important words from your searchable clinical question and/or synonyms of those words. Ideally, an article that has your key words in the title and abstract will be relevant to your searchable clinical question.

Each article entered into the MEDLINE database (that PubMed searches) is also identified with a list of Medical Subject Headings (MeSH). **MeSH terms** are designed to provide a common and consistent language across published articles. Within PubMed you can enter key words from your question into a MeSH database to determine the best MeSH term for that topic. However, therapists often discover that MeSH terms are somewhat limited in appropriately describing the therapy topic of interest. In this case it is best to use key words rather than MeSH terms.

Table 2.4 illustrates an example of our discovery of search terms from our searchable clinical question.

TABLE 2.4 **Selecting Search Terms**

Searchable Clinical Question:

"For a 17-year-old female swimmer with neck pain, is a combination of manual therapy and exercise effective for reducing pain and improving function?"

TERMS	EXPLANATION
Start with terms from the question: ■ 17-year-old ■ Female ■ Swimmer ■ Neck pain ■ Manual therapy ■ Exercise ■ Pain ■ Function	Choose the terms or keywords that best describe the information that you are seeking. In this case, we chose all of the nouns in the sentence except *combination*. *Combination* was not chosen because we expect that the concept of combining the two interventions will be captured by putting both interventions in the search box. It should be noted, however, that this will also result in studies that compare manual therapy and exercise therapy. The terms "reducing" and "improving" were not chosen. We expected that the studies that we would be looking for would inherently address improvement on our outcomes of interest.
Next, reorder terms from most to least important: ■ Neck pain *(most important)* ■ Manual therapy ■ Exercise ■ Pain ■ Function ■ 17-year-old ■ Swimmer ■ Female *(least important)*	After selecting the terms that you feel are most important, reorder the terms from most to least important. Determining which terms are important requires practice and a willingness to take a guess. We have placed the terms that we feel best describe an article that tells us how to treat our patient at the top of the list. For example, an article about people with neck pain has a better chance of being related to our question than an article about females. The order is only a guess. Any term can ultimately be prioritized in a search.
Refine your terms using the MeSH database: • Neck pain (same) • Musculoskeletal manipulations • Exercise therapy • Recovery of function • Adolescent (identified through term "teenager") • Swimming • Female	When you are new to searching in a particular topic area, it is helpful to check your keyword list against the Medline MeSH headings. In this case, we anticipated that the term "17-year-old" would need to be modified. Most papers would not be so specific to list "17-year-old" in the title or abstract. We used the MeSH search to identify the more appropriate term of "adolescent." Additional terms were also modified or added based on our MeSH database search. We found that some keyword terms were the same as the MeSH term.
Finally, order all terms from most to least important: 1. Neck pain 2. Musculoskeletal manipulations 3. Manual therapy 4. Exercise therapy 5. Recovery of function 6. Adolescent 7. Swimming 8. Female	The final list provided is our best guess of order of importance.

After you have identified your most important terms, enter each of the top four terms individually into PubMed's Advanced Search. This will determine the number of articles identified with each term. Searches #1 through #4 under Search History in Figure 2.10 illustrate this step.

Combining Terms

The next step is to combine terms using OR and AND. The term "manual therapy" (Search #3) and the MeSH term "musculoskeletal manipulation" (Search #2) address the same topic. Therefore, they should be combined using the Boolean operator OR. Using OR retrieves a list of all the articles that have *either* the term "musculoskeletal manipulation" OR the term "manual therapy." This can be done using the terms themselves (manual therapy OR musculoskeletal manipulation) or using the search number to the left of each term (#3 OR #4). Note that PubMed requires that you use the number sign (#) when identifying search numbers (see Fig. 2.10A, Search #5).

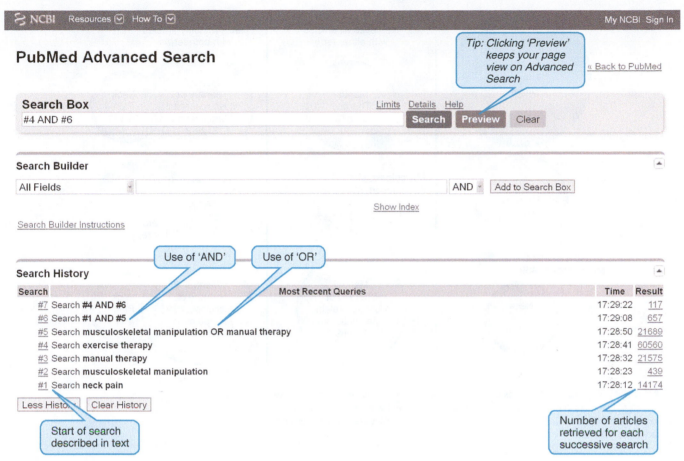

FIGURE 2.10A The concept of the pool of articles that is created through combining and narrowing.

The operator AND is used when you want only articles that contain both (or more than two) terms. In this search, the concepts of "neck pain" and "manual therapy OR musculoskeletal manipulation" were combined using AND (see Fig. 2.10A, Search #6.). Using this strategy retrieved a list of all the articles that contained *both* terms. In this case it is easiest to use the search numbers (see Fig. 2.10A, Search Box). Finally, combine the results from Search #6 with the term "exercise therapy." Figure 2.10B illustrates how the search strategy in Figure 2.10A narrowed the search to relevant articles. Column A illustrates the number of articles retrieved when each separate term is used in the search (Exercise Therapy, Manual Therapy, Musculoskeletal Manipulation, and Neck Pain). The number of articles retrieved is approximated by the size of the circle. Column B illustrates the number of articles retrieved when two terms, Manual Therapy and Musculoskeletal Manipulation, are combined using OR; PubMed retrieves all articles containing *either* of these terms. Hence, the number of articles is greater than either term retrieved separately. Column C illustrates the number of articles retrieved when terms (or combinations of terms) are combined using AND; PubMed retrieves only the articles that contain *all* of the terms. Hence the number of articles is steadily reduced. With all terms combined, 117 articles remain.

Limiting Your Search

Finally, the *Limits* page (see link in Fig. 2.9) can be used to limit the results of a search to the types of articles in which you are interested. An efficient way to search for best evidence is to start by searching for clinical practice guidelines. Then, if necessary (as is frequently the case), proceed down the levels of the pyramid. In our example, the initial *limits* we used restricted the results to recent (the past 5 years) clinical practice guidelines in English (Fig. 2.11).

This search produced "zero" results. Therefore, look for Systematic Reviews. On the Limits page, Systematic Reviews and Narrative Reviews are combined (Review). Look at the titles and abstracts to determine which are systematic and which are narrative. The Review limit plus the Meta-analysis limit (usually a systematic review, see Chapter 8) produce 16 results, 7 of which are systematic reviews. Then choose one by Miller et al[12] to appraise for applicability and quality (see Chapters 3 through 10 for appraisal skills):

Miller, J, Gross, A, D'Sylva J, et al: Manual therapy and exercise for neck pain: A systematic review. Man Ther 15: 334–354, 2010.

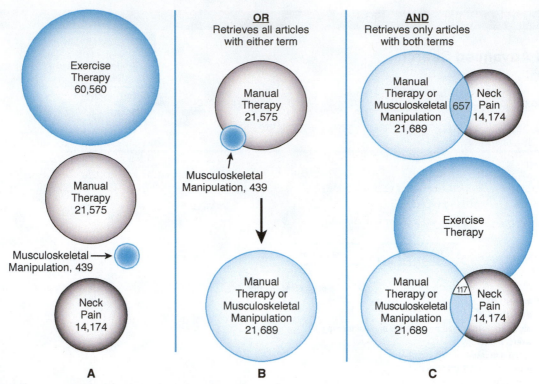

FIGURE 2.10B Column (A) illustrates the number of articles retrieved when each separate term is used in the search. Column (B) illustrates the number of articles retrieved when two terms, Manual Therapy and Musculoskeletal Manipulation, are combined using OR. Column (C) illustrates the number of particles retrieved when terms are combined using AND.

Because the systematic review appraised numerous studies, you also want to review an individual study that might provide more detailed information about the specific treatment strategies. To do this, limit the search to randomized controlled trials; this retrieves 18 articles. You could then choose one article to appraise for applicability and quality (Fig. 2.12).[13]

Search History

The final search strategy used to find the best available research evidence to answer our question is illustrated in Figure 2.13.

This example is one of many search examples for PubMed. Additional suggestions are provided in Digging Deeper 2.2. For self-study, consult the PubMed tutorial page and tutorial pages from other individual online databases and search engines.

DIGGING DEEPER 2.2

Additional tools for searching in PubMed

The PubMed search engine has numerous tools designed to make searching easier. This section highlights Clinical Queries, Single Citation Matcher, MyNCBI, and Related Articles.

CLINICAL QUERIES: The Clinical Queries tool is the best place to start searching if you have a good idea of what terms to use (Fig. 2.14). The page has two components that therapists find useful. First, Search by Clinical Study Category allows the searcher to enter terms and then select the type of clinical question of interest (etiology, diagnosis, therapy, prognosis, and clinical prediction guides). The search can be broad (capturing as many articles as possible) or narrow (capturing a more specific selection of articles). PubMed uses your terms with pre-established search criteria to retrieve articles. The second clinical queries tool is the Find Systematic Reviews tool. This tool allows you to type your terms into a search box designed to retrieve only systematic reviews.

SINGLE CITATION MATCHER: The Single Citation Matcher is useful when you know something about a specific article that you want to find. You can enter information about the article's journal,

DIGGING DEEPER 2.2 — cont'd

date, volume, author, or title words, and PubMed will search for matches. A note of caution—experience suggests that it is best to fill in just one or two of the potential fields (even if you know all of them). Filling all of the fields increases the potential for a mismatch with the article's PubMed entry and may result in "No items found."

MYNCBI: The MyNCBI tool (see link in Fig. 2.9) supports the development of your private library within PubMed. With your personal account you can permanently save collections of articles and searches. One favorite tool initiates an automatic e-mail of new results when you save a search. For example, if

you decide to save the search for questions about interventions for June Wilson, you could request an e-mail of any new articles published that fit that search. That search is automatically performed, and the results are sent to you. MyNCBI is detailed in Chapter 11.

RELATED CITATIONS: The Related Citations tool (see the link in Fig. 2.12) is helpful when you locate a high-quality article and want to retrieve similar articles. The top five related citations are listed in the right-hand column of a given article abstract page. Click "See all" to retrieve a longer list of all related articles.

Limits

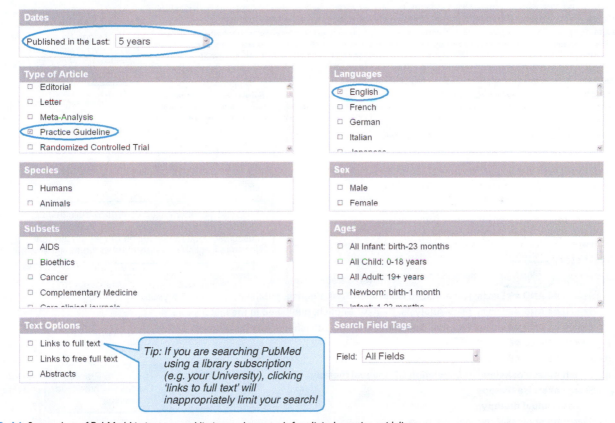

FIGURE 2.11 Screenshot of PubMed Limits page and limits used to search for clinical practice guidelines published in the past five years in English.

Special Considerations for Background Questions

Background questions ask about fundamental, factual information that is often not easily found in recently published journal articles. The list below contains examples of helpful Web sites for accessing credible background information. These

types of resources can also be helpful for patients and clients who want to conduct their own search.

- *Examples of Credible General Medical Information Web Sites*
  - MedlinePlus[14] (www.medlineplus.gov)
  - National Institute of Neurologic Disorders and Stroke[15] (www.ninds.nih.gov)

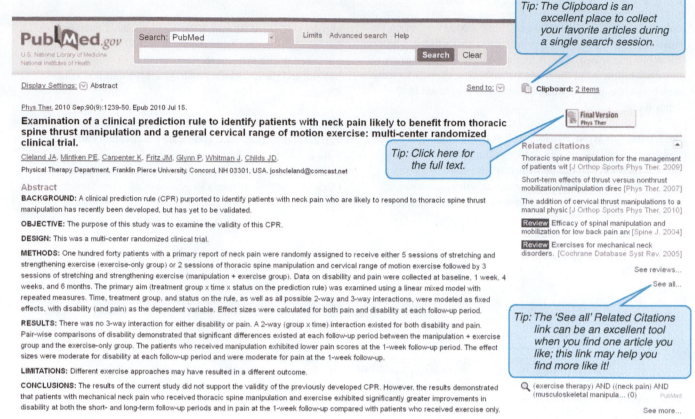

FIGURE 2.12 Screenshot of the PubMed abstract page.

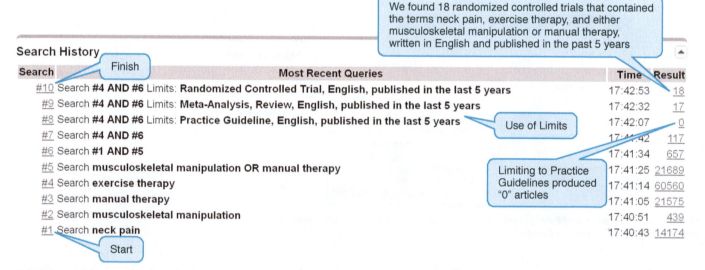

FIGURE 2.13 Final search history in PubMed for the following clinical question: "For a 17-year-old swimmer with neck pain, is a combination of manual therapy and exercise effective for reducing pain and improving function?"

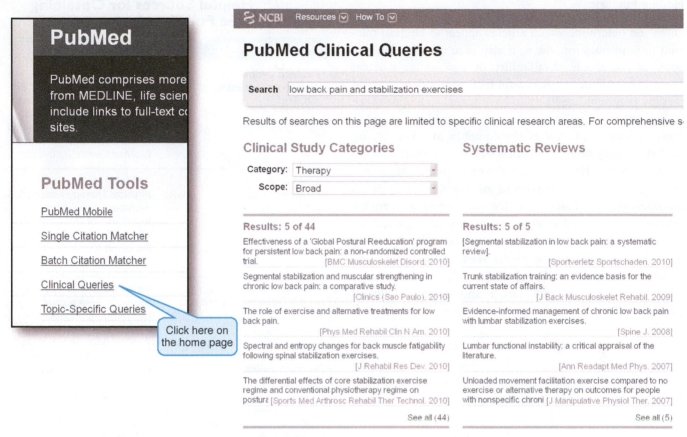

FIGURE 2.14 Screenshot of the location on the PubMed home page to find the Clinical Queries link *(left)* and a search for "low back pain and stabilization exercises" using the tool *(right)*.

• National Institute of Arthritis and Musculoskeletal and Skin Diseases (www.niams.nih.gov/)
• Mayo Clinic (www.mayoclinic.com)
▪ *Examples of Condition-Specific Government and Advocacy Societies*
  • Arthritis Foundation (www.arthritis.org)
  • American Diabetes Association (www.diabetes.org)
  • Multiple Sclerosis Society[16] (www.nationalmssociety.org)
  • National Stroke Association[17] (www.stroke.org)
▪ *Examples of Narrative Reviews in Scientific Journals and Book Chapters*
  • To learn about rehabilitation for persons with cancer: Gilchrist, LS, Galantino, ML, Wampler, M, Marchese, VG, Morris, GS, and Ness, KK: A framework for assessment in oncology rehabilitation. Phys Ther 89:286–306, 2009.
  • To learn about multidisciplinary care for persons with amylotrphic lateral sclerosis: Mayadev, AS, Weiss, MD, Jane Distad, B, Krivickas, LS, and Carter, GT: The amyotrophic lateral sclerosis center: A model of multidisciplinary management. Phys Med Rehabil Clin N Am 19:619–631, xi, 2008.

Choosing and Retrieving Evidence

Choosing the article that is likely to be the *best* available research evidence is not an easy task. Before we discuss retrieving the full text of research articles, we will address a common misperception that often leads to frustration for new searchers.

Let Close be Good Enough!

One of the most challenging tasks for new searchers is to know when they have found the best available evidence. It is import to recognize the emphasis on best rather than perfect. Because each one of your patients is unique, it is improbable that you will find a research article that exactly addresses your clinical question with research participants who are a perfect match to your patient.

For example, review the abstracts from the articles that we found to address our question for June Wilson. None of the articles are specifically about 17-year-olds, or swimmers, or women. In subsequent chapters you will learn how to decide if an article is similar enough to your patient to make it useful. During the search process, look for the closest match you can find and move on to Step 3.

Finding Full Text

Once you determine which articles appear to be most relevant to your question, the next step is to obtain a full-text copy of the article. Availability of free online medical journals contributes to successful EBP. Students in physical therapy programs are likely to have access to a wide range of free online texts through their university library. In addition, the halls of the library should not be avoided because the library may offer hard copies of more journals than are available online. However, access to online texts while working in the clinic is important to making the EBP process manageable. The challenge for the evidence based therapist is to ensure continued access to online texts after graduation. In 2007, Congress passed a law to ensure the availability of research papers to the public from research that was conducted using U.S. taxpayer dollars. These are available within one year of publication and through PubMed Central (effective April 2008; www.pubmedcentral.gov; Fig. 2.15).

Unfortunately, for therapists not associated with a medical library that pays for many journal licenses, many articles are still not available without a substantial fee. Information about how to access PubMed Central and other online text resources are provided in Table 2.5.

■ Pulling it all Together: Your First Search

Now that you have had the opportunity to follow along on our search for information to inform our question about June Wilson, it is time for you to practice searching. Self-Test Box 2.3 will guide you through a PubMed Search for Jose Lopez (Case Study 2.1).

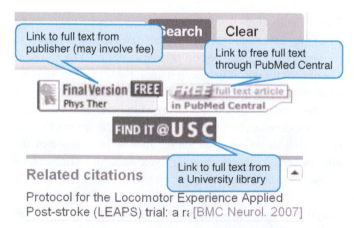

Protocol for the Locomotor Experience Applied Post-stroke (LEAPS) trial: a ra[BMC Neurol. 2007]

FIGURE 2.15 An article in PubMed that has several resources for full text, including free full text through PubMed Central.

TABLE 2.5 **Helpful Sources for Obtaining Free Full-Text Articles**

ONLINE RESOURCE	COMMENTS
PubMed Central www.pubmedcentral.nih.gov	All NIH- funded studies published after April 2008 are available but may have up to a 12-month release delay. PubMed searches link to full text available through BioMed Central.
Open Door www.apta.org	Available to American Physical Therapy Association members. Provides access to full text of Cochrane Library, journals in the ProQuest Nursing and Allied Health database.
Free Medical Journals http://highwire.stanford.edu	Lists free journal titles by specialty. Free access may be limited to articles >1 year old.
HighWire Press www.highwire.stanford.edu	Maintained by Stanford University. Claims to have the largest library of free full-text articles anywhere.
Public Library of Science www.plos.org	Online scientific journals built around a core principle of unrestricted access to research articles.

■ SELF-TEST 2.3 Pulling It All Together

Searchable Clinical Question:

"For a 52-year-old male with knee osteoarthritis, what types of exercise are most effective for reducing pain and improving standing tolerance?"

Step-by-step search:

1. List important terms from the question.
2. Reorder those terms from most to least important (remember that this is your best guess; you can always reorder them again).
3. Use the MeSH database within PubMed to search for MeSH terms that might be more effective for searching.
4. Add any other synonyms that you think are important descriptors of the question.
5. Enter each of your top four or five terms separately in PubMed. Use the "History" tab to see how many articles are associated with each term.

6. Combine similar terms with the operator OR.
7. Combine the two most important concepts with the operator AND.
8. Keep combining until you narrow to less than 300 and greater than 0 articles.
   a. If you get to less than 15 to 20 articles, click on that result and look at the articles that you found.
9. As needed, limit your search to get to your goal of 15 to 20 articles. Remember that study type, language, and time since publication are good limiters to use.
10. Scan your articles' titles and abstracts—how do they look?
    a. Are there any clinical practice guidelines?
    b. Are there any systematic reviews?
    c. Are there any randomized clinical trials?

11. Pick the three articles that are the highest evidence level and are close to the topic of exercise for persons with knee osteoarthritis.
12. Do your best to find a printable (.pdf file) copy of each article.

A final bit of advice: think of searching as learning to ride a bike. It probably isn't as easy as it looks. However, just like riding a bike, with practice you become good at it. Don't get discouraged—you will get it, we promise!

SUMMARY

In Step 1 of the EBP process we identify a need for information and develop a clinical question. Clinical questions can be divided into two types: background and foreground. Background questions seek general information and are more commonly asked when a topic or diagnosis is unfamiliar. Foreground questions are specific to an individual patient or group of patients. Foreground searchable clinical questions have three important parts: patient characteristics, patient management (etiology, diagnosis, intervention, or prognosis), and outcome measures of interest. Outcome measures can address three different levels of the International Classification of Function model: body structures and functions, activity, and participation. A well-designed and focused searchable clinical question improves the efficiency of Step 2.

Step 2, searching for research evidence, is conducted using online databases. Search engines are the user interfaces that allow us to efficiently search a database for the best available research evidence to inform a clinical question. PubMed is a freely available search engine that accesses MEDLINE, a comprehensive database of research evidence. Learning to use a search engine takes practice. Determining the best terms to use and how to narrow and broaden a search with Boolean operators such as OR and AND are examples of those skills. With practice, you can become an efficient user of your favorite search engines. Finally, accessing full-text articles is important for moving to Step 3, appraising research evidence. It is important to be familiar with the resources that you have available as a student and clinician to access free or low-cost full-text articles.

REVIEW QUESTIONS

1. Think of a person with a medical condition . The person might be a physical therapy patient you have encountered or a friend or family member. What questions do you have about that person's medical condition? Can you think of a question for each of the four areas of clinical questions: etiology, diagnosis, intervention, and prognosis?

2. Choose one of the questions that you identified for question 1. Formulate that question into both a background (general) and foreground (patient-specific) question. Check to make sure that the foreground question contains all three important components.

3. Using a computer with access to PubMed, search for the best available research evidence to inform the following

question: "For a 62-year-old grandmother 2 months' post-stroke, is body-weight–supported treadmill training an effective modality for improving gait speed and balance?"

Follow these steps to make the search more manageable:

- First write out all of the search terms that you think might be helpful for this question. Don't forget to think of synonyms (e.g., stroke and cerebrovascular accident).
  - Use the MeSH terms database in PubMed to check your terms list against the terms used to index articles in the MEDLINE database.
  - Prioritize your terms from most to least important.

Continued

REVIEW QUESTIONS—cont'd

- On the "History" tab in PubMed, enter your first four to six terms individually. How many articles came up for each term?
- Combine any synonym terms with OR to find all of the articles that contain *either* term.
- Now, one at a time, use AND to look for articles that contain two important terms (or concepts combined with OR).
- Combine terms to find between 5 and 20 articles, and scan the article titles and abstracts to assess the quality of the results. Use the "Limits" tab to limit articles to the past five years and the "English language" tab to limit your search to those published in English.
- Use the "Limits" tab to search for different types of articles.
  - How many applicable clinical guidelines did you find?
  - How many applicable systematic reviews did you find?
  - How many applicable randomized controlled trials did you find?
    - Review the abstracts of the best articles and the best single article.

- Review the first 10 "Related Articles" in PubMed—can you identify anything better?
- Describe at least one method you can use to access full text for the article you chose and print it out.
  - Finally, use the "Clinical Queries" PubMed tool as an alternate search method for your question. Compare the articles you found with the first search to the "Clinical Queries" results. Are the articles similar? Which search method worked best?

4. Practice using the "Single Citation Matcher" tool to find the following article. After you have found it, use PubMed Central to access and print the article's full text: Wolf, SL, Winstein, CJ, Miller, JP, et al: Effect of constraint-induced movement therapy on upper extremity function 3 to 9 months after stroke: The EXCITE randomized clinical trial. *JAMA* 296(17):2095, 2006.

ANSWERS TO SELF-TESTS

■ SELF-TEST 2.1

Two sample questions:

What types of knee problems cause pain with prolonged standing? (Background question, diagnosis)

For a 52-year-old male with knee osteoarthritis, is water or land exercise more effective for improving standing and walking tolerance? (Foreground question, intervention, three question parts are underlined)

- For a 55-year-old truck driver with low back pain, is physical therapy care or chiropractic care more effective for improving trunk strength?

- For a 55-year-old male with low back pain, are stabilization exercises or strength training exercises more effective for improving sitting tolerance?

- For a 55-year-old male with low back pain, is bedrest or a walking program more likely to improve likelihood to return to work as a truck driver?

■ SELF-TEST 2.2

Body Structure and Function	Activity	Participation
Example: Lumbar Spine Range of Motion	Example: Prolonged Sitting	Example: Occupation—Truck driver
1. Lumbar range of motion	1. Sitting tolerance	1. Truck driver
2. Average pain on 0–10 scale	2. Standing tolerance	2. Tractor mechanic
3. Trunk muscle strength	3. Lifting capacity	3. Spouse
4. Active hip flexion range of motion	4. Driving tolerance	4. Grandfather
5. Balance	5. Climb ladder	5. Handyman

REFERENCES

1. American Physical Therapy Association: Guide to Physical Therapist Practice, ed 2. Author, Alexandria, VA, 2001.
2. International Classification of Functioning, Disability and Health: ICF. Paper presented at World Health Organization, Geneva, Switzerland, 2001.
3. http://medline.cos.com/ MEDLINE, 2008.
4. www.ncbi.nlm.nih.gov/sites/entrez/
5. www.tripdatabase.com, Turning Research Into Practice (TRIP) database, 2008.
6. www.guidelines.gov, National Guideline Clearinghouse, 2008.
7. www.pedro.fhs.usyd.edu.au/, PEDro, 2008.
8. www.pedro.fhs.usyd.edu.au/scale_item.html, Criteria for inclusion on PEDro: PEDro scale, 2008.
9. Maher, CG, Sherrington, C, Herbert, RD, Moseley, AM, and Elkins, M: Reliability of the PEDro scale for rating quality of randomized controlled trials. Phys Ther 83:713–721, 2003.
10. www.hookedonevidence.com, Hooked on evidence, 2008.
11. www.cochrane.org/reviews, Cochrane Collaboration, Cochrane Reviews, 2008.
12. Miller, J, Gross, A, D'Sylva, J, et al: Manual therapy and exercise for neck pain: A systematic review. Man Ther 15:334–354, 2010.
13. Cleland, JA, Mintken, PE, Carpenter, K, et al: Examination of a clinical prediction rule to identify patients with neck pain likely to benefit from thoracic spine thrust manipulation and a general cervical range of motion exercise: Multi-center randomized clinical trial. Phys Ther 90:1239–1250, 2010.
14. http://medlineplus.gov, MedlinePlus, 2008.
15. www.ninds.nih.gov, National Institute of Neurological Disorders and Stroke, 2008.
16. www.nationalmssociety.org, National Multiple Sclerosis Society, 2008.
17. www.stroke.org, National Stroke Association, 2008.

3

Critically Appraise the Applicability and Quality of an Intervention Research Study

PRE-TEST

Read the clinical questions and abstract below[1]:

Searchable Clinical Question:

"For a 6-year-old girl with hemiplegia resulting from cerebral palsy, is constraint-induced movement therapy efficacious for improving the functional use of her hemiparetic arm?"

CHAPTER-AT-A-GLANCE

This chapter will help you understand the appraisal of the following:

- Applicability of research evidence

- Quality of research evidence

Abstract

Background and Purpose: This single-blinded randomized controlled trial compared the efficacy of a reimbursable, outpatient, modified constraint-induced therapy (mCIT) protocol (half-hour therapy sessions occurring 3 days per week in which subjects used the more affected arm combined with less affected arm restriction 5 days per week for 5 hours; both of these regimens were administered during a 10-week period) with that of a time-matched exercise program for the more affected arm or a no-treatment control regimen.

Subjects: Thirty-five subjects with chronic stroke participated in the study.

Methods: The Action Research Arm Test (ARAT), Fugl-Meyer Assessment of Motor Recovery After Stroke (FM), and Motor Activity Log (MAL) were administered to the subjects.

Results: After intervention, significant differences were observed on the ARAT and MAL Amount of Use and Quality of Movement scales, all in favor of the mCIT group.

Discussion and Conclusion: The data affirm previous findings suggesting that this reimbursable, outpatient protocol increases more affected arm use and function. Magnitude of changes was consistent with those reported in more intense protocols, such as constraint-induced therapy.

Page, S., Levine, P., Leonard, A., Szaflarski, J., Kissela, B. Modified Constraint-Induced Therapy in Chronic Stroke: Results of a Single-Blinded Randomized Controlled Trial
PHYS THER March 2008 88:333-340

PRE-TEST—cont'd

1. How will you determine if this study is applicable to your patient?

2. State one major threat to the quality of this study.

■ Introduction: The Process of Study Appraisal

This chapter and Chapter 4 support your knowledge and skill development for the third step of evidence based practice (EBP):

Step 3: Critically **appraise** the research evidence for applicability and quality

Step 3 in the EBP process is study appraisal. The appraisal process is summarized in the four parts in Figure 3.1. The first two parts are detailed in this chapter including appraising the:

A. *Applicability and*
B. *Quality of* a research study.

The third part, appraising study *results,* and fourth part, formulating a *clinical bottom line,* are detailed in Chapter 4. High-quality studies produce valid results. Chapters 3 and 4 focus on the appraisal of intervention studies. When results of an intervention study are valid, they can more confidently be applied to inform patient care.

Part A: Determining Applicability of an Intervention Study

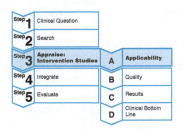

Using Research Evidence to Inform Care for Your Patients

You may have a specific patient in mind when you search the literature, or you may have a more general question about types of patients with shared problems and what interventions are most effective for these types of patients. In both situations, you will examine the research you locate to determine if it applies to your patient or group of patients with a similar problem.

The search engine PubMed was used to locate a randomized clinical trial (RCT) for 17-year-old swimmer June Wilson (Case Study 1.1). This article addressed the specific clinical question regarding a type of treatment and its effects on pain:

Searchable Clinical Question:

"For a 17-year-old swimmer with neck pain, is a combination of manual therapy and exercise effective for reducing pain and improving function?"

Article from search:

Walker MJ, Boyles RE, Young BA, et al. The effectiveness of manual physical therapy and exercise for mechanical neck pain a randomized clinical trial. *Spine.* 2008;33:2371-2378.[2]

The explanatory sections that follow are organized by questions to consider when appraising the applicability of an intervention study. (Questions 1 through 5 are in Table 3.3.)

QUESTION 1: *Is the study's purpose relevant to my clinical question?*

As a first step in the appraisal, you determine if this study could apply to June. The article may be an example of excellent research with valuable results, but June is a unique person with unique circumstances, and this article may or may not be applicable to her. The first step is to review the abstract from the Walker et al[2] study (Fig. 3.2). Read the notes in the abstract, and determine if this study would apply to June Wilson (Case Study 1.1).

QUESTION 2: *Is the study population (sample) sufficiently similar to my patient to justify the expectation that my patient would respond similarly to the population?*

Questions 2 and 3 should be appraised together.

QUESTION 3: *Are the inclusion and exclusion criteria clearly defined, and would my patient qualify for the study?*

You want to know the characteristics of the people studied. Are they similar enough to June or just too different for the results

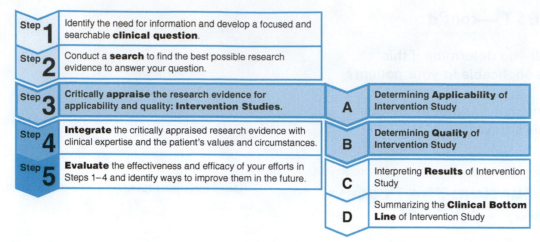

FIGURE 3.1 Four parts of study appraisal.

Note 3.3

The study identifies a treatment that resulted in significant reduction in pain which is one of June's goals.

Note 3.1

The number and characteristics of the subjects in a study will be described in the Method section of a RCT. There were 94 subjects from 3 physical therapy clinics and the subjects' primary complaint was mechanical neck pain with or without upper extremity pain. So far this study could apply to June. She has mechanical neck pain without upper extremity pain.

Note 3.2

The outcome measures include June's goal of reducing pain. The neck disability index may measure some aspects that will apply to June's other goal of continuing competitive swimming.

Study Design: Randomized clinical trial.

Objective: To assess the effectiveness of manual physical therapy and exercise (MTE) for mechanical neck pain with or without unilateral upper extremity (UE) symptoms, as compared to a minimal intervention (MIN) approach.

Summary of Background Data: Mounting evidence supports the use of manual therapy and exercise for mechanical neck pain, but no studies have directly assessed its effectiveness for UE symptoms.

Methods: A total of 94 patients referred to 3 physical therapy clinics with a primary complaint of mechanical neck pain, with or without unilateral UE symptoms, were randomized to receive MTE or a MIN approach of advice, motion exercise, and subtherapeutic ultrasound. Primary outcomes were the neck disability index, cervical and UE pain visual analog scales (VAS), and patient-perceived global rating of change assessed at 3-, 6-, and 52-weeks. Secondary measures included treatment success rates and post-treatment healthcare utilization.

Results: The MTE group demonstrated significantly larger reductions in short- and long-term neck disability index scores (mean 1-year difference −5.1, 95% confidence intervals (CI) −8.1, to −2.1; $P = 0.001$) and short-term cervical VAS scores (mean 6-week difference −14.2, 95% CI −22.7 to −5.6; $P = 0.001$) as compared to the MIN group. The MTE group also demonstrated significant within group reductions in short- and long-term UE VAS scores at all time periods (mean 1-year difference −16.3, 95% CI −23.1 to −9.5; $P = 0.000$). At 1-year, patient perceived treatment success was reported by 62% (29 of 47) of the MTE group and 32% (15 of 47) of the MIN group ($P = 0.004$).

Conclusion: An impairment-based MTE program resulted in clinically and statistically significant short- and long-term improvements in pain, disability, and patient perceived recovery in patients with mechanical neck pain when compared to a program comprising advice, a mobility exercise, and subtherapeutic ultrasound.

Key Words: mechanical neck pain, cervical pain, radicular pain, radiculitis, manual therapy, manipulation, mobilization, exercise.
Spine 2008;33:2371-2378.

FIGURE 3.2 Abstract from Walker MJ, Boyles RE, Young BA, et al. The effectiveness of manual physical therapy and exercise for mechanical neck pain: a randomized clinical trial. *Spine.* 2008;33:2371-2378; with permission.

to be applicable to June? Recall that you will most likely not find a study of people who are exactly like June, but they may have characteristics that are close enough for the results to have relevance for June. The inclusion and exclusion criteria for subjects are typically listed in the Methods section of a research paper. These criteria affect the applicability of the study. A treatment may be thought to be most effective in a restricted sample of patients with very specific criteria. To determine if

the treatment is effective, a study may limit the subjects to these specific inclusion criteria. For example, a treatment intended for patients with cervical pain but without radiculopathy would most likely exclude any patient with radiculopathy. This limits the applicability of the study, but it identifies the specific patient group that will benefit from the treatment.

What other information might you want to know about the subjects in this study? June is a teenager, but the abstract (see Fig. 3.2) does not include the ages of the study subjects. Subject characteristics are typically listed in tables within articles. Table 3.1 (from the Walker et al[2] study) lists the participant characteristics, including the average age and variation in age (standard deviation) of subjects in the study. Subjects were middle-aged and did not include a teenage range. In thinking about the applicability of this research to June, you would ask, "Are there specific characteristics of the teenage period that would make research with older adults less applicable to June?"

The search in Chapter 2 also identified a case series article that might include subjects that are more applicable to June (Case Study 1.1) (Fig. 3.3).

The abstract in Figure 3.3 includes the age of the subjects, but these subjects also are middle-aged. Remember, you will not find the perfect study, but more typically you will find studies that are close enough to be applicable at least to some degree for your patient.

When determining the applicability of a study to your patients, consider the following questions:

1. Is my patient in an age range that has special considerations, for example, children, teenagers, late elderly? What aspects of their age range are relevant? For example, children will respond differently in comparison to adolescents or elders to a strength-building program because the physiology of their muscles and their motivational characteristics are different.

2. Does my patient have a social, ethnic, cultural, or religious background that might constrain a particular type of treatment? For example, your patient might have limited insurance coverage for physical therapy, which might constrain an extended treatment period.

3. Are the treatments under study feasible in my clinical setting? Is special equipment or skill necessary to duplicate the treatment effectively? For example, to use the results from the Walker et al[2] study, you would need manual therapy skills.

QUESTION 4: *Are the intervention and comparison/control groups receiving a realistic intervention?*

The title of the study indicates that the study purpose included treatment of mechanical neck pain, a symptom reported by June. The two treatments that were compared, manual therapy and exercise, are also common physical therapy interventions that you might consider including in June's plan of care.

TABLE 3.1 Baseline Characteristics of 94 Participants

VARIABLE	MANUAL THERAPY AND EXERCISE (n = 47)	MINIMAL INTERVENTION (n = 47)
Age (yr)	48.8 (14.1)	46.2 (15.0)
Female gender	31 (66)	32 (68)
Symptom duration (d)*	1082 (365)	521 (70)
Medications use	31 (66)	31 (66)
Range of motion (degrees)		
Flexion	45.0 (14.1)	46.2 (14.4)
Extension	42.7 (14.3)	40.4 (13.8)
Rotation	50.9 (14.6)	51.9 (15.0)
Sidebending	32.9 (12.6)	31.9 (10.0)
Headache symptoms	27 (57)	32 (68)
Upper extremity symptoms	31 (66)	27 (57)

Data are mean (SD) for continuous variables or No. (%) for categorical variables, unless otherwise stated.
*Data are mean (median).
From Walker MJ, Boyles RE, Young BA, et al. The effectiveness of manual physical therapy and exercise from mechanical neck pain: a randomized clinical trial. *Spine.* 2008;33:2371-2378; Table 1; with permission.

Study Design: A case series of consecutive patients with cervical radiculopathy.

Background: A multitude of physical therapy interventions have been proposed to be effective in the management of cervical radiculopathy. However, outcome studies using consistent treatment approaches on a well-defined sample of patients are lacking. The purpose of this case series is to describe the outcomes of a consecutive series of patients presenting to physical therapy with cervical radiculopathy and managed with the use of manual physical therapy, cervical traction, and strengthening exercises.

Case Description: Eleven consecutive patients (mean age, 51.7 years; SD, 8.2) who presented with cervical radiculopathy on the initial examination were treated with a standardized approach, including manual physical therapy, cervical traction, and strengthening exercises of the deep neck flexors and scapulothoracic muscles. At the initial evaluation all patients completed self-report measures of pain and function, including a numeric pain rating scale (NPRS), the Neck Disability Index (NDI), and the Patient-Specific Functional Scale (PSFS). All patients again completed the outcome measures, in addition to the global rating of change (GROC), at the time of discharge from therapy and at a 6-month follow-up session.

Outcomes: Ten of the 11 patients (91%) demonstrated a clinically meaningful improvement in pain and function following a mean of 7.1 (SD, 1.5) physical therapy visits and at the 6-month follow-up.

Discussion: Ninety-one percent (10 of 11) of patients with cervical radiculopathy in this case series improved, as defined by the patients classifying their level of improvement as at least "quite a bit better" on the GROC. However, because a cause-and-effect relationship cannot be inferred from a case series, follow-up randomized clinical trials should be performed to further investigate the effectiveness of manual physical therapy, cervical traction, and strengthening exercises in a homogeneous group of patients with cervical radiculopathy.
J Orthop Sports Phys Ther 2005;35:802-811.

Key Words: *cervical spine, manipulation, mobilization, thoracic spine.*

FIGURE 3.3 Abstract from Cleland JA, Whitman JM, Fritz JM, Palmer JA. Manual physical therapy, cervical traction, and strengthening exercises in patients with cervical radiculopathy: a case series. *J Orthop Sports Phys Ther.* 2005;35:802-811; with permission. [8]

QUESTION 5: Are the outcome measures relevant to the clinical question, and were they conducted in a clinically realistic manner?

Study outcomes include a pain measure and a pain index, which may relate to June's goal to resume competitive swimming.

Summary of Applicability

Deciding the applicability of a study to your specific patient is a process of weighing the similarities and differences between the study participants and your patient and the intervention proposed and the feasibility of this intervention for you and your clinic. As you read research studies, you can keep track of answers to the questions regarding applicability by using the checklist in Table 3.3.

Part B: Determining Quality of an Intervention Study

Is This a Useful Study?

Appraising the quality of a study focuses on understanding if the study was conducted with sufficient rigor that you can use the study results for making clinical decisions. Appraising study rigor is also referred to as appraising the *internal quality,* or *validity,* of a study.[3] A study might have high applicability, but it may not have been conducted with sufficient rigor to be useful for clinical decisions. Appraisal requires the balancing of the applicability of a study and the quality of the study. Your goal is to have both applicability and quality rate as highly as possible (Fig. 3.4).

The explanatory sections that follow are organized by questions to consider when appraising the quality of an intervention study. Following are questions 6 to 11, which are also included in Table 3.3.

Two Independent Scales for Research Evidence Appraisal:

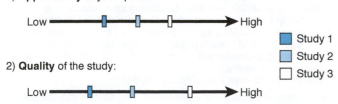

1) **Applicability** to your question:

Low ──────────→ High

☐ Study 1
☐ Study 2
☐ Study 3

2) **Quality** of the study:

Low ──────────→ High

One study can have very different rankings on the two scales.

FIGURE 3.4 Best evidence is a balance between applicability and quality.

QUESTION 6: Were participants randomly assigned to intervention groups?

Study Design

Randomized Controlled Trial or Randomized Clinical Trial

The randomized controlled trial or randomized clinical trial (RCT) is one type of research design. More designs are considered in other chapters; for example, designs that are most appropriate for questions of diagnosis (Chapter 5) and prognosis (Chapter 6). The RCT is often characterized as the gold standard of research designs for intervention studies. It is an experimental design in which treatments are compared. The RCT is considered one of the most valid designs to determine if a particular physical therapy treatment has a positive effect. Types of clinical questions that could be answered with an RCT include the following:

1. Is manual therapy more effective than trunk stabilization for pain reduction and return to activity for people with acute low back pain?
2. What is the efficacy of body weight–supported gait training as an intervention for school-age children with spastic diplegia?
3. What is the efficacy of constraint-induced therapy as an intervention for individuals with a hemiplegia associated with stroke?

Ideally, a random sample of subjects from the entire population of interest would be selected for study. For example, if the entire population of people who have sustained a stroke could be identified, then a sample from the entire population would be chosen randomly for study. Obviously it is not possible to locate or sample from an entire population, but a smaller sample might be selected randomly from a very large sample of people with a particular condition. Often in RCT designs, all *available* subjects are included in a study and then randomly assigned to treatment groups. If the sample is large enough (and this is key), then the random assignment ensures that all groups will be similar in the characteristics that are thought to affect outcome before the treatment begins. This similarity between groups is important to *reduce one potential source of bias* that might affect the outcome of the treatment. **Bias** in a study is any factor that makes you less certain that the results of the study are due to the intervention. Reducing bias increases your certainty that the results are due to the treatment.

For example:

If treatment group A has subjects with more severe disability than treatment group B, then group A might respond with greater change to treatment, regardless of type of treatment.

Conversely, treatment group A might respond more poorly to an intense treatment because the subjects may not have sufficient endurance for the treatment. Randomly assigning subjects to groups *should* even out the groups in terms of severity of disability and reduce this source of bias.

RCTs are typically designed to evaluate the *efficacy* of an intervention.[4,5] Efficacy refers to the effect of treatment under highly controlled conditions. This is in contrast to a study of *effectiveness,* in which the treatment would be evaluated under more typical clinical conditions. Effectiveness speaks to what is likely to happen given a treatment versus efficacy, which determines what could happen in the best possible environment. These are each important but very different questions.

Stratification Within RCTs

Randomization is most effective in reducing potential bias if the sample size is large; however, recruiting enough subjects is often challenging. Stratification of subjects is used in the RCT in situations in which there are potential characteristics that are thought or known to affect outcomes and it is not certain that a sufficient number of subjects with this characteristic will be recruited. For example, if previous research suggests that men and women respond differently to a particular treatment, but the problem is less common in women than it is in men, it may be difficult to recruit enough women to be sure the groups will be similar according to gender. The groups could be stratified on gender and then males and females randomized separately into treatment groups. This gives you more precise applicability of the research to your male and female patients. Figure 3.5 includes an abstract of a study in which subjects are stratified based on locomotor impairment defined as speed of walking.

QUESTION 7: Is the sampling procedure (recruitment strategy) likely to minimize bias?

Samples for Studies

The value of randomization to reduce one source of bias and the need to have subject groups as similar as possible at the beginning of a study have been discussed. There are additional sampling issues that should be considered to minimize bias in the sample of participants chosen for a study.

Sample Size

Study samples in physical therapy are often small. Sometimes samples are too small for the study results to be truly believable (valid). It is difficult and costly to obtain large numbers of subjects with certain types of injury, movement issues, or medical

---

Protocol for the Locomotor Experience Applied Post-stroke (LEAPS) trial: a randomized controlled trial[8]

Pamela W Duncan, Katherine J Sullivan, Andrea L Behrman, Stanley P Azen, Samuel S Wu, Stephen E Nadeau, Bruce H Dobkin, Dorian K Rose, Julie K Tilson for the LEAPS Investigative Team

Abstract

Background: Locomotor training using body weight support and a treadmill as a therapeutic modality for rehabilitation of walking post-stroke is being rapidly adopted into clinical practice. There is an urgent need for a well-designed trial to determine the effectiveness of this intervention. The objective of the Locomotor Experience Applied Post-Stroke (LEAPS) trial is to determine the effectiveness if there is a difference in the proportion of participants who recover walking ability at one year post-stroke when randomized to a specialized locomotor training program (LTP), conducted at 2- or 6-months post-stroke, or those randomized to a home based non-specific, low intensity exercise intervention (HEP) provided 2 months post-stroke. We will determine if the timing of LTP delivery affects gait speed at 1 year and whether initial impairment severity interacts with the timing of LTP. The effect of number of treatment sessions will be determined by changes in gait speed taken pretreatment and post-12, -24, and -36 sessions.

Methods/Design: We will recruit 400 adults with moderate or severe walking limitations within 30 days of stroke onset. *At two months post-stroke, participants are stratified by locomotor impairment severity as determined by overground walking speed and randomly assigned to one of three groups: (a) LTP-Early; (b) LTP-Late or (c) Home Exercise Program-Early.* The LTP program includes body weight support on a treadmill and overground training. The LTP and HEP interventions are delivered for 36 sessions over 12 weeks. Primary outcome measure includes successful walking recovery defined as the achievement of a 0.4 m/s gait speed or greater by persons with initial severe gait impairment or the achievement of a 0.8 m/s gait speed or greater by persons with initial moderate gait impairment. LEAPS is powered to detect a 20% difference in the proportion of participants achieving successful locomotor recovery between the LTP groups and the HEP group, and a 0.1 m/s mean difference in gait speed change between the two LTP groups.

Discussion: The goal of this single-blinded, phase III randomized clinical trial is to provide evidence to guide post-stroke walking recovery programs.

> Each of the three groups in this study will have an equal number of subjects with *moderate* walking limitations and with *severe* walking limitations. Patients may respond differently to locomotor training depending on the severity of their walking limitations.

FIGURE 3.5 Abstract from Duncan PW, Sullivan KJ, Behrman AL, et al. Protocol for the Locomotor Experience Applied Post-stroke (LEAPS) trial: a randomized controlled trial. *BMC Neurol.* 2007;7:39; with permission.

problems. For example, patient characteristics for a hypothetical study are listed in Table 3.2. If your patient is a black female with an affected right side and age 62, this study might be helpful to your clinical decisions. Similarly, if your patient is an Hispanic male with an affected left side and age 83, this study might also be useful for clinical care. The authors of this hypothetical study believed that gender, race, age, and side affected would have an impact on the results of the study. By including all of these characteristics, the applicability of the study is increased.

However, sufficient numbers of subjects are needed in each category in Table 3.2 to make the study valid. Imagine that the study in Table 3.2 has 8 white males with an affected left side who are in the 60-to-70 age range and 232 black males with an affected right side also in this age range. This imbalance in the number of subjects in the study creates problems in interpreting the results of the study and applying the results to specific patients.

Study Power

Without sufficient numbers of subjects, a study may lack power. Power is a statistical term.[6,7] The power of a statistical test is the likelihood that the test will detect a difference between groups if there is a difference. The bigger the difference between treatment groups, the more likely that the difference will be statistically significant. The size of a sample affects power. If a sample is too small, it is possible for the results of a study to suggest that there is no difference between treatments when in fact there is a difference. The study conclusions are not helpful for clinical decisions if the study lacks power. Statistical quality is discussed more thoroughly in Chapter 4, but the important message here is that if samples are too small (study is underpowered) it may not be a good enough study to help you make decisions.

Recruiting a Study Sample

There are different methods used to recruit participants for a study. For example, a study of physical therapy for postsurgical anterior cruciate ligament (ACL) repair might include all patients who are referred to one physical therapy clinic. A consecutive sample[6] (Fig. 3.6) includes all patients referred to this clinic with this problem. Because people with many different characteristics (e.g., age, athletic ability, gender) are referred for physical therapy post ACL surgery, the sample from this clinic might represent this broad sampling. When consecutive sampling is used, *every* patient post ACL surgery who is referred to the clinic is a potential subject. Each patient is then considered in terms of inclusion or exclusion criteria for the study. Selective sampling (see Fig. 3.6) is an alternative method. If orthopedic surgeons and other professional colleagues are asked to refer their patients post-ACL surgery, then most likely a selective sample is recruited. Not all patients will be referred. The surgeons or colleagues may suggest the study only to patients who they believe are likely to participate, or they might remember to refer patients after first hearing about the study, but forget referrals later on. Selective sampling is less ideal than consecutive sampling, but it is common and practical.

TABLE 3.2 **Example Patient Characteristics**

PATIENT CHARACTERISTICS		ACTIVITIES OF DAILY LIVING	WALKING SPEED	QUALITY OF LIFE
Gender	Male			
	Female			
Race	White			
	Black			
	Hispanic			
	Other			
Side Affected	Left			
	Right			
Age	60–70			
	71–80			
	81–90			

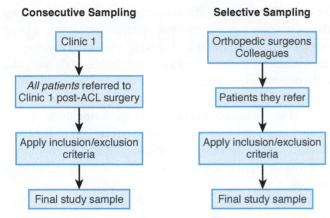

Consecutive Sampling

Clinic 1

↓

All patients referred to Clinic 1 post-ACL surgery

↓

Apply inclusion/exclusion criteria

↓

Final study sample

Selective Sampling

Orthopedic surgeons Colleagues

↓

Patients they refer

↓

Apply inclusion/exclusion criteria

↓

Final study sample

FIGURE 3.6 Consecutive and selective sampling methods typically results in different final study samples.

■ Results

Of the 255 subjects, there was missing data for 31 patients. For 30 subjects, Spurling test results were missing, and 1 subject had a missing score for the likelihood of cervical radiculopathy being present. Therefore, the analysis was performed on the 224 remaining subjects.

Of the 20 patients for whom the electrodiagnostic evaluation was thought to show "fairly specific abnormalities" or "very strong evidence" for cervical radiculopathy, the Spurling test yielded positive results for 6 patients. Therefore, the sensitivity was shown to be 6/20 (30%).

Of the 172 patients for whom the electrodiagnostic evaluation was thought to show no evidence for radiculopathy, the Spurling test yielded negative results for 160 patients. The specificity was therefore shown to be 160/172 (93%). The odds ratio for a patient with positive Spurling test results if there is an electrodiagnostically confirmed radiculopathy is 5.71 (95% confidence interval, 1.86–17.5).[15]

FIGURE 3.7 A section of the results from Tong HC, Haig AJ, Yamakawa K. The Spurling test and cervical radiculopathy. *Spine.* 2002;27:156-159; with permission.[9]

QUESTION 8: *Are all participants who entered the study accounted for?*

Losing Subjects in the Sample

Maintaining all subjects in a study is challenging. It is particularly important if the sample is small. Details about who dropped out of a study and reasons for dropout are important considerations in your appraisal. Subjects might have a higher dropout rate from one group in comparison to the other, leaving the groups unbalanced in size, and possibly not the same (or at least similar) on important characteristics. If subjects drop out because they could not complete a type of intervention, this tells us about the characteristics of patients who could tolerate the treatment.

As a part of your appraisal, compare the number of subjects reported in tables and statistical results with the number of subjects originally enrolled in the study. If these are different, the authors should provide details on subject attrition and how they analyzed the potential impact on the study results. For example, in the Results section in Figure 3.7 there were 255 subjects originally enrolled in the study as reported in the first sentence. However, test results for only 192 subjects are reported (20 patients reported in the second paragraph and 172 reported in the third paragraph). The authors account for 31 dropouts and then state that the analysis was conducted on the final sample of 224 subjects. There are 32 subjects without reported results. These subjects must be accounted for in order to fully appraise the quality of this study.

QUESTION 9: *Was a comparison made between groups with preservation of original group assignments?*

Subject attrition is a potential threat to the quality of the results of a study. It is usually reported in the analysis or the results section of a paper. A common statistical analysis that considers subject attrition is the **intention-to-treat (ITT)** analysis.[6] This procedure is used in randomized controlled trials. In an ITT analysis, all subjects are analyzed in the groups to which they were initially assigned even if they did not receive their assigned treatment.

The ITT, however, assumes that subjects' measurements are available even if the subjects did not complete treatment according to the study protocol. If data are not available, it may be estimated. What is essential is that the authors report subject attrition, explain reasons for the attrition, and at least attempt to analyze the impact of subjects leaving the study on the study results.

■ Determining Threats and Strengths of a Research Study

We want to be as certain as possible that the treatment and not other factors caused the change in the study participants. All studies will have threats and strengths in relation to internal quality. A **threat** is a factor that is not controlled in a study that might affect the outcome. Threats create uncertainty that intervention caused the change in patient results. If there are too many threats to internal quality, the study becomes useless to us for making clinical decisions because too many uncontrolled factors may be responsible for the results. Some example threats to a study are small samples, no randomization, and groups having different characteristics before intervention began that might affect outcomes. A **strength** is a factor that is well controlled and contributes to the conclusion that the treatment was responsible for the change in the patients and not other uncontrolled factors. Strengths of a study include randomization, intention to treat analysis, and masking of evaluators as to which treatment each subject received, thus potentially biasing the outcome evaluations.

Testers and Treaters: The Importance of Masking

QUESTION 10: *Was blinding/masking optimized in the study design? (evaluators, participants, therapists)*

The person giving the treatment during an intervention study should not be the person who measures the patients' results from the intervention. The "treaters" should not be the "testers." Ideally, the testers should not know which treatment a patient received during the study and they should know as little as possible about the study goals (Fig. 3.8). This is referred to as masking or blinding.[6] Neither the treaters nor the testers may consciously bias the results, but their opinions and clinical experiences with specific treatments may influence their measurements. If the treating therapist also measures the results of the intervention, this is a serious threat to the quality of the results. It reduces your certainty that the study results were due to the specific intervention and thus reduces the usefulness of the results for your clinical decisions.

Equivalent Treatment

QUESTION 11: *Aside from the allocated treatment, were groups treated equally?*

When two or more treatments are compared or when a treatment is compared with that of a control group, all other interventions must be stopped or held constant for the duration of the study. For example, if some subjects in a treatment group also participated in another type of intervention (e.g. adding therapy, taking medications, or seeking alternative treatments), this reduces the certainty that the results of the study were due to the original intervention. Patients may be taking medications that should not be stopped during a study, but these must be reported and held as constant as possible during the study duration. Study participants are asked to refrain from other interventions during the study, but this should also be monitored periodically during a study, especially if study duration is lengthy.

Treatments should also be equivalent in intensity (Fig. 3-9). One type of treatment may involve longer periods of therapy; for example, manual therapy plus exercise versus exercise alone. The length of therapy and the intensity or dose (once a week, twice a week, etc.) must be equivalent. An equal amount of exercise may be used for both study groups and while one group receives manual therapy, the exercise-only group may receive an educational session or other form of intervention to make the time in therapy equivalent.

Summary of Research Study Quality

The above content is summarized as a checklist in Table 3.3. These questions are used to appraise the *quality* of a study. As you read the study, you can keep track of answers to the questions by checking "Yes" or "No." This is a partial checklist,

Treatment A

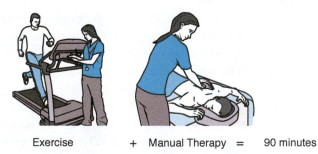

Exercise   +   Manual Therapy =   90 minutes

Treatment B

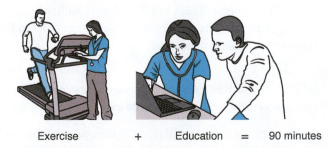

Exercise   +   Education   =   90 minutes

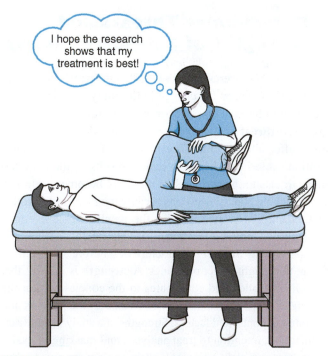

I hope the research shows that my treatment is best!

FIGURE 3.8 The therapist giving treatment in a research study should not measure outcomes in the study.

FIGURE 3.9 Treatments A and B must be equivalent in length of treatment.

TABLE 3.3   **Key Questions to Determine an Intervention Research Study's *Applicability* and *Quality***

QUESTION	YES/NO	WHERE TO FIND THE INFORMATION	COMMENTS AND WHAT TO LOOK FOR
1. Is the study's purpose relevant to my clinical question?	__ Yes __ No	Introduction (usually at the end)	The study should clearly describe its purpose and/or hypothesis. Ideally, the stated purpose will contribute to answering your clinical question.
2. Is the study population (sample) sufficiently similar to my patient to justify the expectation that my patient would respond similarly to the population?	__ Yes __ No	Results section	The study should provide descriptive statistics about pertinent study population demographics. Ideally, the study population would be relatively similar to your patient with regard to age, gender, problem severity, problem duration, co-morbidities, and other sociodemographic and medical conditions likely to affect the results of the study.
3. Are the inclusion and exclusion criteria clearly defined and would my patient qualify for the study?	__ Yes __ No	Methods section	The study should provide a list of inclusion and exclusion criteria. Ideally, your patient would have characteristics that meet the eligibility criteria or at least be similar enough to the subjects. Remember, you will not find "the perfect study"!
4. Are the intervention and comparison/control groups receiving a realistic intervention?	__ Yes __ No	Methods (some post-study analysis about the intervention may be found in the Results)	The study should clearly describe the treatment regimen provided to all groups. Ideally, the intervention can be reproduced in your clinical setting and the comparison/control is a realistic contrasting option or well-designed placebo. Consider the quality of the dose, duration, delivery method, setting, and qualifications of the therapists delivering the intervention. Could you implement this treatment in your setting?
5. Are the outcome measures relevant to the clinical question and were they conducted in a clinically realistic manner?	___ Yes ___ No	Methods	The study should describe the outcome measures used and the methods used to ensure their reliability and quality. Ideally, the outcome measures should relate to the clinical question and should include measures of quality of life, activity, and body structure and function. For diagnostic studies, it is important that the investigated measure be realistic for clinical use.
6. Were participants randomly assigned to intervention groups?	__ Yes __ No	Methods	The study should describe how participants were assigned to groups. **Randomization** is a robust method for reducing **bias.** Computerized random-ization in which the order of group assignment is concealed from investigators is the strongest method.
7. Is the sampling procedure (recruitment strategy) likely to minimize bias?	__ Yes __ No	Methods	The study should describe how and from where participants were recruited. **Consecutive recruitment,** in which any participant who meets eligibility criteria is invited to join the study, is the strongest design. Studies in which the authors handpick participants may demonstrate the best effects of a specific treatment, but they will lack applicability across patient types.
8. Are all participants who entered the study accounted for?	__ Yes __ No		The study should describe how many participants were initially allocated to each group and how many finished the study. Ideally, >80% of participants complete the study and the reason for any participants not finishing is provided.

Continued

TABLE 3.3 **Key Questions to Determine an Intervention Research Study's** *Applicability* **and** *Quality*—cont'd

QUESTION	YES/NO	WHERE TO FIND THE INFORMATION	COMMENTS AND WHAT TO LOOK FOR
9. Was a comparison made between groups with preservation of original group assignments?	__ Yes __ No	Methods will describe the planned analysis. Results will report findings.	The study should make comparisons between groups (not just a comparison of each group to itself). Ideally, an **intention-to-treat analysis** is conducted to compare groups' participants according to their original group assignment.
10. Was blinding/masking optimized in the study design? (evaluators, participants, therapists)	__ Yes __ No	Methods	The study should describe how/if **blinding** was used to reduce bias by concealing group assignment. Most physical therapy–related studies cannot blind therapists or participants due to the physical nature of interventions. Bias can be reduced, however, by blinding the evaluators (who conduct the outcome measures).
11. Aside from the allocated treatment, were groups treated equally?	__ Yes __ No	Methods will describe the treatment plan. Results may report adherence to plan.	The study should describe how equivalency, other than the intended intervention, is maintained between groups. Ideally, all participants will have exactly the same experience in the study except for the difference between interventions.

with the remaining questions to appraise study quality included in a checklist in Chapter 4.

■ Research Notation

When you first read a study, you want to understand *what* was done and then determine *how* it was done. Research notation, first described by Campbell and Stanley,[7] is a helpful shorthand to diagram the design of an intervention study and give you the big picture of the overall study. Research notation will be used to diagram what was done in the example studies and identify the type of design used in the study. Different clinical questions are best answered with specific study designs. For example, the RCT is an excellent design for intervention research but not for prognostic studies. Thus research notation is used to depict intervention studies.

There are four symbols used in research notation with the following definitions:

R subjects were randomly assigned to treatment groups
– – – subjects were not randomly assigned
X intervention
O observation (time of measurement)

Using Research Notation for Example Study Designs

The studies diagrammed in Figure 3.10, Examples 1 and 2, have less potential bias than the study diagrammed in Example 3. In Example 1 two treatments are compared, and in Example 2 one treatment is compared with a no-treatment condition. The design in Example 1 helps to determine which treatment might have a greater effect. The design in Example 2 helps to determine if treating the patient with a particular treatment is better than doing nothing. If there are positive results from Example 3, you may determine that subjects improved, but it does not help you to understand how to choose among treatments or if time alone might have been sufficient for the subjects to improve. Studies in which a control (no treatment) or comparison (an alternate treatment) are used have higher quality than studies with only one treatment group.

■ SELF-TEST 3.1

Using research notation, diagram the study in the abstract found in Figure 3.2. Compare your answers with those in Answers to Self-Test.

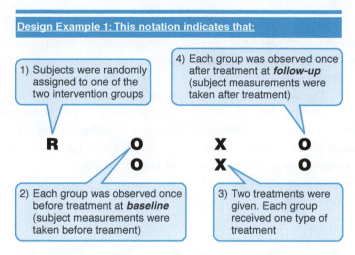

Treatment may have been given once or multiple times. The X merely indicates that treatment was given but not the type or amount of treatment. Research notation does not specify what measures were taken at each observation point. We have a general diagram of what was done in this study, but no specifics about treatments or outcome measures.

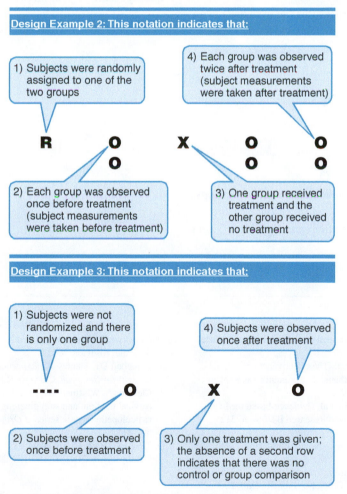

FIGURE 3.10 Diagrams of example research designs using research notation.

SUMMARY

Appraising the applicability of research evidence: After identifying your clinical question, searching for evidence, and then locating research evidence, you determine if the research is appropriate for your particular patient. The *applicability* of research is a first step in appraising research. Applicability is determined by comparing the study participants' characteristics to your patient (e.g., age, rehabilitation potential, gender). Then you determine if the intervention is appropriate for your patient and if you have the skills and necessary equipment in your clinic to implement the treatment intervention

Appraising the quality of research evidence: Once you have determined that a research study is applicable to your patient, you will appraise the quality of the research. You will determine if a study has been conducted with sufficient rigor for you to use the results in the care of your patient. Appraising the rigor or *internal quality* of a research study includes an understanding of sampling of subjects, measurement, and sources of bias in a study.

REVIEW QUESTIONS

1. State the three most important characteristics of a high-quality intervention study.

2. Why should the person who measures the outcomes in an intervention study not administer the intervention?

3. What is more relevant to the application of a study to your clinical question, the applicability of the study or the study quality? Defend your answer.

ANSWERS TO SELF-TEST

■ SELF-TEST 3.1

R   O   X   O   O   O

O   X   O   O   O

Explanation: Subjects were randomized into two groups, MTE or MIN, and measurements were taken once before interventions began and three times after treatment (at 3, 6, and 52 weeks).

REFERENCES

1. Page S, Levine P, Leonard A, et al. Modified constraint-induced therapy in chronic stroke: results of a single-blinded randomized controlled trial. *Phys Ther.* 2008;88:333–340.
2. Walker MJ, Boyles RE, Young BA, et al. The effectiveness of manual physical therapy and exercise for mechanical neck pain: a randomized clinical trial. *Spine.* 2008;33:2371-2378.
3. Sackett DL, Rosenberg WM, Gray JA, et al. Evidence-based medicine: what it is and what it isn't. *BMJ* [Clinical Research Ed.]. 1996;312:71-72.
4. Domholdt B. *Physical Therapy Research.* 2nd ed. Philadelphia, PA: Saunders; 2000.
5. Portney LG, Watkins MP. *Foundations of Clinical Research: Applications to Practice.* 2nd ed. Englewood Cliffs, NJ: Prentice Hall; 2000.
6. Straus SE, Richardson WS, Glasziou P, Haynes RB. *Evidence-Based Medicine: How to Practice and Teach EBM.* 3rd ed. Edinburgh, Scotland: Elsevier; 2005.
7. Campbell DT, Stanley JC. *Experimental and Quasi-Experimental Designs for Research.* Chicago, IL: Rand McNally; 1971.
8. Cleland JA, Whitman JM, Fritz JM, Palmer JA. Manual physical therapy, cervical traction, and strengthening exercises in patients with cervical radiculopathy: a case series. *J Orthop Sports Phys Ther.* 2005;35:802-811.
9. Tong HC, Haig AJ, Yamakawa K. The Spurling test and cervical radiculopathy. *Spine.* 2002;27:156-159.

4

Critically Appraise the Results of an Intervention Research Study

PRE-TEST

1. What are the differences between descriptive statistics and inferential statistics?

2. How do you determine if the results of a research study are clinically important?

3. The median income in the United States is $44,000, but the mean income is $60,500. Why are these values different? Which value is likely to best describe incomes in the United States?

4. Why is 0.05 typically chosen as the alpha value in a research study?

5. Which value represents the difference between two treatments in a randomized clinical trial: alpha level, p value, effect size, or number needed to treat?

CHAPTER-AT-A-GLANCE

This chapter helps you understand the following:

- Interpretation of the results of a intervention research study

- Reliability of measures

- Reasons to use statistics

- Types of statistics: descriptive, inferential, clinically relevant

■ Introduction

Chapters 3 and 4 support your knowledge and skill development for the third step of evidence based practice (EBP):

STEP 3: Critically appraise the research evidence for applicability and quality

Chapter 3 included parts A, Determining applicability, and B, Determining quality of a research study. This chapter includes parts

C. Interpreting study results and
D. Summarizing the clinical bottom line (Fig. 4.1).

Reading and interpreting study results can be challenging. If you develop a systematic approach to reading through the results of a study, it becomes easier and faster to interpret the study findings. This chapter describes a process for appraising results and guides you through the appraisal, including the interpretation of statistics.

Part C: Interpreting Results of an Intervention Study

Locating and Appraising the Results of a Research Study

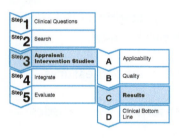

Tables have it all! The results of intervention research studies are summarized in tables. A helpful habit to develop is to read through the tables in a paper and reflect on the information contained in them before trying to understand the text in the results section. The title of a table indicates what will be included in the main part of the table. Figure 4.2 illustrates a typical table describing the demographic and clinical characteristics of the study sample for each group.[1]

Data are summarized using **descriptive statistics.** Descriptive statistics give you an overall impression of the typical values for the group as well as the variability within and between the groups.[2,3] First, look at the demographic data. Compare the control and the two training groups on average age, height, weight, and body mass index (see Fig. 4.2, Note 4.1). The numerical values within the table are reported as means and standard deviations for each characteristic and each group. The details for the units of expression for each characteristic are added under the table as a table footnote (Fig. 4.2, Note 4.2).

DIGGING DEEPER 4.1

Descriptive statistics

A. MEASURES OF CENTRAL TENDENCY: Measures of central tendency are measures of the "average" or "most typical" and are the most widely used statistical description of data.

Many variables that are measured in rehabilitation research fall into a normal (bell-shaped) curve in the normal population (Fig. 4.3A). The logic of a **normal distribution** is based on repeated measures in a large sample of people. When variables such as weight or range of motion are measured in a large sample of people, the distribution of these variables takes on a bell shape.

Non-normally distributed data (skewed) (Fig. 4.3B) is common with clinical populations. It is expected that the subjects in a research study on people with disease or injury may not have the typical distribution of values that are seen in a healthy population.

The results of measurement are reported using terms that are associated with specific types of distributions. For example, mean and standard deviation are typically reported if a variable has a normal (bell-shaped) distribution. Median and mode are typically reported for variables with a non-normal (skewed) distribution.

1. **Mean** – the arithmetic average – the mean of a set of observations is simply their sum, divided by the number of observations.
2. **Median** – the median is the 50th percentile of a distribution – the point below which half of the observations fall.
3. **Mode** – the mode is the most frequently occurring observation – the most popular score of a class of scores.

B. MEASURES OF VARIABILITY OR DISPERSION: Measures of variability reflect the degree of spread or dispersion that characterizes a group of scores and the degree to which a set of scores differs from some measure of central tendency.

DIGGING DEEPER 4.1 — cont'd

1. **Range** – the range is the difference between the highest and lowest scores in a distribution.
2. **Standard deviation** – the standard deviation is the most commonly used measure of variability. The standard deviation is the average amount that each of the individual scores varies from the mean of the set of scores.

C. EXAMPLE CLINICAL VALUES: *What is the average range of motion of the subjects before treatment?*

The arithmetic *mean*, the sum of values of range of motion divided by the number of values of range of motion, would answer this question. When it is associated with a normal distribution, then it occurs at the middle of the distribution, with half of the scores above and half below. With a normal distribution

you also know that approximately 64% of the sample is 1 standard deviation (SD) either above or below the mean, and approximately 92% will be 2 SD above or below the mean. But the mean value is only one number. The mean may adequately represent the values of range of motion for a sample, or it may be less adequate. To further understand the characteristics of this sample, you need to ask another question.

What is the variability in the range of motion of the subjects before treatment?

The SD gives a measure of the variability in a sample. It is the square root of the variance. The variance is also a measure of the variability in a sample. If you assume a variable that is normally distributed, then each increment of the SD captures a known percentage of your sample.

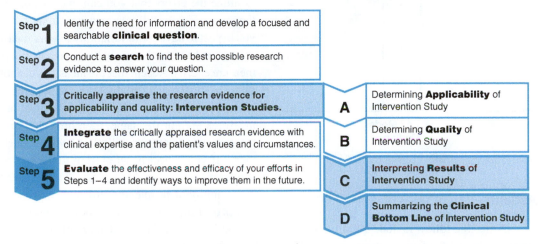

FIGURE 4.1 Appraising the results of a study and the clinical bottom line.

Table 1. Demographic and Clinical Data of the Patients in the Intervention and Control Groups*

Variable	Control Group (n = 60)	Training Groups — Endurance (n = 59)	Training Groups — Strength (n = 60)
Demographics			
Age, y	46 (5)	46 (6)	45 (6)
Height, cm	164 (5)	165 (6)	165 (5)
Weight, kg	69 (12)	68 (10)	67 (11)
Body mass index†	26 (4)	25 (3)	25 (3)
Clinical			
Duration of neck pain, y	8 (5)	9 (6)	8 (6)
Short depression inventory score‡	6 (3)	6 (4)	5 (3)
Grip strength, right hand, N§	293 (54)	299 (50)	299 (54)
Grip strength, left hand, N§	266 (46)	270 (53)	286 (52)
Maximum oxygen uptaken, mL/kg per min	31 (5)	32 (4)	33 (5)
Smoking, No. (%)	10 (17)	12 (20)	10 (17)

Abbreviation: N, Newton, which is a measure of force.
*Data are presented as mean (SD) unless otherwise indicated.
†Body mass index is calculated as weight in kilograms divided by the square of height in meters.
‡Mood is assessed on a theoretical range of 1 to 21, with a lower score indicating a better mood.
§Grip strength was measured using a hand-held Jamar grip-strength device while the participant was in a seated position and the elbow supported in a right angle.

Note 4.1
Means and standard deviations for age are listed by group.

Hypothetical Ages:
Control = 52 (6)
Endurance = 46 (6)
Strength = 42 (3)

Note 4.3
Grip strength has a wide variability among groups

Note 4.2
Units of measure and comments

FIGURE 4.2 Typical table describing the demographic and clinical characteristics of the study sample for each group. *From: Ylinen J, Takala EP, Nykanen M, et al. Active neck muscle training in the treatment of chronic neck pain in women: a randomized controlled trial. JAMA. 2003;289:2509–2516; with permission.*

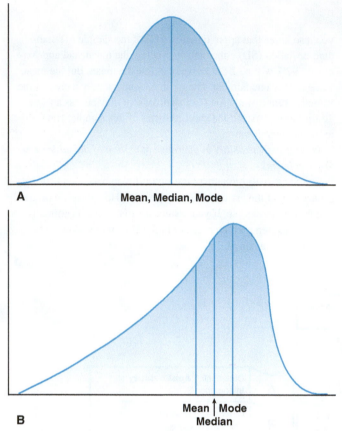

FIGURE 4.3 (A) Normal distribution; (B) non-normal (skewed) distribution.

Appraisal Questions

The explanatory sections that follow include questions to consider when appraising the quality of an intervention study. Five questions are included that form Table 4.5. Combining the checklists found in Tables 3.3 and 4.5 gives a complete list of questions to use when appraising the applicability an intervention study (Appendix).

QUESTION 1: *Were the groups similar at baseline?*

The groups should be as similar as possible at the beginning of an intervention study, that is, before treatment. Randomization of subjects should ensure that groups are at least similar if not exactly the same. But how similar should they be? What if they are "somewhat" different? How different can samples be at the start of a study and still be acceptable? Now look at the "Hypothetical Ages" (see Fig. 4.2, Note 4.1). There is a 10-year mean age difference between the control and the strength groups. Are these ages similar "enough," or could the difference in age contribute somehow to the subjects' responses to treatment and thus to the results?

Recall that you want to be as certain as possible that the results of a study are due to the intervention and not to other sources

of bias (sometimes referred to as error). Group differences at the beginning of a study are potentially a source of errors that could contribute to the results of a study and thus reduce your certainty that the intervention led to the results. Groups may have different values on the pre-intervention characteristics because:

- Groups really are different and randomization was not successful
- They have been measured differently by different people
- The instruments or tests used introduce error

Grip strength reported in Figure 4.2, Note 4.3, was measured with a dynamometer, a device that when squeezed registers the amount of force generated. The *Strength Group* started the study with a mean value that was 20 newtons greater than that of the *Control Group*. Is this a "real" difference or the result of bias introduced by the dynamometer or by the people measuring? First, examine the errors that you can make as *measuring* physical therapists (Fig. 4.4). If you measure strength twice in a patient, you expect to have some variability in your measures. This variability can be termed *error* because you are not replicating your measure exactly. Accept that the measures cannot be exactly the same, but how much variability (error) is acceptable? If you expect that the treatment will improve strength, but your repeated measures are not the same, then how can you know what is measurement error (variability) and what is an effect from treatment? If you expect benefits from treatment to be small, then any error can confound the results. The **reliability** of measures is the ability of people and instruments to produce consistent values over time. The tests and devices used and the measuring physical therapist should reliably reproduce measurements.

Reliability of Testers and Participants

QUESTION 2: *Were outcome measures reliable and valid?*

To have high-quality data and results from a study, the data must be valid and reliable. Reliable data are reproducible by one or more people (therapists) and are stable within a defined time period. **Intra-rater reliability** is the repeatability of a measure by the same therapist on the same patient at two or more time points. For example, if you measure a patient's knee flexion range of motion as 120 degrees, you should be able to obtain that same score of 120 degrees the second and third time. **Inter-rater reliability** is the repeatability between two or more therapists measuring the same patient. Both therapists should obtain the score of 120 degrees from the example above. The therapists who are testing study participants and the tools and instruments they use must be reliable (Fig. 4.4).

Patients also introduce variability into measurements. This variability may be the result of the natural fluctuations of the disease or normal physiological processes, day/night changes, emotional state, state of alertness, and the myriad of other factors that influence human performance. Repeated measures of the variables of interest, termed *intra-subject variability* (for example, before an intervention begins) provide a quantitative method for establishing the true range of the variable. One pre-intervention measurement, similar to one mean value, has limited value without an understanding of the normal variability of what one is measuring. If intra-subject variability is high, it might mean that what you are measuring is high variability OR your measuring technique needs to improve and become more reliable.

Reliability of Measures is Determined by Instruments and Machines

The dynamometer in the example would need to be tested for measurement accuracy and reproducibility over time. A valid

The Person or Persons Completing the Measures

Intra-rater reliability

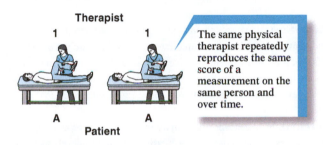

Inter-rater reliability

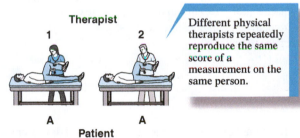

The Person Who is Measured

Intra-subject reliability

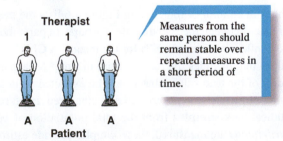

FIGURE 4.4 Multiple forms of reliability.

instrument measures the constructs it was intended to measure. A reliable instrument is one that yields repeatable results when administered correctly by reliable testers. Studies that investigate test and instrument reliability are presented in detail in Chapter 10.

Reliability within and between people is typically expressed by association (correlation) of the values obtained in repeated measurements. Both intra-rater and inter-rater reliability should have high values of association, that is, values should be similar. The type of correlation that is performed depends on the measurement scale that is used, as the scale determines the form of the data.

Reliability should be established within a research study, and it should be high. Studies have higher validity when high reliability has been established between the raters actually conducting the study. Authors may cite other research in which reliability has been established, but this is not as valid as conducting reliability testing among raters actually performing the tests. The fact that two or more raters can achieve high reliability does not support the fact that the testers in the study you are appraising were similarly reliable.

Methods to Analyze Reliability

The Pearson product-moment coefficient of correlation is sometimes used to report reliability.[2] Figure 4.5 illustrates why this is an insufficient measure of the reliability of measures. The Pearson correlation between these two testers is a perfect 1.0; however, the actual measures are very different. The range-of-motion values recorded by Physical Therapist 1 change in the same way as the values recorded by Physical Therapist 2, but the absolute values in the two series are not the same. A measure such as the intraclass correlation coefficient (ICC) takes into account both the nature of the change

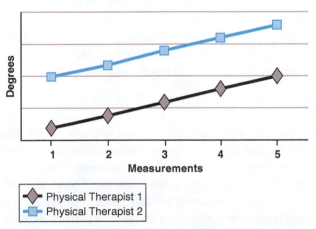

FIGURE 4.5 Range-of-motion values from two physical therapists.

DIGGING DEEPER 4.2

Scales of measurement and types of data

DATA: Data are measured variables; variables become data. The variables below—height, missed workdays, a score on a functional scale—are represented by numerical data. Different types of scales yield different types of data.

Height = 74 inches
Missed workdays = 12
Pediatric Evaluation of Disability Score = 36

SCALE OF MEASUREMENT: The type of data is defined by the measurement tool that is used. All measurement tools have a specific scale that is used to describe the variable of interest. There are at least four scales of measurement you will encounter in research and in clinical practice:

- Nominal
- Ordinal
- Ratio
- Interval

NOMINAL SCALES: Variables in a nominal scale are in categories. Nominal scales are also termed *categorical,* and there is no order of the categories in nominal scales. If there are only two categories, then the nominal scale is a *dichotomous* scale. Gender is on a dichotomous scale, male or female.

ORDINAL SCALES: Variables on an ordinal scale are in categories that are ordered. The ranking within the scale typically indicates most to least, but the distance between ranks is not uniform within the scale. The Modified Rankin Scale[4] below is an example of an ordinal scale. A person with a score of 2 has less disability than a person with a score of 4, but not "one-half" the disability.

Modified Rankin Scale

Score	Description
0	**No symptoms at all**
1	**No significant disability:** despite symptoms, able to carry out all usual duties and activities
2	**Slight disability:** unable to carry out all previous activities but able to look after own affairs without assistance
3	**Moderate disability:** requiring some help, but able to walk without assistance
4	**Moderately severe disability:** unable to walk without assistance, and unable to attend to own bodily needs without assistance
5	**Severe disability:** bedridden, incontinent and requiring constant nursing care and attention

With permission from: Bonita R, Beaglehole R. Recovery of motor function after stroke. *Stroke.* 1988;19:1497.

RATIO SCALES: Variables on a ratio scale are ordered precisely and continuously. The measured intervals on the scale are equal. A value of 4 on a ratio scale is twice the value of 2 on the same scale. Range of motion as measured with a goniometer is on a ratio scale. Ratio level variables do not have a meaningful zero value.

INTERVAL SCALES: Variables on an interval scale are also measured precisely and share the properties of equal intervals as with ratio scales. Temperature recorded on a Fahrenheit or Celsius scale is the typical example of an interval scale. Interval scales have a meaningful zero value in that temperature can have a value below zero. Meaningful measures in physical therapy typically do not use interval scales.

Note: Ratio and Interval data are also referred to as *continuous data.*

and the absolute values and thus is a preferred statistic to evaluate the reliability of continuous data (ratio or interval).

There are various statistical methods to compute reliability for both instruments and people (Table 4.1). The choice of statistic reflects the type of data that is analyzed.

Appraising Statistical Results

Tables are also used to display the result of interventions. Reading through tables before reading the results section can give you an overall impression as to the study outcomes. The table in Figure 4.6 is from a study by Santamato et al[5] comparing two interventions for the treatment of subacromial impingement syndrome. The first three columns of the table list the tests, the baseline (before treatment) scores, and post-treatment scores on the tests used in the study for each of the two intervention groups.

These results are expressed as means and standard deviations for each of the treatment groups (HILT and US Therapy).

QUESTION 3: *Were confidence intervals reported?*

The fifth column of the table in Figure 4.6 lists the mean differences between the two treatment groups. In parentheses are the confidence intervals (CI) for the means. A CI is a range of values that includes the real (or true) mean.[3,6] Means are *estimates* of the true values that would be expected from a population of people who are treated and measured. In all research studies, only **samples** from the total population of *possible participants* are measured; these samples provide estimates of what might be expected from the larger group. You want an idea of how accurately the means represent the population

TABLE 4.1   **Statistical Methods for Analysis of Reliability**

METHOD	STATISTIC REFLECTS	TYPE OF DATA	INTERPRETATION
Intraclass correlation coefficient (ICC)	Association of two or more measures and amount of association	Continuous	Value of zero = no association between variables; value of 1 = there is perfect association; most commonly used statistic for more than two measures; different variables can be compared or different people's scores can be compared
Spearman's rho	Association of two measures; comparable to Pearson's in that it does not reflect the sameness of the scores, only the nature of how they change	Ordinal	Value of zero = no association between variables; value of 1 = there is perfect association
Kappa (κ)	Association of two measures but accounting for "chance" agreements	Nominal	Value of zero = no association between variables; value of 1= there is perfect association; values tend to be lower than other measures of association; contribution of chance is removed
Kendall's tau	Association of two measures; comparable to Pearson's in that it does not reflect the sameness of the scores, only the nature of how they change	Nominal	Value of zero = no association between variables; value of 1 = there is perfect association
Chronbach's alpha	Internal consistency of an instrument or scale	Continuous Categorical Ordinal	Internal consistency should be close to 1; all items relate to each other and to the construct being measured by the scale
Standard error of measurement (SEM)	Variability of the standard deviation (SD) of a measure against probabilities of this variation	Continuous	High values indicate large variability of SD implying a lack of reliability.

because means are only estimates. CIs can give you this information, and they are typically expressed at the 95th percentile or the 90th percentile (see Fig. 4.6, Note 4.4). The CI is expressed as the 90th or 95th.[6]

Guyatt et al[6] offer the example of a coin toss to illustrate the concept of CIs. The larger the sample (coin tosses), the better the estimate you have of the true value, that is, the smaller the CI.

 DIGGING DEEPER 4.3

Interpreting CIs

CIs can be calculated for many different statistics. One common and useful CI is computed for the difference between means from two treatment groups in an intervention study. Research is based on the behavior of samples of people, but you are trying to apply this research to your patients. In a typical intervention study comparing two different treatments, the mean differences between groups are computed to determine which treatment was more affective. The difference between means from the sample is used to infer to a population of people, and the CI helps you determine the value of this mean. CIs must be reviewed and interpreted. If the CI crosses zero, meaning that the CI range includes

negative and positive values, then the result of the intervention cannot be considered statitistically significant. Consider the following: If the results of an intervention are expressed as a positive change (for example, increased strength on a dynamometer), then the estimated mean difference in the change between groups should be positive following intervention if the treatment group had greater strength than the comparison group. If the CI range includes negative values, then this finding suggests that the true mean (recall that the means of the samples in the study are *estimates* of the population mean) may be negative. Negative values suggest that the comparison group performed better after intervention.

Continued

DIGGING DEEPER 4.3 — cont'd

Some measures, such as a pain scale, might be expected to have lower values after intervention. In this example, an improvement would be expressed as a negative value between group means. The CI for this result should only include a range of scores with negative values.

Regardless of what type of measure is used or whether a positive or negative range is expected, *if the CI crosses zero,* then the result is not statistically significant. This means that both a positive and a negative result are possible given the difference between means. However, further interpretation of CIs is warranted. Guyatt et al[6] suggest looking at the low and high values in the CI to evaluate the sample size of a study further and thus what you can take away from the study. In a study with a positive result for a treatment, if the lowest value in a CI is greater than the smallest difference that is clinically important, then you know that the sample size was adequate in demonstrating a positive effect above the minimal threshold. Even if the CI is somewhat wide, the lowest value would still indicate a positive effect, albeit small, of the treatment. In a study with a negative result for a treatment, if the highest value in a CI is less than the smallest difference that is clinically important, then you know that the sample size was adequate in demonstrating a negative effect above the minimal threshold.

CIs are typically expressed at the 90th and 95th percentile. This reflects the degree of certainty from the CI. You can be 90% or 95% certain that the "true" (population) mean (in this example) is within the range given for the CI.

Table 3.

Change in Test Performance Over Time From Baseline for Participants with Subacromial Impingement Syndrome in High-Intensity Laser Therapy (HILT) and Ultrasound (US) Therapy Groups: Evaluation Between Groups[a]

Variable	Both Groups (n=70)	HILT Group (n=35)	US Therapy Group (n=35)	Difference in Means (95% CI)	Actual *P* Value	Bonferroni-Corrected *P* Value[b]
VAS score						
$\overline{X}$ (SD)	−3.01 (1.46)	−3.86 (1.53)	−2.17 (0.75)	−1.69 (−2.27 to −1.12)	<.001	<.01
%	−48.89	−61.36	−33.04			
CMS score						
$\overline{X}$ (SD)	10.86 (3.68)	12.69 (3.64)	9.03 (2.70)	3.66 (2.13 to 5.19)	<.001	<.01
%	17.19	20.06	14.31			
SST score						
$\overline{X}$ (SD)	2.14 (0.98)	2.46 (1.17)	1.83 (0.61)	0.63 (0.18 to 1.08)	.006	<.05
%	30.30	33.99	26.45			

[a] CI-confidence interval, VAS-visual analog scale, CMS-Constant-Murley Scale, SST-Simple Shoulder Test.
[b] The statistical inferences were adjusted according to Bonferroni inequality (0.05/6-0.008 and 0.01/6-0.002).

Note 4.4 Confidence Interval
We can be 95% confident that the true mean lies between −2.27 to −1.12

Note 4.5
Is this a difference that we should consider in our clinical decisions?

Note 4.6
The *P* value is .006 (p<.05) for the difference between the HILT and US Therapy groups.

FIGURE 4.6 Comparison of two interventions for the treatment of subacromial impingement syndrome.
From: Santamato A, Solfrizzi V, Panza F, et al. Short-term effects of high-intensity laser therapy versus ultrasound therapy in the treatment of people with subacromial impingement syndrome: a randomized clinical trial. Phys Ther. 2009;89:643–652; with permission.

Interface of Descriptive and Inferential Statistics

QUESTION 4: Were descriptive and inferential statistics applied to the results?

Descriptive statistics help summarize information about groups before and after intervention. However, these summary scores must be interpreted to understand their implications for clinical decisions. Should you be concerned about the difference in the mean values of the demographic or clinical characteristics in Figure 4.2? The descriptive statistics, in this case the mean values, indicate that the differences exist in these samples. However, this type of statistic does not help you sort out whether these differences threaten the validity of the study, with the consequence that the study is less useful for your clinical decision. Could the differences in subject characteristics affect or explain the outcomes of the study sufficiently, such that you are less certain that the outcomes are due to the treatment? In addition, it is not certain as to how to interpret the change in mean scores from before to after treatment (see Fig. 4.6, Note 4.5). You can see from the data in columns 3 and 4 that both treatment groups made positive changes on all three variables that were measured (VAS, CMS, and SST) but that the HILT group made larger positive changes. From this data, would you accept that the HILT is more effective than US Therapy?

Descriptive statistics are useful but insufficient for making conclusions about the differences between groups. **Inferential statistics** [2,3,7,8] are helpful in making these conclusions. Inferential statistics are tools that use the mathematics of probability to interpret the differences observed in research studies. These statistics focus on the following question:

Is the outcome due to the intervention, or could it be *due to chance*?

Role of Chance in Communicating Results

Inferential statistics are based on the mathematics of probability; they can be expressed as probability, or *p* **values.** The

sixth column in the table in Figure 4.6 includes *p* values. A *p* value is an expression of the probability that the difference that has been identified is due to chance. If there is a high probability that the results are due to chance (large *p* value), then you cannot conclude that the treatment was the reason for the difference observed between the two groups. What are values that represent high or low probability? The consensus among researchers is that most want the probability of chance in explaining the results of a study to be as low as possible. This agreed-upon value is termed the **alpha level,** and it is typically 5%.

The results of an analysis using inferential statistics are expressed as *p* values, and these values are evaluated as either below or above the agreed-upon alpha level ($<p = 0.05$ or $>p = 0.05$) (see Fig. 4.6, Note 4.6). If you were comparing groups, then you would infer that the groups are statistically significantly different and that the HILT group improved significantly more than the US Therapy group, although both groups improved following treatment.

DIGGING DEEPER 4.4

Hypothesis testing

Using inferential statistics to test the role of probability in determing differences between groups relies on an understanding of hypothesis testing, which is fundamental to statistical analyses. In what is referred to as the *null hypothesis*, groups are considered (in statistical terms) to be equal; that is, there is no difference between groups. A given statistical test supports either acceptance or rejection of the null hypothesis. If the null hypothesis is rejected (the groups are different), then the *p* values express the probability that chance contributed to this result.

TYPE I ERROR: The results of a study may conclude falsely that there is a statistically significant difference when there is actually no difference. You might assume falsely that the intervention under study was effective when in fact it was not. This is a type I error, because the result was actually due to chance. This is one reason for the decision among scientists to use the conservative alpha level of 0.05; there is only a minimal percent that chance could account for the result. As the alpha level increases (0.08 or 0.10), the chances of type I errors increase.

TYPE II ERROR: The result of a study may also conclude falsely that there is no statistically significant difference between groups when there is actually a difference. This is a type II error. From this conclusion, we might not use a treatment that might indeed be effective with our patients. Small samples are important contributing factors to type II error. The difference between groups may not have been large enough to detect with only a small sample.

The last column in the table in Figure 4.6 includes the Bonferroni-corrected *p* values, which are the values to accept in terms of statistical significance. The Bonferroni correction takes into account the number of statistical comparisons that are made in an analysis. Recall that inferential statistics are based on probability, and if there are many comparisons in an analysis, then there is the probability that one or more will be significant. For example, if 20 statistical comparisons were made at an alpha level of 0.05, then you would expect that one of the comparisons would show a statistically significant difference between groups even if one does not exist. The Bonferroni statistics correct for these multiple comparisons.

Should you be concerned about the difference in the distribution of demographic or clinical characteristics at baseline? Figure 4.6 includes characteristics of the participants in the two treatment groups, HILT and US Therapy, at baseline prior to intervention (please see Table 1 in Santamato, et al[5]). The means, standard deviations, and range are given for age, onset of pain, and the stage in the diagnostic process. How do you interpret these values? All

of the *p* values are greater than 0.05, the conventional alpha level. This supports the statement that the groups are *not* statistically significantly different. This is interpreted to mean that the groups are similar at baseline and that subject characteristics included in the baseline measures will not likely bias the results of the study. This increases the certainty that the treatments, and not an imbalance between groups at baseline, are responsible for the results.

What does it mean to approach significance? Recall that the alpha level of 0.05 is a convention, the amount of error that researchers are willing to accept. What if the *p* value is in the range of 0.05 to 0.10 or slightly higher? Do you automatically assume that the difference between groups is due only to chance? A *p* value of 0.06 indicates that there is a 6% chance that the difference is due to chance. A bit of common sense must prevail. You do not want to ignore important findings because the *p* values are above the conventional 0.05 threshold. Carefully review all *p* values in a study, and consider the relevance of values between 0.15 and 0.05. There may be a pattern of results that should be considered even if the *p* values are above 0.05.

There are many inferential statistical tools, but there are some statistics that are typically used in the rehabilitation literature. A list of these statistics and their uses is included in Digging Deeper 4.5. Familiarity with these statistics assists you in interpreting the results of a study.

Part D: Summarizing the Clinical Bottom Line of an Intervention Study

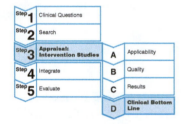

Statistics to Evaluate Clinical Relevance

QUESTION 5: Was there a treatment effect? If so, was it clinically relevant?

Descriptive and inferential statistics are two categories of statistical tools that are used to analyze the data in a research study. Readers sometimes conclude (and authors sometimes imply) that a finding of statistical significance from a valid study (e.g., a result of *p* <0.05 in a well-designed intervention study) means that the study's results must be *important*. However, this is not the case: *statistically* significant results may not be *clinically* important.

For example:

Suppose you try a new intervention with a patient who has severely limited range of motion in several fingers of her dominant hand. After a reasonable trial period, the patient increases her ability to move her fingers by about a quarter of an inch. If you replicated this intervention with a very large sample of patients and achieved the same outcome, a statistical analysis might show the significance of this change is *p* <0.05. However, this change is not very likely to improve the functional use of the hand.

To be clinically important, the results must:

- Show change on a measure that has **value** to the patient in terms of his or her daily life (patient values). In the example, a measure of functional use of the hand as well as range of motion might help evaluate the value of the change for the patient.
- Show change of a **magnitude** that will make a real difference in the patient's life (in terms of function, satisfaction, comfort, etc.)

Therefore, you need some measures other than *p* values to answer the following question: Are the results of this valid study important?

Effect Size

The *p* values help to establish the role of chance in the results of a study. However, you also need to know how big a difference occurred between the treatments. One approach to evaluating the magnitude of the difference following treatments is to calculate the **effect size,** the most common form of which is **Cohen's *d*.**[9] The effect size *d* provides a measure of just how distinct the samples are, or specifically, how far apart the two means are, relative to the variability, as you can see from looking at the following formula:

$$d = \frac{\text{Mean}_{\text{group 1}} - \text{Mean}_{\text{control group}}}{\text{SD}_{\text{control group}}}$$

A large *d* value indicates a big difference between the two groups. Papers do not always include the effect sizes, but descriptive statistics (means and standard deviations) of the results are usually given in tables. You can readily calculate *d* to help you evaluate the magnitude of the differences that are reported. Interpretation of the *d* statistic as suggested by Cohen[9] is included in Table 4.2.

Number Needed to Treat

Many discussions in the medical EBP literature about examining the importance of results focus on dichotomous outcomes. A dichotomous outcome has two categories; for example, healthy or sick, admitted or not admitted, or relapsed or not relapsed. Effect size can be computed only on results

TABLE 4.2 **Interpretation of Effect Size Values**

Large	>0.8
Medium	0.5–0.8
Small	0.2–0.5

From: Cohen J. *Statistical Power Analysis for the Behavioral Sciences.* Hillsdale, NJ: Erlbaum; 1988.

that have continuous results; for example, range of motion, a score on a functional measure, or strength on a dynamometer. There are some important examples in physical therapy in which outcomes are dichotomous. For example, intervention success may be measured by comparing the number of patients who do or do not return to work or to a sport, who do or do not walk independently, or who are classified (by some criterion) as improved or not improved.

It is unlikely that a new intervention helps everyone, but the significant ($p < 0.05$) statistical result indicates that a greater proportion of patients who received the new intervention had a positive outcome than would not be expected by chance. Now what is needed is a statistic that could answer the following question: If I use the new intervention for all new patients of this type, how many would I have to treat in order to see a positive benefit for *one* additional patient (compared with using the old treatment)?

This question is answered by the statistic **number needed to treat (NNT)**.[10,11] NNT is a ratio of the rate of the desired outcome in the experimental group and the rate of the desired outcome in the control or comparison group. This ratio is expressed in terms of persons, and it makes the NNT statistic applicable to the results of your practice. Globally, the NNT is captured by the formula:

$$\frac{\text{Desired outcome in the experimental group}}{\text{Desired outcome in the control group}} = \text{NNT}$$

It is hoped that the authors of the journal articles you read provide enough details in their reports (e.g., number or percentage improved in each group) to make calculating the NNT a simple matter.

TABLE 4.3 The Number of Patients Hospitalized After Two Different Treatments

TREATMENT	NO HOSPITALIZATION	HOSPITALIZATION
New (Exp. Group)	a (95)	b (5)
Usual care (Control group)	c (85)	d (15)

For example:

You find a study investigating the efficacy of a new intervention to reduce hospitalization for persons with Parkinson's disease. The study included 200 patients divided into the control or new interventions groups. It reports that, in the control condition, 15 of 100 participants experienced a hospitalization within the 6-month follow-up period, whereas in the new intervention condition 5 of 100 participants had a hospitalization (Table 4.3). (Note that the "event" or "desired outcome" in this example is "no hospitalization").

How would the results of the NNT computation be stated?

For every 10 people with Parkinson's disease who receive the new intervention, hospitalization will be avoided in 1 additional person.

On average, the new intervention would need to be provided to 10 people in order to prevent hospitalization of 1 person (Table 4.4). In this example, the "desired outcome" is no hospitalization, so you are hoping that the experimental event rate is *higher* than the control event rate. Therefore, the negative relative risk reduction (RRR) and

TABLE 4.4 Computing Number Needed to Treat

	CER	EER	ARR	RRR	NNT
Definition of term	Control event rate	Experimental event rate	Absolute risk reduction (risk difference)	Relative risk reduction	Number needed to treat
Calculation of statistic (letters refer to Table 4.2)	c/c + d	a/a + b	CER – EER	$\frac{\text{CER} - \text{EER}}{\text{CER}}$	1/ARR
Answers	85/100 = 0.85	95/100 = 0.95	–0.10, or the intervention reduced the rate of hospitalizations by 10%	0.85 – 0.95/0.85 = –0.12 or the new intervention caused a 12% relative reduction in hospitalizations compared to the control	10

DIGGING DEEPER 4.5

The most commonly used statistical procedures

Chi-square (χ^2): a statistic that can be used to analyze nominal (categorical) data. It compares the observed frequency of a particular category with the expected frequency of that category.

Example: Are there more men than women in a study?

The result is written as: $\chi^2(df) = 289.3$, $p < 0.05$

The result is reported as: A chi-square analysis found that there were significantly more men than women in the study. [$\chi^2(150) = 289.3$, $p < 0.05$].

The degrees of freedom, the number of values in a calculation that are free to vary, is expressed as (df) in statistical reporting.

t-test: a statistical analysis that is used to compare the means of *two* groups.

Example: Do elderly men and women differ in speed of walking?

The result is written as: $t(df) = 3.86$, $p < 0.05$.

The result is reported as: The mean speed of walking in the two groups was compared with a *t*-test and found to be significantly different [$t(df) = 3.86$, $p < 0.05$].

The authors must add a statement for you to determine which group was faster. You can also see this in the descriptive statistics if they are included.

Analysis of variance (ANOVA): used to compare results for *more than two groups*.

Example: Are there differences in walking speeds among elderly men, elderly women, middle-aged men, and middle-aged women?

The result is written as: $F(df) = 9.82$, $p < 0.01$.

The result is reported as: There was a significant difference in walking speeds between groups [$F(df) = 9.82$, $p < 0.01$].

The single *F* value tells you only that there is a difference between groups, but you do not know which groups just by looking at the *F* value. *Post hoc* tests (e.g., *t*-test, Tukey's) are used to compare each group pairs to determine which groups have a difference (see below).

A repeated measure (ANOVA) (univariate): used to compare *multiple measures* from the *same subjects*. The multiple measures may be taken within a shorter or longer period.

Example: Are there differences in functional use of the arm for individuals with a hemiparesis from stroke immediately after 4 weeks of constraint-induced manual therapy compared with differences sustained at 3 months and at 6 months after therapy?

The result is written as: $F(df) = 19.12$, $p < 0.001$. This is the *F* value for the time differences. (There may also be an *F* value for the subjects' variability, but this does not reflect the research question.) The *F* value for means between time points only indicates that there is a significant difference between means, but not which specific means. To determine where the difference(s) occurred (e.g., immediately after therapy and at 3 months), pairs of means are compared. Statistics termed post hoc tests are used. Common post hoc tests are the Tukey's honestly significant difference method, Scheffeé's comparison, and *t*-test.

The result is reported as: There was a significant difference between means [$F(df) = 19.12$, $p < 0.001$]. Significant differences were found for functional arm movements immediately after treatment ($p = 0.001$) and at 3 months ($p = 0.01$) but not at 6 months ($p = 0.45$) after treatment.

There are many repeated measures designs and statistics. In the above example, if a comparison was made between two treatments at three times points, then this is a multivariate design and requires a multivariate repeated ANOVA for analysis. An analysis of covariance (ANCOVA) is used to compare means and to remove the contribution of a factor that is present during treatment that was not controlled in the experimental design.

Examples: Medication usage while receiving an intervention may vary widely for patients in a study. ANCOVA can statistically account for the contribution of medication to the outcomes of interest.

absolute risk reduction (ARR) indicate that this was, indeed, the direction of the results. In this case, the negative sign is not relevant when interpreting the NNT. However, if the desired outcome was a *decrease* in rate, a negative RRR and ARR would indicate that your intervention had the *opposite* result; that is, that the control condition was more successful than the experimental condition. Think through the desired outcome when computing NNT, and interpret the results accordingly.

Even a "better" intervention will not necessarily result in a better outcome for 100% of patients (i.e., most NNTs are greater than 1). Better interventions merely increase the likelihood of success. There is no rule defining a "good" NTT; it depends on the context. You must use your clinical reasoning and expertise to determine the answer. Typically, NNT is used to

evaluate a program of intervention rather than to make an intervention decision for a single patient. It may be used to determine if a change in treatment should occur for a particular type of problem. For example, if an intervention program to prevent falls in the elderly has an NNT of 5, then for every 5 elderly people who receive the new intervention, a fall will be avoided in one additional person.

The questions in Table 4.5 should be used when interpreting the results of an intervention study and determining the clinical bottom line. Full details for question 2 are given in Chapter 10. Combining the checklists of key questions from Chapter 3 (Table 3.3) with the key questions in Table 4.5 from this chapter completes the key questions for appraising all aspects of an intervention research study.

TABLE 4.5 **Key Questions to Interpret the Results and Determine the Clinical Bottom Line for an Intervention Research Study**

QUESTIONS	YES/NO	WHERE TO FIND INFORMATION	COMMENTS AND WHAT TO LOOK FOR
1. Were the groups similar at baseline?	__ Yes __ No	Results (occasionally listed in Methods)	The study should provide information about the baseline characteristics of participants. Ideally, the randomization process should result in equivalent baseline characteristics between groups. The authors should present a statistical method to account for baseline differences.
2. Were outcome measures reliable and valid?	__ Yes __ No	Methods will describe the outcome measures used. Results may report evaluators' inter- and/or intra-rater reliability.	The study should describe how **reliability** and **validity** of **outcome measures** were established. The study may refer to previous studies. Ideally, the study will also provide an analysis of rater reliability for the study. Reliability is often reported with a kappa or intraclass correlation coefficient score—values >0.80 are generally considered to represent high reliability (Table 4.1).
3. Were CIs reported?	__ Yes __ No	Results	The study should report a 95% CI for the reported results. The size of the CI helps the clinician understand the precision of reported findings.
4. Were descriptive and inferential statistics applied to the results?	__ Yes __ No	Methods and Results	Descriptive statistics will be used to describe the study subjects and to report the results. Were the groups tested with inferential statistics at baseline? Were groups equivalent on important characteristics before treatment began?
5. Was there a treatment effect? If so, was it clinically relevant?	__ Yes __ No	Results	The study should report whether or not there was a statistically significant difference between groups and if so, the magnitude of the difference (effect sizes). Ideally, the study will report whether or not any differences are clinically meaningful.

SUMMARY

It is useful to follow a series of steps in interpreting the results of a study. Practicing these steps ensures that your appraisal skills improve and that the clinically meaningful application of the results of a study become a part of your clinical practice. A first step is to read through the tables and figures in the results section of a study before reading the author's conclusions or the statistical methods used for analyses. This gives you an impression of the results of the study and the form of the results. There should be a table that includes the characteristics of the subjects in the treatment groups. Typically, these characteristics are represented with descriptive statistics. The groups should be similar in the characteristics that might influence their responses to treatment. Then read the tables of results after the study was completed. These typically include descriptive statistics and may also include *p* values, which express the role of chance in the study results. Look for CIs. These assist you in interpreting the *p* values, the sample size of the study, and what to conclude from study results. Look for clinically meaningful statistics such as effect size and number needed to treat. Only after careful inspection of the tables and graphs should you read through the text of the results. The authors should take you step by step through each table and graph with the process used for their analyses and conclusions. Reflect on what you believe are the results of the study and then read through the authors' conclusions. Assess if you agree with the conclusions and how these conclusions are applied to the clinic or could be applied. Repeated practice pays off!

REVIEW QUESTIONS

Read the abstract (Fig. 4.7) and answer the following questions:

1. State what you would tell your patient with low back pain and sciatica about the first sentence in the results of this abstract.

2. Your patient is a 65-year-old female. Is this study applicable to your patient? Defend your answer.

3. Diagram this study using research notation.

A Pilot Study Examining the Effectiveness of Physical Therapy as an Adjunct to Selective Nerve Root Block in the treatment of Lumbar Radicular Pain From Disk Herniation: A Randomized Controlled Trial

Anne Thackeray, Julie M. Fritz, Gerard P. Brennan, Faisel M. Zaman, Stuart E. Willick

Background: Therapeutic selective nerve root blocks (SNRBs) are a common intervention for patients with sciatica. Patients often are referred to physical therapy after SNRBs, although the effectiveness of this intervention sequence has not been investigated.

Objective: This study was a preliminary investigation of the effectiveness of SNRBs, with or without subsequent physical therapy, in people with low back pain and sciatica.

Design: The investigation was a pilot randomized controlled clinical trial.

Setting: The settings were spine specialty and physical therapy clinics.

Participants: Forty-four participants (64% men; mean age=38.5 years, SD=11.6 years) with low back pain, with clinical and imaging findings consistent with lumbar disk herniation, and scheduled to receive SNRBs participated in the study. They were randomly assigned to receive either 4 weeks of physical therapy (SNRB+PT group) or no physical therapy (SNRB alone [SNRB group]) after the injections.

Intervention: All participants received at least 1 SNRB; 28 participants (64%) received multiple injections. Participants in the SNRB+PT group attended an average of 6.0 physical therapy sessions over an average of 23.9 days.

Measurements: Outcomes were assessed at baseline, 8 weeks, and 6 months with the Low Back Pain Disability Questionnaire, a numeric pain rating scale, and the Global Rating of Change.

Results: Significant reductions in pain and disability occurred over time in both groups, with no differences between groups at either follow-up for any outcome. Nine participants (5 in the SNRB group and 4 in the SNRB+PT group) underwent surgery during the follow-up period.

Limitations: The limitations of this study were a relatively short-term follow-up period and a small sample size.

Conclusions: A physical therapy intervention after SNRBs did not result in additional reductions in pain and disability or perceived improvements in participants with low back pain and sciatica.

FIGURE 4.7 Abstract from the journal article "Pilot Study Examining the Effectiveness of Physical Therapy as an Adjunct to Selective Nerve Root Block in the Treatment of Lumbar Radicular Pain From Disk Herniation: A Randomized Controlled Trial." *Abstract from: Thackeray A, Fritz JM, Brennan GP, et al. Pilot study examining the effectiveness of physical therapy as an adjunct to selective nerve root block in the treatment of lumbar radicular pain from disk herniation: a randomized controlled trial. PhysTher. 2010;90:1717–1729; with permission.*

REFERENCES

1. Ylinen J, Takala EP, Nykanen M, et al. Active neck muscle training in the treatment of chronic neck pain in women: a randomized controlled trial. *JAMA.* 2003;289:2509–2516.
2. Domholdt B. *Physical Therapy Research.* 2nd ed. Philadelphia: Saunders; 2000.
3. Portney LG, Watkins MP. *Foundations of Clinical Research: Applications to Practice.* 2nd ed. Englewood Cliffs, NJ: Prentice Hall; 2000.
4. Bonita R, Beaglehole R. Recovery of motor function after stroke. *Stroke.* 1988;19:1497–1500.
5. Santamato A, Solfrizzi V, Panza F, et al. Short-term effects of high-intensity laser therapy versus ultrasound therapy in the treatment of people with subacromial impingement syndrome: a randomized clinical trial. *Phys Ther.* 2009;89:643–652.
6. Guyatt G, Jaeschke R, Heddle N, et al. Basic statistics for clinicians. 2. Interpreting study results: confidence intervals. *CMAJ.* 1995;152:169–173.
7. Guyatt G, Jaeschke R, Heddle N, et al. Basic statistics for clinicians. 1. Hypothesis testing. *CMAJ* 1995;152:27–32.
8. Greenhalgh T. How to read a paper: statistics for the non-statistician. I: Different types of data. *BMJ.* 1997;315:364–366.
9. Cohen J. *Statistical Power Analysis for the Behavioral Sciences.* Hillsdale, NJ: Erlbaum; 1988.
10. Straus SE, Richardson WS, Glasziou P, et al. *Evidence-Based Medicine: How to Practice and Teach EBM.* 3rd ed. Edinburgh, Scotland: Elsevier; 2005.
11. Glasziou P, Del Mar C, Salisbury J. *Evidence-Based Practice Workbook.* 2nd ed. Malden, MA: Blackwell Publishing; 2007.

5

Appraising Diagnostic Research Studies

PRE-TEST

1. How does the appraisal process change when considering diagnostic research in comparison with intervention research?

2. What are typical study designs for diagnostic research?

3. What impact might a false-positive test result have on your clinical decision?

4. What would be the clinical application of a negative likelihood ratio?

CHAPTER-AT-A-GLANCE

This chapter will help you understand the following:

- Application of diagnostic literature for specific tests and measures

- Appraising the quality of diagnostic studies

- Interpretation of the statistics most relevant to the diagnostic process

■ Introduction

The Diagnostic Process in Physical Therapy

The physical therapy diagnostic process includes patient history, systems review, and informed use of tests and measures. This chapter focuses on the processes of appraising the diagnostic literature of tests and measures and the clinical application of diagnostic research results (Fig. 5.1). Understanding evidence regarding diagnostic tests and integrating diagnostic test results, clinical experience, and patient goals are essential to best practice. Communicating results of the diagnostic process to patients and other professionals requires thorough knowledge of valid and reliable diagnostic tests and the correct interpretation of those tests.

Physical therapists examine patients and evaluate the results of the examination, yielding a diagnosis, plan of care, and likely prognosis.[1] The diagnostic process in physical therapy has been discussed and debated in the literature.[2,3–6] When you engage in the diagnostic process, you are determining appropriate (if any) physical therapy interventions and any need for referral to another professional. With direct access to physical therapy comes increased professional responsibility. Part of this responsibility is accurate diagnosis of conditions within the scope of physical therapy practice and appropriate referral to other professionals.

Prior to direct access, physical therapists may have relied on a prescription or referral from a physician. Physician referrals continue as the primary referral source for physical therapists, but the majority of these referrals have nonspecific diagnoses.[7] For example, a referral may be written as "elbow pain," "improve aerobic capacity," or "post-stroke," without a diagnosis concerning the purported etiology of the problem or its relation to movement. It is the physical therapist's responsibility to correctly diagnose the movement problem and determine the appropriate intervention, possible prognosis, and, if necessary, referral to other professionals.

A fundamental tenet of any diagnostic test used in physical therapy is that it can distinguish between people who have a movement disorder and people who do not. Although this sounds obvious, it is more complex.

If you have a sore throat, your physician may use a rapid antigen throat culture for the streptococcal bacteria to diagnose a strep infection. You most likely assume that the results of this test determine that you either have a strep throat or you do not. However, every diagnostic test has a range of values that is positive and a range of values that is negative. This quick test for strep throat detects 80% to 90% of strep infections, thus missing 10% to 20% of cases.[8] This test might miss the strep infection even if it is present (false-negative). However, some of the positive tests may also be inaccurate (false-positives). No diagnostic test is 100% accurate in either ruling in or ruling out a diagnosis. Your medical health-care provider uses the rapid antigen throat culture along with your history and clinical symptoms to determine whether you require treatment for strep infection and if additional testing is necessary.

Each question in the history, each observation during a systems review, and each choice of a test or measure should be guided by an initial hypothesis about the likely problem. Therefore, the information you seek should rapidly move from general to specific. You determine what tests and measures will be most helpful when you are clear about the nature of the information you are seeking. For example, consider a patient presenting with the nonspecific diagnosis of shoulder pain. The patient reports a history and symptoms that are consistent with, for example, a labral tear, supraspinatus tear, or supraspinatus tendonitis. Your hypothesis concerning the movement problem is shaped by the patient's report and then tested with your examination. A positive anterior slide test may support the hypothesis of a labral tear. The results of each test chosen in

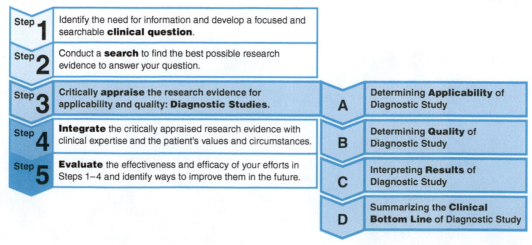

FIGURE 5.1 Appraising diagnostic research studies.

your examination should be directly relevant either to ruling in or to ruling out a particular diagnosis. An efficient diagnostician will ask, "To what extent will the result of this test assist my decision?" To fully determine the answer to this self-imposed question, you need to know what constitutes a clinically valid and reliable test. In the example of the possible labral tear, you should consider the question, "What is the accuracy of the anterior slide test in ruling in or ruling out a labral tear?" The answer to this question is determined from research results on this test.

DIGGING DEEPER 5.1

Reference intervals

Diagnostic tests typically have what Riegelman[9] refers to as **reference intervals.** A reference interval is a range of scores that captures individuals without a movement problem. Individuals with a movement problem would fall outside of this reference interval.

Of course, not all diagnostic tests yield a normal distribution as depicted in Figure 5.2. The important aspect of Figure 5.2 is the overlap in the distributions of people with and without a movement problem. This is the gray zone that captures the expected variation present in individuals with and without movement problems. This zone affects the accuracy of a diagnostic test and its usefulness in the diagnostic process. If you falsely categorize a person with a specific movement problem, then the plan of care that follows from the categorization or diagnosis may not help the patient. If the patient does not improve from the chosen intervention, then both the intervention and the original diagnosis must be reevaluated. Riegelman states, "Knowing how to live with uncertainty is a central feature of good clinical judgment."[9] This underscores that diagnosis is a *process* during which the physical therapist uses patient reports, valid and reliable tests and measures, clinical experience, and a constant evaluation of the patient's progression.

Diagnostic Questions in the Clinic

A diagnosis in physical therapy results from the integration of examination and evaluation processes. A correct diagnosis forms the basis for the choice of intervention and the potential prognosis for our patients. However, many of the tests used in physical therapy may not have been fully evaluated for quality and reliability. A test's quality is established for specific purposes and often with consideration of a specific patient problem. For every diagnostic test that you use in an examination, you should know the answers to the following questions:

- What diagnostic information am I seeking?
- Will this test assist me in confirming or refuting my clinical hypothesis regarding my patient's movement problem?
- How will this test result affect my treatment recommendations?
- What *do* I know about the characteristics of the test I am using?
- What *should* I know about the characteristics of the test I am using?

Searching the Literature: Research Designs Specific to Diagnostic Tests

Cohort designs are the most common study designs for the development of a diagnostic test. The same principles for searching the literature described in Chapter 2 also apply to searching the diagnostic literature. However, the types of designs that are used in the studies of diagnostic tests and measures will be cohort designs, not randomized clinical trials (RCTs). Prospective cohort designs are preferable to retrospective designs for the evaluation of diagnostic tests.[10] Although

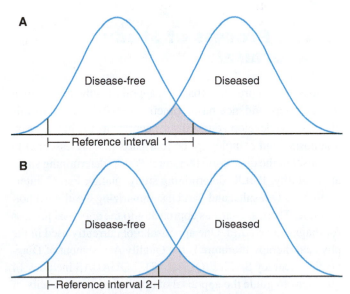

FIGURE 5.2 A. The disease-free group and the disease group have an area of overlapping values. B. Deciding the values that will distinguish between these two groups is defined as a "reference interval." Reference interval 1 will include some people who have the disease, but are labeled as disease free (false-negative). Reference interval 2 will include some people who are disease free, but are labeled with disease (false-positive).

it is possible to use a retrospective design, these designs present challenges in terms of the validity of the information. An example of a hypothetical retrospective design will help elucidate the need for prospective designs. Suppose that researchers want to know if results of the Lachman test[10] that is typically used in the clinic for patients with suspected anterior cruciate ligament (ACL) tear yields the same results as magnetic resonance images (MRIs) of these patients. They consult the patients' medical records to determine the results of these two tests. However, not all subjects may have had the Lachman test, the test may not have been recorded, or it may not be obvious in the record. In addition, it is not likely that reliability among clinicians performing the tests was established for the Lachman or the MRI, making it impossible to determine if the tests were administered correctly and reliably.

Prospective studies of diagnostic tests are *planned* to collect data on both the clinical test under study (the Lachman test in the example) and a gold standard comparison test (the MRI). Development of a valid and reliable diagnostic test requires the use of two tests, the index test and the gold standard test, for each subject. In a research study, the data collection procedures have typically been completed to meet the rigors of a valid study design, for example, reliability of testers for both tests. Study participants agree to both procedures as a part of the research. The important feature is the forward planning that is inherent in a prospective study. Subjects could be sampled at one time point (prospective and cross-sectional) and data obtained once and within a short time frame or sampled at one time point and followed over a longer time frame to determine if the target condition is confirmed (prospective and longitudinal).

■ The Process of Study Appraisal

As discussed in previous chapters, appraisal is the third step in the five-step evidence based practice (EBP) process. In this chapter, you develop your skills for appraising the literature on diagnosis; and completing the four parts that are essential to appraisal of the diagnostic literature: Part A: determining study applicability; Part B: determining study quality; Part C: interpreting study results; and Part D: summarizing the clinical bottom line. There are various approaches to the appraisal process for diagnostic studies. One appraisal tool currently used in the physical therapy literature is the Quality Assessment of Diagnostic Accuracy Studies (QUADAS).[11] QUADAS includes 14 questions to guide the appraisal of applicability and quality of a diagnostic study. Each question is recorded as "yes," "no," or "unclear." The total number of "yes" answers can be summed for a quality score for each diagnostic study appraised. Although a quality scoring process for the use of diagnostic studies in systematic reviews is not recommended,[12] some

authors suggest that these total scores can be used to obtain an estimate of diagnostic study quality.[13] Another tool that has been cited in the physical therapy literature is the Standards for Reporting of Diagnostic Accuracy (STARD).[14,15] This tool, however, is used to systematically report diagnostic study research for publication and is not directly applicable to the appraisal process for individual diagnostic studies described in this chapter.

We have organized the explanatory sections that follow according to eight questions that provide a useful and somewhat abbreviated process for appraising the applicability and quality of a diagnostic study. These eight questions form a checklist found in Table 5.7.

Part A: Determining Applicability of a Diagnostic Study

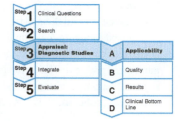

Study Sample

QUESTION 1: Is the entire spectrum of patients represented in the study sample? Is my patient represented in this spectrum of patients?

The spectrum of the impact of disease, disability, or injury should be represented in a study of a diagnostic test. If the entire spectrum is not represented, then the applicability of the test will be limited and this should be acknowledged by the authors.

The study must include a clinical population that is relevant to the test, but also relevant to your patient. This question then is important to both the applicability (to your patient) and quality of a study. For example, the Berg scale[16] has been validated in a sample of people who have movement disorders as the result of a stroke as well as a sample of people without movement disorders and without stroke. The same scale has not been validated with people with Parkinson's disease (PD). Although people with PD have movement and balance disorders, it has not been determined how they might perform on this scale. The test would not be correctly used in the diagnostic process with people with PD; if it is, then this limitation must be acknowledged when test results are interpreted.

The test should be used for its intended purpose and as stated above, with the types of patients for which the test was developed. As discussed in Chapter 10, the outcome measures used in an intervention research study should be valid measures of the expected outcomes. For example, if improvement in activities of daily living (ADL) is the goal of intervention, then using a measure of strength would not give insight into the expected impact of the intervention. Diagnostic tests must be similarly evaluated and applied. For example, a standardized, norm reference developmental motor scale may be appropriately used to decide eligibility for an early intervention program. However, this type of test is not useful in determining the classification of a child for a specific intervention. For example, a child with Down syndrome and a child with cerebral palsy may both score two standard deviations below the mean on the Bayley Scales of Infant Development-II[17] and this criterion may make each child eligible for early intervention services. However, this score will not assist the physical therapist in determining the specific recommendations for intervention for each child, nor will it confirm the diagnosis of either Down syndrome or cerebral palsy.

Part B: Determining Quality of a Diagnostic Study

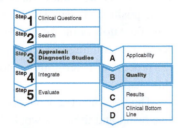

Ideally, the tests and measures used in physical therapy should be validated with clinical research. Although this is not yet always the reality, the science on diagnostic tests in physical therapy is increasing.[18,19] There are essential features of a research study of diagnostic tests that should be considered when appraising study applicability. Just as with intervention, or any other type of research study, the quality of studies must be appraised before a diagnostic test can be appropriately applied in the clinic. There are common aspects of study quality for diagnostic, prognostic, and intervention studies. However, there are aspects of validity that are unique to diagnostic studies.

QUESTION 2: *Was there an independent, blind comparison with a reference (gold) standard of diagnosis?*

As stated previously, the quality (sometimes referred to as validity) of a test or measure is established through the comparison of the diagnostic test (referred to as the index test or test of interest) results to the results of another test, referred to as the gold standard. Both the index and gold standard tests must have the same purpose. A gold standard is a test that is widely accepted as being the best available. Many tests developed in physical therapy that are used for musculoskeletal diagnoses have been compared and validated against imaging tests, for example, an MRI.[20,21] Valid tests given by a physical therapist might save the patient both time and money if this testing yields the same or similar information to more costly tests or tests that are not available in all settings.

QUESTION 3: *Were the diagnostic tests performed by one or more reliable examiners who were masked to results of the reference test?*

Research on test validity should include a masked (also referred to as *blinded*) application of both the test of interest and

the gold standard test. This requires at least two examiners, each completing only one of the tests. Each test should be completed without knowledge of the other test result and ideally without knowledge of the study goals.

One essential characteristic of a useful test is that it is reliable. Test reliability is affected both by the stability of the phenomenon being tested (e.g., balance, quality of life) and by the ability of the raters to repeat the test in the absence of any true change. Reliability is discussed in Chapter 4. There is abundant reliability research on many of our clinical tests; however, much of the reliability testing is conducted with samples that do not have movement problems. Establishing reliability on healthy, typically moving people is not adequate for studies of diagnostic tests designed for patient populations.

Both intra-rater (within rater) and inter-rater (between raters) reliability must be established for both the test of interest and the gold standard test. Reliability should be established with the types of patients that are appropriate to the test and the range of severity of the test problem should be included in the reliability sample.

QUESTION 4: *Did all subjects receive both tests (index and gold standard tests) regardless of test outcomes?*

Both tests should be completed regardless of the outcome of each test. As mentioned above, two or more masked professionals perform this comparison and then test results are analyzed. For example, the physical therapist would complete the Lachman test on participants in a clinical research study, and the results would be compared with the same subjects' results from the MRI (gold standard) that was interpreted by a radiologist. Ideally, both tests would result in the same diagnostic information. This means, for example, that even though a person has a negative Lachman test, indicating an intact ACL, this person must complete the MRI to confirm the negative test.

Part C: Interpreting Results of a Diagnostic Study

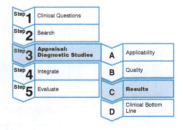

QUESTION 5: *Was the diagnostic test interpreted independently of all clinical information?*

Physical therapists use tests and measures in conjunction with patient history and clinical experience. When a test is developed, however, this additional information must not be available to the people conducting the index and gold standard tests. Physical therapists want to know what the test under study will contribute to the diagnostic process in addition to the history and circumstances of the patient. This information is determined from carefully controlled diagnostic research. For example, if a clinical balance test is compared with a gold standard test, then each test much be administered without knowledge of the results of the other test and without knowledge of additional clinical characteristics of the subjects.

QUESTION 6: *Were clinically useful statistics included in the analysis and interpreted for clinical application?*

Comparing a diagnostic test to a gold standard involves the computation of diagnostic statistics. There are many different statistics that can be used to reflect the accuracy and usefulness of a test for physical therapy diagnosis. Some of the statistics included in this chapter are also used in prognostic research. Statistics have been included that can be applied to your clinical diagnostic process.

Common Statistics in Diagnostic Research

This section focuses on the following diagnostic statistics:

- Sensitivity
- Specificity
- Receiver operating curves
- Positive and negative predictive values
- Positive and negative likelihood ratios
- Pre-test/post-test probabilities

Computing some of these tests relies on the logic of 2×2 tables (Table 5.1). Understanding 2×2 tables gives you a clearer understanding of sensitivity, specificity, predictive values, and likelihood ratios. Table 5.1 includes the participants' results of the clinical test under investigation (positive or negative) and the same participants' results on the gold standard (comparison) test. The gold standard is effectively used to establish the "truth" about the presence or absence of the condition. "Truth" then, is only as good as the gold standard. For example, a study might include a sample of 60 patients who presented with a history of trauma and symptoms compatible with an ACL tear. All patients have both the results of the Lachman test performed and graded by a physical therapist and an MRI of the knee evaluated by a radiologist. The results from these two tests can then be entered into the table, and you can determine the agreement or lack of agreement between these two tests (Table 5.1). As is evident in Table 5.1, to compute these diagnostic statistics, both test results must be expressed as dichotomous variables, that is, determined to be positive or negative. This requires that the test have a specific cutoff point for determining a positive and negative result. Determining this cutoff point requires thoughtful study; the process of determining cutoff points is discussed later in this chapter.

The Lachman test would be reduced to a positive or negative result and the MRI would be reduced to ACL tear or no tear (or injury/no injury). The radiologist needs to determine the criteria defining a positive versus a negative MRI. Each patient's data would be coded into one of the four boxes in the table. The columns in the 2×2 table are the results of the gold standard test, in this example the MRI. The rows in the 2×2 table are the results of the clinical test under study.

Ideally, *all* patients should be true positives (see Table 5.1A) or true negatives (see Table 5.1D). A true positive indicates that the person *definitely has* the condition, whereas a true negative indicates that the person *definitely does not have* the condition. This rarely happens even with the best of diagnostic tests. A false-positive (see Table 5.1B) suggests that the person *does not* have the condition as tested with the gold standard, but does test positive on the clinical test. A false-negative (see Table 5.1C) suggests the opposite; the person tests positive on the gold standard, but negative on the clinical test. The diagnostic statistics of sensitivity and specificity should be considered as estimates of a test's quality.[22] These tests merely quantitatively express the agreement between the test of interest and the gold standard.

Sensitivity

Sensitivity expresses a clinical test's accuracy in correctly identifying a problem as established by the gold standard. Using the example of the Lachman test and MRI for the diagnosis of ACL rupture, each subject is assigned to the appropriate box depending on his or her combination of test results (Table 5.2). The sensitivity of the test is then the total number of patients who have both a positive Lachman and a positive MRI test (true positives; Table 5.2 divided by the total number of patients with a positive MRI [A/(A + C)]. The following question is asked:

Of all the patients with a positive MRI, how many (what percentage) have a positive Lachman test?

TABLE 5.1 **Table Comparing Two Test Results**

	GOLD STANDARD POSITIVE	GOLD STANDARD NEGATIVE
Clinical test Positive	A True positive	B False-positive
Clinical test Negative	C False-negative	D True negative

Table cell A = Patients with positive Lachman and positive MRI tests are true positives

Table cell B = Patients with positive Lachman and negative MRI tests are false-positives

Table cell C = Patients with negative Lachman and positive MRI tests are false-negatives

Table cell D = Patients with negative Lachman and negative MRI tests are true negatives

TABLE 5.2 **Examples of an Index Test (Lachman) and a Gold Standard Test (MRI)**

	MRI POSITIVE	MRI NEGATIVE
Lachman test Positive	A True positives	B False-positives
Lachman test Negative	C False-negatives	D True negatives

A = Patients with positive Lachman and positive MRI tests are true positives
B = Patients with positive Lachman and negative MRI tests are false-positives
C = Patients with negative Lachman and positive MRI tests are false-negatives
D = Patients with negative Lachman and negative MRI tests are true negatives

TABLE 5.3 **Subject Values Summed for Each Test**

	MRI POSITIVE	MRI NEGATIVE
Lachman test Positive	A True positives n = 39	B False-positives n = 10
Lachman test Negative	C False-negatives n = 3	D True negatives n = 8
	Sensitivity A/(A + C) 39/39 + 3 = 0.93	*Specificity* D/(B + D) 8/8 + 10 = 0.44

An alternate expression is the following:
How sensitive is the Lachman test to the presence of a ruptured ACL as determined by an MRI?

Assuming the MRI yields an accurate diagnosis of either ACL rupture or no rupture, you are determining the sensitivity of the Lachman test in determining an ACL rupture. If the Lachman and the MRI both correctly diagnose the same problem, then you only need one or the other test, but not both. You could confidently use the less expensive and less time-consuming Lachman test to establish the integrity of the ACL and eliminate the need for an MRI for this diagnosis. However, before you can make this choice of test, you must know the specificity of these tests; that is, does it correctly identify all negative results as well as positive? The specificity of a test is described later in the chapter.

Computing the math for sensitivity using the column numbers from Table 5.3, you obtain a sensitivity of 0.93.

$$A/(A + C)$$
$$39/(39 + 3)$$
$$39/42 = 0.93$$

What type of clinical statement can you make about this sensitivity value?

For example:

"A positive Lachman test correctly identified 93% of the patients with a torn ACL."

We can then infer from this statistic only that a positive Lachman test incorrectly identified 7% of patients as having a torn ACL when there was no tear diagnosed on the MRI.

Specificity

Specificity expresses the test's ability to correctly identify the absence of a problem. It is the number of patients with a negative Lachman test and a negative MRI or true negatives (see Table 5.3D) divided by the total number of patients with a negative MRI

$$D/(B + D)$$

This helps us answer the following question:
"Of all the patients with a negative MRI, how many (what percentage) have a negative Lachman test?"

An alternate expression is the following:
"How specific is the Lachman test in identifying a nonruptured ACL as determined by an MRI?"

In the clinic, a major advantage of a highly specific test is that the patient would not need further referral for MRI for a diagnosis if the Lachman test is negative (using the above example).

To complete the math for specificity using the numbers in Table 5.3, you obtain a specificity of

$$D/(B + D)$$
$$8/(10 + 8)$$
$$8/18 = 0.44$$

What statement can you make about this specificity value?

For example:

"A negative Lachman test correctly identified 44% of the patients without a torn ACL."

We can then infer from this statistic only that a negative Lachman test incorrectly identified 56% of the patients as not having a torn ACL when there was a tear identified on the comparison gold standard test (MRI).

Sensitivity and specificity are diagnostic statistics that may assist you in choosing useful clinical tests for your practice. These two statistics are not directly dependent on the relative frequency of the problem in the population, but they are dependent on the spectrum of the problem represented in the samples that are used in the research.[9]

The samples used to establish sensitivity and specificity are crucial in determining the obtained values and in determining the test's usefulness for a particular patient. Cleland[18] lists a wide range of Lachman test values reported in the literature for sensitivity (0.65–0.99) and specificity (1.0–0.42). A review of two of the studies cited by Cleland investigating the Lachman test's utility in detecting an ACL rupture illustrates the importance of study sample, method, and application when considering the value of the sensitivity and specificity of a test. In a study by Katz and Fingeroth,[23] patients were recruited when they were referred for arthroscopy. A positive Lachman in this study was the lack of end point for tibial translation or positive subluxation. They reported high sensitivity (0.82) and specificity (0.97). In comparison, subjects in a study by Cooperman et al[24] were recruited when they were referred to physical therapy for initial evaluation of the knee. The Lachman test was graded on a four-point scale with increments separated by 5 mm or less. Their sensitivity (0.65) and specificity (0.42) values were considerably lower than those reported in the Katz and Fingeroth study. The Lachman might have higher values (better detection) when detecting ACL injuries that have a high pre-test probability of ACL rupture, for example, when subjects were already referred for arthroscopy compared to subjects referred to physical therapy for any knee problem. The test may also be more sensitive and specific when extreme signs on the Lachman test are used to determine a positive finding in comparison to determining a positive finding using more subtle signs.

Receiver Operating Characteristic (ROC) Curve

One crucial decision in computing sensitivity and specificity is the choice of the cutoff score used to define positive and negative test scores. To construct and validate a diagnostic test, a cut point is determined that provides a dichotomous test result (positive or negative).

Clinically useful cut points are best determined by studying the effects of various cut points in the data on the sensitivity and specificity.[25] The receiver operating characteristic (ROC) curve is a graphic representation of the sensitivity and specificity values that are generated from a series of cut points (Fig. 5.3).

The optimal cut point is the highest value for a combination of sensitivity and specificity. It is the value closest to the upper left corner of the ROC. In Figure 5.3, the optimal cut point for the Oswestry Low Back Pain and Disability Questionnaire (modified OSW) and the Quebec Back Pain Scale (QUE) are circled. However, this value is based on the premise that a false-positive (the patient tests positive, but does not have the condition) is equally as important as a false-negative (the patient tests negative, but actually has that condition). An example from medical testing might clarify the important balance between the sensitivity and specificity of a test. If a throat strep test is negative, but the patient actually has strep throat (false-negative), antibiotics may not be prescribed by the physician.

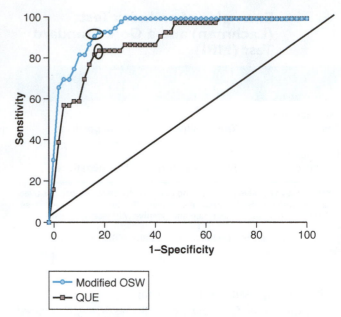

FIGURE 5.3 Receiver operative curve (ROC). From Fritz JM, Irrgang JJ. *Phys Ther.* 2001;81:776-788; with permission.

Although the recovery time may be slower, an otherwise healthy person may recover from a strep throat infection, but there is a risk, although rare, of an undetected strep infection leading to rheumatic fever.[26] A false-negative in an elderly person with many co-morbidities, however, could be life threatening. In this situation, the sensitivity of the test is important to avoid serious consequences. If a patient tests positive for strep, but does not have a strep infection (false-positive) then antibiotics may be prescribed when they are not necessary.

Another example from physical therapy highlights the need to ask, "How important are the results of the testing?" If a patient tests negative for risk of falling, but is actually at risk for falls (false-negative), then important follow-up may not occur. This could be a potentially threatening situation. A false-positive in detecting the risk of falling may unnecessarily alarm a patient, but additional testing using more specific tests may rule out the problem. With testing for the risk of falls, the sensitivity of a test may be stressed over the specificity to identify every person who is at serious risk.

No test will be completely accurate, that is, 100% sensitive and 100% specific. It is critical to identify the repercussions of an incorrect diagnosis given a particular test result.

Positive Predictive Value

Predictive values are computed from the rows in a 2 × 2 table (Table 5.4). A **positive predictive value (PPV)** expresses the proportion (percentage) of people *with a positive result* on the study test that have the problem as determined by the gold standard test. The PPV gives you results on the gold standard for only those people who have tested positive on the test of interest.

TABLE 5.4 **Values for Positive Predictive Value (PPV) and Negative Predictive Value (NPV)**

	MRI POSITIVE	MRI NEGATIVE	
Lachman test Positive	A True positives n = 39	B False positives n = 10	PPV A/A + B 39/39 + 10 = 0.80
Lachman test Negative	C False negatives n = 3	D True negatives n = 8	NPV D/C + D 3/8 + 3

The following is the formula for the PPV:

$$A/(A + B)$$
$$39/(39 + 10)$$
$$39/49 = 0.80$$

In our example, 80% of the patients with a positive Lachman test had a torn ACL as confirmed by MRI (positive MRI).

Negative Predictive Value (NPV)

A **negative predictive value (NPV)** expresses the proportion (percentage) of people *with a negative result* on the study test that does not have the problem as determined by the gold standard test (see Table 5.4). The NPV gives you results on the gold standard for only those people who have tested negative on the test of interest.

The formula for the NPV is the following:

$$D/(C + D)$$
$$3/(3 + 8)$$
$$3/11 = 0.27$$

In our example, 27% of the patients with a negative Lachman test did not have a torn ACL.

One of the major limitations to the use of predictive values is the influence of the prevalence of the problem of interest in the study sample. Lower prevalence in the sample yields a lower PPV. Return to the example of 60 patients in a study of the diagnostic utility of the Lachman test for determining ACL rupture (see Table 5.4). If you change the prevalence of ACL rupture in the sample from 39 true positives to 16 true positives, the PPV drops to 62%. To be valid, research studies must have accurately represented the prevalence of the disorder in the study sample that would be expected in the larger population. In addition, the sample of 60 patients might not include a large percentage of people who tested negative on the Lachman test; thus, the NPV should be interpreted cautiously. Both PPV and NPV are influenced by the prevalence of the condition in the study sample and should typically be interpreted with caution.

Part D: Summarizing the Clinical Bottom Line of a Diagnostic Study

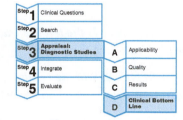

Sensitivity and specificity may help answer the question, "What is the best test to help me rule in or rule out a specific problem?" but only if the values have been calculated on a sample that encompasses the entire spectrum of the disorder or at a minimum in a sample that is similar to your patient. A series of cut points using different values for the distinction between positive and negative results of the test should have been determined before a test can be clinically useful. However, sensitivity and specificity are not useful statistics to communicate to patients; patients assume that the best tests are used. These statistics refer to the test, not directly to the patient.

Sensitivity and specificity are typically more helpful for understanding how a test performs in a population rather than how to interpret the result of a test for a single patient. The concept of SpPin and SnNout may be more helpful for the interpretation of a test result for your patient. These concepts are described in Digging Deeper 5.2.

✦ DIGGING DEEPER 5.2

SpPin and SnNout Definition

SnNout: This abbreviation or mnemonic indicates that a negative test result from a highly sensitive test can assist in ruling out the diagnosis.

SpPin: This abbreviation or mnemonic indicates that a positive test result from a highly specific test can assist you in ruling in the diagnosis.

Reflection

Reflect on the logic of this concept. If a test is highly sensitive, this indicates that the test correctly identifies most people with the problem. The reality might be that the test overidentifies problems, but the specificity of the test will assist you in determining this. However, if your patient has a negative test, then this assists you in ruling *out* the problem (because most people with the problem will have a positive test!).

You typically interpret test *results* of your diagnostic testing to your patients; that is, you interpret the likelihood that a positive test indicates the presence of a specific movement problem or the likelihood that a negative test rules out this problem. In the diagnostic process you choose tests to determine if a specific problem exists or it does not. Your goal is to increase the certainty of your diagnostic hypothesis. You have the patient history and symptoms that help in establishing probabilities of certain problems. A person who is an aggressive skier and heard her knee "pop" when she landed a jump has a high probability of having a damaged ACL. The physical therapist engaged in the diagnostic process uses the hypothesis of a damaged ACL and continues to add information to determine the likelihood that the hypothesis is correct. Each test that is chosen should add to this determination.

QUESTION 7: *Is the test accurate and clinically relevant to physical therapy practice?*

QUESTION 8: *Will the resulting post-test probabilities affect my management and help my patient?*

Diagnostic tests must be accurate in determining a patient's diagnostic status; however, just as important, the tests must be relevant to the patient's goals and the goals of physical therapy. Each test chosen should be not only be accurate but also clinically useful for your decisions.

Likelihood Ratios

Likelihood ratios combine the sensitivity and specificity of a test into one expressed value. The value of the positive likelihood ratio is that it answers the question, "What is the likelihood that my patient with *a positive test* result actually has the problem?" Related to that question, the negative likelihood ratio answers the question, "What is the likelihood that my patient with *a negative test* result has the problem? You have shifted the focus of the results of your diagnostic test from the test to the patient.

Likelihood ratios can assist your diagnostic certainty after you have a test result. These values provide quantitative information that shifts your certainty about your clinical diagnosis. Likelihood ratios can be used to communicate test results to your patients by providing the change in probabilities that a problem is present or absent given their positive or negative test result. That is, given the history, patient symptoms, and your diagnostic testing, you can express to your patients the likelihood that they have a particular movement problem. You can use a general statement: "I believe it is very likely that you have knee instability from a torn ACL." You can give more specific information in the form of a likelihood ratio for a specific test. The likelihood ratio of a test is expressed in relation to the pre-test probability of a diagnosis. For example, if you quantify your patient's likelihood of a ruptured ACL as 60%,

then any diagnostic test you use should affect this probability. After the test, the probability of the patient having an ACL should be either greater or less than 60%.

As mentioned previously, ideally a diagnostic test should have a combination of high sensitivity and specificity. No test is 100% sensitive and specific, but what is an acceptable combination of values? There really are no exact numbers that define good sensitivity or good specificity. Deciding on acceptable values depends on the clinical implications for being wrong in your diagnostic decision. Computing likelihood ratios combines sensitivity and specificity into one diagnostic expression.

Positive Likelihood Ratio

A **positive likelihood ratio** (LR+) expresses the numeric value of a positive test if the movement problem is present versus absent.

$$LR+ = \frac{\text{Probability of a positive test if the movement problem is present}}{\text{Probability of a positive test if the movement problem is absent}}$$

The following formula is used to compute a positive likelihood ratio:

$$LR+ = \frac{\text{Sensitivity (true positive rate)}}{1- \text{Specificity (true negative rate)}}$$

Let's return to the sensitivity and specificity values in Table 5.3. If you use these values, your positive likelihood ratio is the following:

$$0.93/1 - 0.44 = 1.6$$

How would you express this value to a patient?

For example:

> "Your positive Lachman test suggests that you are 1.6 times more likely than your pre-test probability to have a ruptured ACL."

A likelihood ratio of 1 offers no additional information to the positive diagnosis of damaged ACL. The ratio of 1.6 offers a small amount of additional information to the history and symptoms for a positive diagnosis of ACL damage. That is, it only minimally changes the post-test probability of damage to the ACL. This is comparable to the information obtained from the PPV: a positive test is found in 80% of patients with a torn ACL. Neither value may add substantially to our diagnosis of a ruptured ACL. This depends on our level of diagnostic certainty with the patient history and symptoms alone.

Negative Likelihood Ratio

A **negative likelihood ratio** (LR-) expresses the numeric value of a negative test if the movement problem is present.

LR– = Probability of a negative test if the movement problem is present

Probability of a negative test if the movement problem is absent

The formula to compute a negative likelihood ratio is the following:

$$LR- = \frac{1 - \text{Sensitivity (false-negative rate)}}{\text{Specificity (true negative rate)}}$$

Again, using the sensitivity and specificity values in Table 5.3, the following is our negative likelihood ratio:

$$1 - 0.93/0.44 = 0.16$$

The smaller the negative likelihood ratio, the less likely it is that the patient with a negative test has the movement problem. How would we express this value to a patient?

For example:

"Your negative Lachman test supports that you do not have a damaged ACL."

Revising Pre-Test to Post-Test Probability

The value of the tests you choose for improving your diagnosis depends on your estimate of the probability that the person has the problem before you begin testing. This **pre-test probability** can be estimated from prevalence of the problem in the population, but more commonly in physical therapy we estimate the probability of a movement problem from the patient history and report of symptoms. This information should focus the choice of tests and measures. Test results should then sufficiently increase the **post-test probability** that the problem exists to warrant performing the test.

Each diagnostic test we use should help us to rule in or rule out a particular diagnosis of a movement problem. Diagnostic tests should either support or refute our hypothesis about the patient's problem. Estimating pre-test probabilities however, is a challenge for most physical therapy diagnoses. If we *do* have a pre-test estimate, we can plot both positive and negative likelihood ratios on a nomogram[27] (Fig. 5.4) to visualize and quantify our post-test probabilities. In the nomogram, the pre-test probability score is connected with a straight line through the likelihood ratio, either positive or negative, to the post-test probability score.

The nomogram in Figure 5.4 captures the minimal effects of the positive Lachman test results on the post-test probabilities that our patient has a ruptured ACL and the somewhat larger effects of a negative Lachman test on the post-test probability that the patient does not have a ruptured ACL.

Given the patient's history and current symptoms, you may still have confidence in your pre-test clinical impression of a

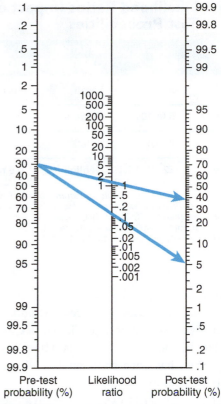

FIGURE 5.4 The ability to plot both positive and negative likelihood ratios on a nomogram to visualize and quantify post-test probabilities. From Fagan TJ. Nomogram for Baye's theorem. *N Engl J Med.* 1975;293:257; with permission.

torn ACL. At this point, you may want to add an additional diagnostic test (e.g., pivot shift test) to assist your diagnosis. You will again want to know the diagnostic statistics on this test.

Cleland[18] summarizes the recommendations of Jaeschke et al[28] for the interpretation of both positive and negative likelihood ratios. These are summarized in Table 5.5. The larger the positive likelihood value, the greater the potential impact will be on post-test probabilities. The smaller the negative likelihood ratio (approaching zero), the greater the potential impact will be on post-test probabilities.

Clinical Prediction Rules for Diagnosis

Clinical predictions rules (CPR), also termed *clinical decision rules,* are sets of validated predictor variables that characterize patients and that are used to make a specific diagnosis, prognosis, treatment recommendation, or referral to another professional. Here we consider a CPR for diagnosis or referral.

CPR for Diagnosis and Prognosis

A CPR can be used as a diagnostic statement that classifies patients for the purpose of treatment and prognosis.[29–31] A CPR

TABLE 5.5 **Likelihood Ratios Impact on Post-Test Probabilities**

POSITIVE LIKELIHOOD RATIOS		NEGATIVE LIKELIHOOD RATIOS	
Large	>10	Large	<0.1
Moderate	5 to 10	Moderate	0.1 to 0.2
Small	2 to 5	Small	0.2 to 0.5
Negligible	<2	Negligible	0.5 to 1.0

Data from: Cleland J. *Orthopedic Clinical Examination: An Evidence-Based Approach for Physical Therapists.* Carlstadt, NJ: Icon Learning Systems; 2005; and Jaeschke T, Guyatt GH, Sackett DL. How to use an article about a diagnostic test: B. what are the results and will they help me in caring for my patients? *JAMA.* 1994;271:703-707.

differs from a clinical practice guideline[32–34] in that a CPR is based on a multi-step research process including a rigorous statistical analysis to generate a prediction. A CPR should be implemented by physical therapists after this thorough research process has been completed. A clinical practice guideline (CPG) describes clinical recommendations that are generated from a panel of experts using evidence from the literature and expert practice to shape the guideline (see Chapter 9).

Patient characteristics obtained through our history and examination and results from other professionals' diagnostic tests can be used to identify who might best benefit from a specific type of treatment. A CPR quantifies the contributions of each of these variables to the diagnostic outcome. A CPR can be used to do the following:

1. Make a specific diagnosis, for example, cervical radiculopathy[35]
2. Use diagnostic criteria to make a prognosis regarding a response to treatment, for example, specific characteristics of patients with low back pain are used to predict their response to spinal manipulation[36]
3. Refer patients to another professional, for example, identifying the risk of lower-extremity deep vein thrombosis[19]

The development of a CPR requires rigorous multistep research to identify the specific patient characteristics that cluster and relate to a specific diagnosis or to positive (or negative) outcomes from a specific physical therapy intervention.[32,36,37] You should appraise the rigor of the developmental process that has been used to validate a CPR before implementing the rule in your clinical practice. McGinn et al[31] offer a three-step process for the development of a valid CPR. This process has been applied by Childs and Cleland[29] to CPR development in physical therapy. The three steps are detailed below.

Development of the CPR

Step 1: Creating the CPR

A CPR is developed through the use of the diagnostic statistics previously described in this chapter: sensitivity, specificity, likelihood values, and confidence intervals. Subjects' outcomes on both the CPR and the gold standard are recorded in a 2×2 table. The index test described previously is typically a set of clinical variables that are associated with a particular type of problem, for example, the clinical characteristics of people with cervical radiculopathy. This cluster of clinical variables is then compared to a gold standard test.

Identifying the best predictive variables is the first step in developing a CPR. Clinical experience and expertise are combined with a thorough appraisal of the available literature to determine the variables that are the best bets to include in a CPR. A clinically useful CPR distills the most predictive variables and does not include all possible variables obtained through the history or examination. The best set of predictor variables that make up the CPR are typically determined through multiple regression analyses[30,31] (see regression in Chapter 6). But before a regression can be computed, the researchers must know the patient's outcome on the gold standard measure: Does the patient have the problem that the CPR is attempting to identify? For example, Riddle and Wells[19] developed a CPR (they term it a clinical decision rule) for identifying lower extremity deep vein thrombosis (DVT) in an outpatient setting. They used ascending venography as the gold standard against which they measured their suggested cluster of clinical risk factors. This decision rule is used to identify patients as belonging to a high, moderate, or low probability group for DVT. The physical therapist can then use this classification to decide on the immediacy of the need for referral.

As described in the CPR for DVT, the cluster of clinical variables chosen for a diagnostic CPR are measured against a gold standard, in this case, venography. Someone who is masked to the outcome of the other diagnostic outcome must administer the gold standard. The choice of the gold standard is critical to the clinical usefulness of the CPR in that it must accurately reflect a clinically important outcome and be related to the comparison test. For example, Wainner et al[35] used neural conduction outcomes as the gold standard in the development of the CPR for cervical radiculopathy defined with a cluster of clinical variables.

Flynn et al[36] used treatment outcome on the Oswestry Disability Questionnaire[38] to determine the predicted treatment outcome from the CPR for low back pain treated with spinal manipulation (Table 5.6). There were five factors that predicted patient success from the treatment: lumbar hypomobility, no symptoms distal to the knee, symptom duration of less than 15 days, lower fear-avoidance beliefs, and hip internal rotation range of motion of greater than 35 degrees. The presence of any four of these five factors increased the probability of

TABLE 5.6 **Constructing a Clinical Prediction Rule**

	50% IMPROVEMENT ON OSWESTRY POSITIVE	LESS THAN 50% IMPROVEMENT ON OSWESTRY NEGATIVE
Four clinical factors present *Positive*	True positives	False-positives
Four clinical factors not present *Negative*	False-negatives	True negatives
	Sensitivity	Specificity

Data from: Flynn TW, Fritz JM, Whitman J, et al. A clinical prediction rule for classifying patients with low back pain who demonstrate short-term improvement with spinal manipulation. *Spine*. 2002;27:2835-2843.

success from short-term spinal manipulation from 45% (estimated pre-treatment probability) to 95%. Patients with four of these five variables were 25 times more likely to benefit from this treatment. This is a powerful predictive statement that gives therapists clear guidelines as to who would benefit from a specific physical therapy intervention. These five factors could then be a valid part of the diagnostic process during the examination of patients who present with acute low back pain.

In developing a CPR, the possible errors in decision making, for example, missing a diagnosis or falsely diagnosing a problem, again must be evaluated in light of the seriousness of the problem. For example, the CPR for cervical radiculopathy developed by Wainner et al[35] must be highly accurate to avoid, for example, misdiagnosing cervical radiculopathy and recommending manipulation for someone with spinal cord compression. Treatment with manipulation could cause serious injury.[29]

Step 2: Validating the CPR

The applicability of a CPR also must be systematically evaluated. In the second step of creating a CPR, the proposed CPR must be replicated with a different set of patients and in one or more different settings of practice. Obviously, for a CPR to have maximum impact, it should be applicable across different groups of patients and settings. The validation study should implement the CPR and outcome measures precisely as was done in the first step of the development of the CPR.

Step 3: Conducting an Impact Analysis

The clinical utility of a CPR relies on the accuracy of the CPR in diagnosing patients correctly and the generalizability of the diagnostic process across patient groups and practice settings. A useful CPR improves patient outcomes and is cost effective. The Ottawa Ankle Rules[39,40] are detailed by Childs et al,[29] and this CPR is an excellent example of the importance of an impact analysis as a final step in developing and implementing a clinically useful CPR.

The Ottawa Ankle Rules are clinical prediction rules that are used to identify ankle fractures. Only patients with specific characteristics identified by the prediction rule are considered to require referral for radiographs. The use of the Ottawa rules by emergency personnel led to a decrease in use of ankle radiography, a decrease in emergency room waiting times, and a decrease in costs without patient dissatisfaction or missed fractures. It is estimated that the use of these rules could save substantial health-care dollars.

The impact of a CPR should be measured in the quality of outcomes for patients and also for the effect on utilization and cost of care.

Table 5.7 is a summary of the appraisal questions for diagnostic studies.

TABLE 5.7 **Key Questions for Appraising Studies of Diagnosis***

QUESTION	YES OR NO	WHERE TO FIND THE INFORMATION	COMMENTS AND WHAT TO LOOK FOR
1. Is the entire spectrum of patients represented in the study sample? Is my patient represented in this spectrum of patients?	__ Yes __ No	Methods	The study should report specific details about how the sample of participants was selected. It is important that participants are at a similar stage in the event of interest (or recovery process) prior to starting the study. Finally, it is important that all participants are measured at study outset on the primary outcome that will be used to detect change in status.
2. Was there an independent, blind comparison with a reference (gold) standard of diagnosis?	__ Yes __ No	Methods	Development of a valid and reliable diagnostic measure requires the use of two tests, the index test and the gold standard test for each subject.
3. Were the diagnostic tests performed by one or more reliable examiners who were masked to results of the reference test?	__ Yes __ No	Methods	Because all outcome measures are subject to bias, when possible, it is ideal for evaluators to be blinded to the primary hypothesis and previous data collected by a given participant.

Continued

TABLE 5.7 **Key Questions for Appraising Studies of Diagnosis*—cont'd**

QUESTION	YES OR NO	WHERE TO FIND THE INFORMATION	COMMENTS AND WHAT TO LOOK FOR
4. Did all subjects receive both tests (index and gold standard tests) regardless of test outcomes?	__ Yes __ No	Methods	Even if the gold standard test is completed first and indicates the best diagnosis in current practice, the comparison test must be completed for each subject.
5. Was the diagnostic test interpreted independent of all clinical information?	__ Yes __ No	Methods	The person interpreting the test should not know the results of the other test or other clinical information regarding the subject.
6. Were clinically useful statistics included in the analysis and interpreted for clinical application?	__ Yes __ No	Methods and results	Have the authors formed their statistical statement in a way that has application to patients?
7. Is the test accurate and clinically relevant to physical therapy practice?	__ Yes __ No	Methods, results, and discussion	Accuracy is estimated by comparison to the gold standard. Does the test affect practice?
8. Will the resulting post-test probabilities affect my management and help my patient?	__ Yes __ No	Results and discussion	This requires an estimate of pre-test probabilities. If the probability estimates do not change, then the test is not clinically useful.

*The key questions were adapted from Sackett DL, Straus SE, Richardson WS, Rosenberg W, Haynes RB. *Evidence-Based Medicine.* 2nd ed. New York, NY: Churchill Livingstone; 2000 [41]; and Straus SE, Richardson WS, Glaszious P, Haynes RB. *Evidence Based Medicine.* 3rd ed. Philadelphia, PA: Elsevier; 2003 [42], and applied to physical therapy.

SUMMARY

The diagnostic literature has specific types of designs and statistical analyses. The research designs most typically applied to diagnostic questions are prospective, cohort designs. Statistical analyses of diagnostic studies assist you in determining the clinical usefulness of the test. A valid, clinically useful test should improve your diagnostic outcomes. Diagnostic studies can assist you in making statements about expected outcomes for a patient or patient group and provide estimates of the likelihood of certain outcomes. Just as with all other study types, the clinical usefulness of a study of diagnosis is dependent on both the applicability to your patient and to the rigor of the study.

REVIEW QUESTIONS

1. What are the differences between likelihood ratios and sensitivity and specificity statistics?

2. How would you interpret a positive likelihood ratio of 12.5 for a patient with a positive test result?

3. What are important disadvantages to a retrospective diagnostic study?

4. What are factors that influence the pre-test probabilities of a movement problem for a patient?

REFERENCES

1. American Physical Therapy Association. Guide to Physical Therapy Practice. 2nd ed. *Phys Ther.* 2001;81:9-744.
2. Rose SJ. Physical therapy diagnosis: role and function. *Phys Ther.* 1989;69:535-537.
3. Delitto A, Snyder-Mackler L. The diagnostic process: examples in orthopedic physical therapy. *Phys Ther.* 1995;75:203-211.
4. Sahrmann S. Are physical therapists fulfilling their responsibilities as diagnosticians? *J Orthop Sports Phys Ther.* 2005;35:556-558.
5. Davenport TE, Kulig K, Resnik C. Diagnosing pathology to decide the appropriateness of physical therapy: what's our role? *J Orthop Sports Phys Ther.* 2006;36:1-2.
6. Zimmy NJ. Physical therapy management from physical therapy diagnosis: necessary but insufficient. *J Phys Ther Educ.* 1995;9:36-38.
7. Davenport TE, Watts HG, Kulig K, et al. Current status and correlates of physicians' referral diagnoses for physical therapy. *J Orthop Sports Phys Ther.* 2005;35:572-579.

8. Pierce SR, Daly K, Gallagher KG, et al. Constraint-induced therapy for a child with hemiplegic cerebral palsy: a case report. *Arch Phys Med Rehabil.* 2002;83:1462-1463.

9. Riegelman RK. *Studying a Study and Testing a Test: How to Read the Medical Literature.* 4th ed. Philadelphia: Lippincott Williams & Wilkins; 2000.

10. Cooperman JM, Riddle DL, Rothstein JM. Reliability and validity of judgments of the integrity of the anterior cruciate ligament of the knee using the Lachman's test. *Phys Ther.* 1990;70:225-233.

11. Whiting P, Rutjes AW, Dinnes J, et al. Development and validation of methods for assessing the quality of diagnostic accuracy studies. *Health Technol Assess.* 2004;8:1-234.

12. Whiting P, Harbord R, Kleijnen J. No role for quality scores in systematic reviews of diagnostic accuracy studies. *BMC Med Res Methodology.* 2005;5.

13. Cook CE, Hegedus EJ. *Orthopedic Physical Examination Techniques: An Evidence Based Approach.* Upper Saddle River, NJ: Pearson/Prentice Hall; 2008.

14. Bossuyt PM, Reitsma JB, Bruns DE, et al. Towards complete and accurate reporting of studies of diagnostic accuracy: The STARD Initiative. *Ann Intern Med.* 2003;138:40-44.

15. Bossuyt PM, Reitsma JB, Bruns DE, et al. The STARD statement for reporting studies of diagnostic accuracy: explanation and elaboration. *Ann Intern Med.* 2003;138:W1-12.

16. Wood-Dauphinee S, Berg K, Brave G, Williams JL. The Balance Scale: responding to clinically meaningful changes in patients with stroke. *Can J Rehabil.* 1997;10:35-50.

17. Bayley N. *Bayley Scales of Infant Development.* New York; 1993.

18. Cleland J. *Orthopedic Clinical Examination: An Evidence-Based Approach for Physical Therapists.* Carlstadt, NJ: Icon Learning Systems; 2005.

19. Riddle DL, Wells PS. Diagnosis of lower-extremity deep vein thrombosis in outpatients. *Phys Ther.* 2004;84:729-735.

20. Rubinstein RA Jr, Shelbourne KD, McCarroll JR, et al. The accuracy of the clinical examination in the setting of posterior cruciate ligament injuries. *Am J Sports Med.* 1994;22:550-557.

21. Lee JK, Yao L, Phelps CT, et al. Anterior cruciate ligament tears: MR imaging compared with arthroscopy and clinical tests. *Radiology.* 1988;166:861-864.

22. Campo M, Shiyko MP, Lichtman SW. Sensitivity and specificity: a review of related statistics and controversies in the context of physical therapist education. *J Phys Ther. Educ.* 2010;24:69-78.

23. Katz JW, Fingeroth RJ. The diagnostic accuracy of ruptures of the anterior cruciate ligament comparing the Lachman test, the anterior drawer sign, and the pivot shift test in acute and chronic knee injuries. *Am J Sports Med.* 1986;14:88-91.

24. Cooperman JM, Riddle DL, Rothstein JM. Reliability and validity of judgments of the integrity of the anterior cruciate ligament of the knee using the Lachman's test. *Phys Ther.* 1990;70:225-233.

25. Fetters L, Tronick EZ. Discriminate power of the alberta infant motor scale and the movement assessment of infants for infants exposed to cocaine. *Pediatric Physic Ther.* 2000;12: 16-23..

26. Del Mar CB, Glasziou PP, Spinks AB. Antibiotics for sore throat. *Cochrane Database Syst Rev.* 2006:CD000023.

27. Fagan TJ. Nomogram for Baye's theorem. *N Engl J Med.* 1975;293:257.

28. Jaeschke T, Guyatt GH, Sackett DL. How to use an article about a diagnostic test: B. what are the results and will they help me in caring for my patients? *JAMA.* 1994;271:703-707.

29. Childs JD, Cleland JA. Development and application of clinical prediction rules to improve decision making in physical therapist practice. *Phys Ther.* 2006;86:122-131.

30. Laupacis A, Sekar N, Stiell IG. Clinical prediction rules: A review and suggested modifications of methodological standards. *JAMA.* 1997;277:488-494.

31. McGinn TG, Guyatt GH, Wyer PC, et al. Users' guides to the medical literature: XXII:How to use articles about clinical decision rules. *JAMA.* 2000;284:79-84.

32. Fritz JM, Delitto A, Erhard RE. Comparison of classification-based physical therapy with therapy based on clinical practice guidelines for patients with acute low back pain. *Spine.* 2003;28:1363-1372.

33. Ottawa panel evidence-based clinical practice guidelines for therapeutic exercise and manual therapy in the management of osteoarthritis. *Phys Ther.* 2005;85.

34. O'Neil ME, Fragala-Pinkham MA, Westcott SL, et al. Physical therapy clinical management recommendations for children with cerebral palsy—spastic diplegia: achieving functional mobiltiy outcomes. *Pediatr Phys Ther.* 2006;18:49-72.

35. Wainner RS, Fritz JM, Irrgang JJ, et al. Reliability and diagnostic accuracy of the clinical examination and patient self-report measures for cervical radiculopathy. *Spine.* 2003;28:52-62.

36. Flynn TW, Fritz JM, Whitman J, et al. A clinical prediction rule for classifying patients with low back pain who demonstrate short-term improvement with spinal manipulation. *Spine.* 2002;27:2835-2843.

37. Hicks GE, Fritz JM, Delitto A, et al. Preliminary development of a clinical prediction rule for determining which patients with low back pain will respond to a stabilization exercise program. *Arch Phys Med Rehab.* 2005;86:1753-1762.

38. Fairbank JC, Pynsent PB. The Oswestry Disability Index. *Spine.* 2000;25:2940-2952; discussion 2952.

39. Stiell IG, McKnight RD, Greenberg GH, et al. Implementation of the Ottawa Ankle Rules. *JAMA.* 1994;271:827-732.

40. Auleley GR, Ravaud P, Giraudeau B, et al. Implemention of the Ottawa Ankle Rules in France: a multicenter randomized controlled trial. *JAMA.* 1997;277:1935-1939.

41. Sackett DL, Straus SE, Richardson WS, et al. *Evidence-Based Medicine.* 2nd ed. New York: Churchill Livingstone; 2000.

42. Straus SE, Richardson WS, Glaszious P, et al. *Evidence Based Medicine.* 3rd ed. Philadelphia: Elsevier; 2003.

6 Appraising Prognostic Research Studies

PRE-TEST

1. How does the appraisal process change when considering prognostic research in comparison to intervention research?

2. What are typical study designs for prognostic research that one is likely to find in the literature?

3. What is the flaw in the following statement about a regression analysis? It appears that subject weight, previous injuries, and type of profession were all causes of low back pain.

CHAPTER-AT-A-GLANCE

This chapter will help you understand the following:

- Application of prognostic literature to specific patients and patient groups

- Appraising the validity of prognostic studies

- Interpretation of the results of prognostic studies

■ Introduction

Prognostic Questions in the Clinic

Patients, families, and physical therapists have many questions about prognosis. Prognostic questions may be about the impact of a disease or event on a patient's long-term outcome. For example, a patient may ask, "Will I be able to ski after back surgery?" or "When can I expect to go back to work?" Prognostic questions may also guide discharge planning. You may ask, "What is the prognosis for my patient to return home versus a rehabilitation facility at discharge?" or "What are the odds that this intervention will benefit my patient's independent ambulation?" Many factors influence the answers to prognostic questions such as the severity of the patient's problem, gender, age, home environment, and co-morbidities. Valid prognostic studies can assist in answering these types of questions, and they assist in weighing the various factors that may contribute to specific outcomes. The prognostic literature has specific types of designs and statistical analyses. This chapter begins with design descriptions for prognostics studies, as these will be different from the types of designs used for intervention studies (Fig. 6.1).

Research Designs That are Specific to Prognostic Studies

The same principles for searching the literature described in Chapter 2 also apply to searching the prognostic literature. However, the research designs most typically applied to prognostic questions are observational studies that used associations between or among variables. These typically include cohort and case control designs (Fig. 6.2), which can be either longitudinal (subjects are followed over time) or cross-sectional (subject data are collected at one point in time).

Cohort Studies

In a cohort study, a group of subjects who are likely to develop a certain condition or outcome is followed into the future (prospectively) for a sufficient length of time to observe if the subjects develop the condition. Cohort studies can provide data concerning the timing of the development of the outcome within the group and assist in defining possible causal factors in developing the condition. The factors, or risks, for a particular outcome are identified, and the effect is observed.

For example:

All athletes in one high school are followed throughout the season to determine who sustains anterior cruciate ligament (ACL) injuries. Data on gender, type of sport, previous injury, play time, and so on may also be collected and analyzed at the end of the season to determine the association of these factors to ACL injury.

For example:

Individuals post-stroke are evaluated once to investigate factors that contributed to a stroke (cross-sectional, retrospective, or historic design).

For example:

Following a group of infants of very low birth weight, prematurely born, to determine who develops cerebral palsy (longitudinal, prospective design).

Case Control Studies

Case control studies are conducted *after* an outcome of interest has occurred. The factors that contributed to the outcome are studied in a group that has the outcome (case group) and compared to a group that does not have the outcome of interest

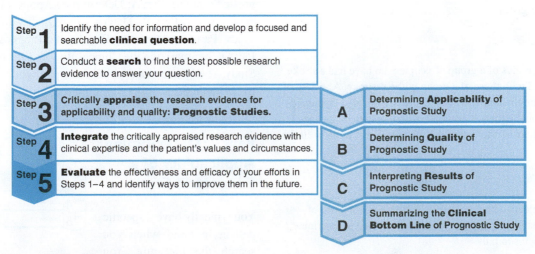

Step 1 Identify the need for information and develop a focused and searchable **clinical question**.	
Step 2 Conduct a **search** to find the best possible research evidence to answer your question.	
Step 3 Critically **appraise** the research evidence for applicability and quality: **Prognostic Studies**.	**A** Determining **Applicability** of Prognostic Study
Step 4 **Integrate** the critically appraised research evidence with clinical expertise and the patient's values and circumstances.	**B** Determining **Quality** of Prognostic Study
Step 5 **Evaluate** the effectiveness and efficacy of your efforts in Steps 1–4 and identify ways to improve them in the future.	**C** Interpreting **Results** of Prognostic Study
	D Summarizing the **Clinical Bottom Line** of Prognostic Study

FIGURE 6.1 Appraising prognostic research studies.

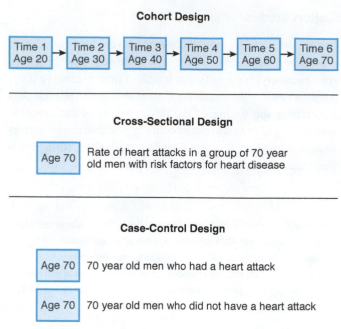

FIGURE 6.2 Cohort, cross-sectional, and case control study designs.

but is similar to the case group in other factors (control group). For example, a group of athletes with repeated ACL tears may be studied in comparison with a group of athletes without ACL tears. The outcome of interest—repeated ACL tears—has already occurred and the researchers are trying to identify the factors that contributed to these repeated injuries. A group without the tears but of the same gender and age range and who play the same sport would be compared on all factors that are thought to contribute to the risk of tears. Notice that this is the same *problem* as given in the example for a cohort design, "What factors contribute to ACL tears?" The difference is that in a cohort study, the event has not yet occurred, whereas in a case control design, the event has occurred and the group with the event (case group) is compared to a group who has not experienced the event (control group), but is similar to the case group.

For example:

The characteristics of a group of people who have had a stroke are compared with those of a group without stroke. A variety of factors that might contribute risk could be collected from medical records and patient reports. These factors would be analyzed in both groups to determine the possible relation to stroke outcome.

For example:

A group of elders with repeated falls and a similar group of elders who have not experienced falls are studied to determine what contributes to falls.

Cohort and case control designs are commonly used in epidemiological research in which very large groups of subjects may be followed over long periods of time. The Framingham Heart Study began as a study of the health of a cohort of people in 1948 and later included two generations of cohorts.[1]

Cross-Sectional Studies

Some authors refer to a cross-sectional *design* rather than the cross-sectional aspect as a part of a cohort or case control design.[2] In cross-sectional studies, data are collected at one point in time. A group of people with an outcome of interest might all be measured during 1 week or over a longer period but at the time of the presenting problem. For example, all subjects in three outpatient clinics with leg fractures could be measured once. All the data might be collected within a short period. However, each patient is measured only once. Another example: all patients with leg fractures presenting to these clinics between January 1 and December 31 of a given year are measured once. The important factor is that subjects are measured once and at the same point in the disease, injury, or rehabilitation process.

Care must be taken in the design of the research that within a longer data collection period important and relevant changes have not occurred that would seriously affect the outcome of the event. For example, if a new medication administered immediately post-fracture is introduced midway in the data collection period, the outcome of patients taking this newly introduced medication might be different from that of subjects who were measured earlier in the year.

■ The Process of Study Appraisal

As discussed in previous chapters, appraisal is the third step in the five-step evidence based practice (EBP) process. In this chapter you will develop your skills at appraising the literature on prognosis, completing all four parts of appraising the prognostic literature: Part A: Determining Applicability of a Prognostic Study, Part B: Determining Quality of a Prognostic Study Part C: Interpreting Results of a Prognostic Study, and Part D: Summarizing the Clinical Bottom Line of a Prognostic Study. The 10 questions within these parts comprise the checklist in Table 6.3.

Part A: Determining Applicability of a Prognostic Study

You typically have a specific patient in mind when you search the literature. You

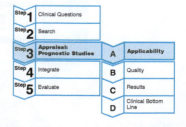

develop a clinical question based on this patient such as, "Will Ms. Smith walk following her stroke?" The type of stroke, Ms. Smith's age, her diabetes, and accessibility to continued therapy will influence her prognosis. For this case, you would search for the studies that are most applicable to Ms. Smith. Alternatively, you may have a more general question about types of patients with similar problems, and you search for common outcomes for these problems. An example question might be, "What determines return to play for female basketball players after an ACL tear?"

Reading the study abstract may give you sufficient information to determine if the subjects were similar enough to your patient or patient group to be useful for clinical decision-making. More subject detail will be included in the Methods section of the paper. Remember, you are not looking for a perfect match of study to patient. You are in search of a valid article that includes subjects that are close enough to your patient to be useful. Refer to Chapter 3 for detail regarding literature applicability.

Part B: Determining Quality of a Prognostic Study

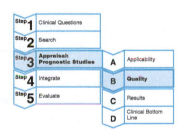

The clinical usefulness of a study of prognosis depends on both the applicability to your patient or patient group and the rigor of the study. Just as with intervention, diagnostic, or any other type of research study, the quality of the study must be appraised before it can be applied in the clinic. There are common aspects of quality for both prognostic and intervention studies. However, there are aspects that are unique to prognostic studies. Consider the following explanatory sections.

Study Sample

QUESTION 1: Is there a defined, representative sample of patients assembled at a common point that is relevant to the study question?

Subjects are not randomly assigned to groups as they would be in a randomized controlled trial (RCT). In prognostic studies, a group is identified that either has the outcome (as in a case control design) or may develop the outcome (as in a cohort design). A sample that sufficiently represents the study event must be identified at a common point. The common point could be relative to the time of an injury; for example, 2 weeks' post-stroke or between 4 and 6 weeks after the onset of acute back pain. Plisky et al[3] studied the association between a balance test and lower extremity injury in a group of high school basketball players. The common point for recruitment and first

measurement for all athletes was the beginning of the athletic season. No subject could join the study after the athletic season began.

The common point that is identified must have relevance to the problem under study. For example, mixing subjects with acute and chronic back pain may confound the prognosis of return to work. Recall that a confounder in an RCT study is a factor other than the treatment under study that could account for the results of the study. Researchers try to control factors other than treatment to increase the chances that the study results are due to the treatment. Another example of a confounder in a study might be that some subjects were recruited 3 months after onset of physical therapy and other subjects were recruited on the first day of therapy. These two groups of subjects would have different treatment experiences, and different outcomes would be expected. Confounders can be controlled by elimination: that is, the study might include only subjects with acute back pain and begin on the first day of treatment. A factor that is thought to potentially affect the study results can be anticipated and planned for in the design as a part of the study; for example, equal numbers of subjects with acute and chronic back pain both at the beginning of treatment and after 3 months of treatment. This creates subgroups within the study that can be statistically analyzed. The number of factors that are hypothesized to affect the outcome will influence both the design of the study and the size of the sample. The more factors that are included, the larger the required sample.

Prognostic studies typically have large samples. The reasons for this depend in part on the multi-factor nature of making prognostic statements. Just like a diagnostic statement, accurate prognostic statements have multiple contributing factors. When many factors affect an outcome, the study must include a sufficient number of subjects and with varying levels of the factors for a valid analysis and prognostic statement. The factors identified as relevant and the common point for recruitment will determine the inclusion and exclusion criteria for the study. For example, if type of work, gender, age, and weight are factors that contribute to acute back pain, then there must be a sufficient number of subjects within specific levels of these categories to determine the impact of each factor or the cluster of factors on the outcome of interest. If age is thought to have an impact, then subjects with a range of ages must be included in the study to determine the prognostic relevance of age. Figure 6.3 depicts age as a factor in back pain (A) and age and gender as factors in back pain (B). As the number of factors increases (e.g., age or gender), the sample size for a study must also increase.

The sample subjects must not already have important aspects of the study outcome. This issue is somewhat clearer when considering a disease. If a study determines that adolescent onset of diabetes is affected by diet during the early years

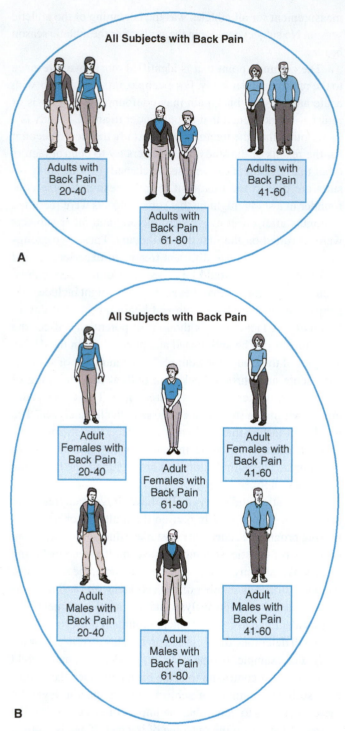

FIGURE 6.3 Multiple factors for back pain here include (A) age and (B) age and gender.

of life, and presence of diabetes by age 15 is the study outcome, then subject participants must be determined to be free of diabetes at the outset of the study. For physical therapy, if a study of low back pain uses the Oswestry Disability Index as the outcome measure, then subject scores on the Oswestry must be determined at the outset of the study.

Outcome Measures and Factors Associated With These Measures

QUESTION 2: Were end points and outcome measures clearly defined?

The systematic and precise measurement points (end points) should be clearly stated in the study. One or more measurement points may be included, but the time points should have relevance to the conditions and course of care. Outcome measures must be both reliable and valid as would be expected for an RCT (Chapter 4; Chapter 10). Reliability should be determined between people who perform measurements within the study that is reported. An outcome measure may have been determined to be reliable in other studies, but this is not sufficient to determine if the people who conducted measures in the reported study could reliably perform the measures in the study sample and under the study conditions. Reliability within and between people is typically expressed by association (correlation) of the values obtained in repeated measurements. Both intra-rater and inter-rater reliability should have high values of association; that is, values should be similar. The type of correlation that is performed depends on the measurement scale that is used, as the scale determines the form of the data. See Chapter 4 for more detail on reliability methods and analysis.

Outcome measures must be explicitly stated, have validity in terms of their relevance to the study question, and should be reliable. The time points for outcome measures should be clear and consistent across subjects. In the Plisky et al study,[3] *lower extremity injury* was the outcome measure. Injury data were systematically collected by coaches and athletic trainers (ATs). Lower extremity injury was operationally defined as " any injury to the limb including the hip, but not the lumbar spine or sacroiliac joint, that resulted from a team-sponsored basketball practice or game that caused restricted participation in the current or next scheduled practice or game" (p 913). Coaches and ATs were trained in systematic data collection, and injury reports were cross-validated among players, coaches, and ATs. The data collection began at the start of the basketball season and ended when the season completed.

QUESTION 3: Are the factors associated with the outcome well justified in terms of the potential for their contribution to prediction of the outcome?

Prognostic studies are studies of association, not studies of causality. An RCT or quasi-experimental design is appropriate to test causal relations. It is tempting to assume that factors that are strongly associated with an outcome actually *cause* the outcome. For example, playing lacrosse may be associated with a type of shoulder injury, but lacrosse does not cause the injuries; it is associated with an increase in this type of injury. Causal factors are factors that might be controlled or eliminated for a patient. You most likely would not recommend that a patient quit playing lacrosse; rather, you would determine the factors of the person and of the sport that contribute to injury. In prognostic studies, factors are identified that are hypothesized to be associated with the outcome of interest. Hypotheses are often derived from previous research and critical clinical observation. Each factor should be justified as being relevant to the study outcome. Many outcomes for our patients have multiple influencing factors. A prognostic study is not likely to include all of the factors that are associated with a particular outcome, but the study should identify the most important factors. The contribution of each factor can be determined with the appropriate statistical analysis. This is detailed later in this chapter in the section "Interpreting Results of a Prognostic Study."

Study Process

QUESTION 4: *Were evaluators masked to reduce bias?*

The members of the research study who conduct the measurements must be objective. This objectivity is best obtained if the "measurers" do not know the study purpose or the group status for the participants they are measuring. Just as with all research, it is not always possible to maintain masking to study purpose, but it is critical that people measuring study outcomes remain masked to as many features of the study and participant characteristics as possible.

QUESTION 5: *Was the study time frame long enough to capture the outcomes of interest?*

Relevant outcomes might take months or even years to determine in a prognostic study. For example, assessing if a group is likely to achieve the goal of independent living following a stroke might take many months and perhaps years to determine. The study must be conducted over a sufficiently long period with a sufficient number of subjects to determine living status. Subject attrition and causes for attrition should be stated. Again, just as in an RCT, a sufficient number of subjects must complete the study to appropriately analyze the study (see Power Analysis in Chapter 3).

If different levels of the International Classification of Function (ICF)[4] are included in the outcome measures, the study should be sufficiently long enough to capture outcomes at all levels. If subject participation in typical life roles is to be determined, the study may include a time point many months or even years after study start.

QUESTION 6: *Was the monitoring process appropriate?*

QUESTION 7: *Were all participants followed to the end of the study?*

Prognostic studies are typically observational studies. The factors that are measured are thought to be important contributors to the prognostic statements that will be derived from the study, but other factors might also influence the study outcomes. Sufficient information should be collected on factors that might influence the outcomes. In the example of the study measuring independent living following stroke, it might be important to monitor medications, compliance in treatment, or interventions added during the study period. These might influence outcome and could be adjusted for later in the statistical analysis.

Part C: Interpreting Results of a Prognostic Study

QUESTION 8: *What statistics were used to determine the prognostic statements? Were the statistics appropriate?*

Measures of association statistics are most appropriate for the analyses of prognostic studies.[2,5,6] Association statistics are based on correlation. Chapter 4 describes correlation statistics that are used in determining intra-rater and inter-rater reliability for various types of data. Here, correlation statistics are applied to the analysis of the association of factors that influence prognostic statements. Common statistics for prognostic research in rehabilitation include correlations, linear and multiple regression, and logistic regression as examples.

In addition to these measures of association, statistics used in epidemiology are used for analysis in prognostics studies. Commonly used statistics are relative risk, expressed as odds ratios, and risk ratios. In medicine, the concept of risk is typically applied to a negative outcome such as the presence of a disease. In physical therapy, these ratios might, for example, assist in understanding the probabilities of an outcome such as "the odds (probability) of being discharged home versus a rehabilitation unit" for a group of patients with specific characteristics following stroke.

Common Statistics in Prognostic Research

Correlation

A correlation is a measure of the extent to which two variables are associated, a measure of how these variables change together. One factor does not necessarily cause the other factor to change but is associated with its change. For example, age does not cause a change in height, but it is associated with a change in height; that is, age and height tend to increase together. The pattern of change or association of the two variables over different levels of the variables can be calculated as a *correlation coefficient* and is represented as *r*. This is a mathematical statement of the extent of association between two variables.

The association *r* varies between -1.0 and +1.0. A value of -1.0 is a negative correlation; as one variable increases, the other variable decreases. For example, a quality of life measure may decrease as a disability measure increases; range of motion decreases as swelling increases. A value of +1.0 is a positive correlation; as one variable increases or decreases, the other variable varies in the same direction; for example, age and height both positively increase in the first year of life; pain may decrease as swelling decreases. The *coefficient of determination* is the square of the correlation coefficient and is expressed in the literature as *r*^{2}. This expresses the percentage of variance that is shared by the two variables. The concept of shared variance is depicted in the Venn diagrams in Figure 6.4, A, B, and C. The shaded, overlapping areas represent the shared variance of (A) gender and incidence of stroke; (B) age and incidence of stroke; and (C) gender, age, and incidence of stroke.

Correlations are evaluated in terms of strength of association and also evaluated in terms of the probability that chance accounts for the value. The strength of correlations as suggested by Munro[5] is expressed in Table 6.1.

Correlations also have an associated probability, or *p*, value. A correlation result may be stated as *r* = .35, *p* < 0.01. The correlation is statistically significant but has low strength. Correlations from large samples may be statistically significant, but have low strength. This is a mathematical contribution from sample size.

Regression

Regression is a statistical analysis that builds on correlation statistics. Regression is used to make *predictions* from one or more variables to an outcome of interest. For example, a

TABLE 6.1 **Strength of Correlation**

r VALUE	STRENGTH
0.00–0.25	Little or no correlation
0.26–0.49	Low
0.50–0.69	Moderate
0.70–0.89	High
0.90–1.0	Very high

From: Munro BH. *Statistical Methods for Health Care Research.* 5th ed. Philadelphia, PA: Lippincott Williams & Wilkins; 2004.

regression analysis to predict falling might include age, visual perception score, a score on a balance test, and a score on a fear of falling questionnaire. The analysis will take into account each of these factors when predicting the likelihood of falling. The results of a regression analysis may be expressed through equations. An *R*^{2} symbol is used to represent the results of a regression. The closer the *R*^{2} is to 1, the better the prediction. The regression equation will have a *p* value, which expresses the amount that chance contributed to the prognostic equation. A significant *p* value does not convey "meaningfulness," and although a regression may be statistically significant, the equation may explain very little of the outcome of interest. Remember that an *R*^{2} value does not indicate a *causal* relationship between the selected variables in the equation and the outcome measure.

Predictive statistics such as regression analyses have errors in the predictions. The results of the analyses are estimates, and you want to know the accuracy of the estimates. Confidence intervals may be included with the regression equation and should be included in your appraisal of the validity of the results. A wide range in the confidence intervals reflects more error in the prediction. See Chapter 4 for a more complete description and interpretation of confidence intervals.

Simple Linear Regression

In simple linear regression, one variable (X) is used to try to predict the level of another variable (Y). The assumption is that the two variables have a linear relationship. The graph in Figure 6.5 relates the velocity of gait to range of motion at the knee. The straight line on the graph is the "best fit" line. This is the straight line that best represents the relation among the *x, y* data points on the graph. Visual inspection of the plotted data suggests that the line does not capture all the scatter of the data. Inspecting the scatter of the data (scatter plot), not just the best fit line, assists in interpreting the data. Each data point is a measured distance from the regression line and is termed the *residual*. With small residuals, the data fit closer to the straight line and better describe the prediction of y from x.

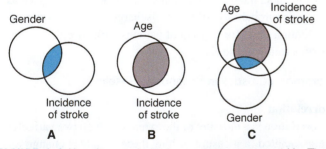

FIGURE 6.4 Venn diagrams depict the associations among variables. The shaded, overlapping areas represent the shared variance of (A) gender and incidence of stroke; (B) age and incidence of stroke; and (C) gender, age, and incidence of stroke.

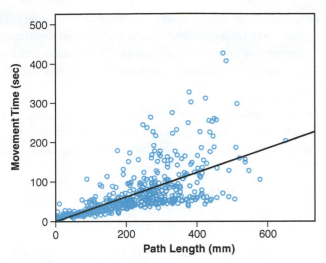

FIGURE 6.5 Plot of a linear regression of path length and movement time for a reach.

A linear regression equation with (X) as the predictor of outcome (Y) is expressed:

$$Y = a + bX$$

Where

Y = outcome
a = intercept of the regression line at Y; this is the value of Y when X is zero
b = is the slope of the line

Multiple Regression

Outcomes of interest to patients and physical therapists are typically associated with more than one variable. Predictions with multiple contributing variables are accomplished with the use of multiple regression techniques. The conceptual idea of shared variance of multiple contributing factors is represented in the Venn diagram in Figure 6.4, in the overlap of age and gender. This is a diagram of multiple correlations. If you are trying to predict incidence of stroke, then age and gender might be used in a prediction equation (regression equation).

Following is a typical regression equation using four predictor variables. The four variables together are used to predict (Y), the outcome of interest.

$$Y = a + b_1X_1 + b_2X_2 + b_3X_3 + b_4X_4$$

Where

Y = outcome
a = a single intercept of the regression line at Y
b = beta-weights for each predictor variable

Each variable contributes some amount to the outcome measure. This amount is expressed through a weighting process. The relations among variables may be linear or nonlinear, but in a multiple regression more than one variable is considered as contributing to the outcome of interest.

Logistic Regression

Multiple regression is typically used when the outcome measure is continuous, even though some of the predictor variables used in the equations are categorical. Examples of continuous outcome measures are scores on various standardized scales, range of motion, or distance walked in 6 minutes. When the outcome measure of interest is categorical, typically dichotomous (two categories) logistic regression is used. Physical therapists might be interested in the dichotomous outcomes that relate to their patients such as "discharge home versus discharge to a nursing home" or "community ambulator versus not a community ambulator." Dichotomous outcomes can be derived from continuous scales after systematically defining the outcome measure as "present or absent." For example, the distanced walked by a patient can be measured using a continuous scale such as feet or miles. These data can then be translated into two categories, patients who can walk a certain distance are considered community ambulators, and those who cannot achieve this distance are not community ambulators. Care must be taken when defining the criterion or criteria that divide groups. Various "cut points" can be used to investigate the most meaningful definitions.

Application of Regression Analysis

Figure 6.6 includes an abstract that describes a prognostic study to estimate the likelihood of falling for older adults with specific characteristics.[7] Characteristics ("factors") that were significantly correlated with falling were used to develop a logistic regression equation. The final equation was used to predict fall/no fall (logistic regression) and included two factors, the score on the Berg Balance Scale and a history of imbalance. In the results, the authors state, "this model, for example, would predict that an individual with no history of imbalance (coded as 0) and a score of 54 on the Berg Balance Scale would have a predicted probability of falling of 5%. In contrast, an individual with a history of imbalance (coded as 1) and a Berg Balance Scale score of 42 would have a predicted probability of falling of 91%."

Part D: Summarizing the Clinical Bottom Line of a Prognostic Study

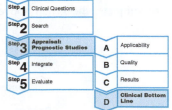

QUESTION 9: Were clinically useful statistics included in the analysis?

Relative Risk

Relative risk ratios (risk ratios and odds ratios) are common statistics used in case control studies.[6] These ratios are used to

Background and Purpose: The objective of this retrospective case-control study was to develop a model for predicting the likelihood of falls among community-dwelling older adults.

Subjects: Forty-four community-dwelling adults (≥65 years of age) with and without a history of falls participated.

Methods: Subjects completed a health status questionnaire and underwent a clinical evaluation of balance and mobility function. Variables that differed between fallers and nonfallers were identified, using *t* tests and cross tabulation with chi-square tests. A forward stepwise regression analysis was carried out to identify a combination of variables that effectively predicted fall status.

Results: Five variables were found to be associated with fall history. These variables were analyzed using logistic regression. The final model combined the score on the Berg Balance Scale with a self-reported history of imbalance to predict fall risk. Sensitivity was 91%, and specificity was 82%.

Conclusion and Discussion: A simple predictive model based on two risk factors can be used by physical therapists to quantify fall risk in community-dwelling older adults. Identification of patients with a high fall risk can lead to an appropriate referral into a fall prevention program. In addition, fall risk can be used to calculate change resulting from intervention.

FIGURE 6.6 Predicting the probability for falls in community-dwelling older adults. Abstract from Shumway, Baldwin, Polissar, et al. Predicting the probability for falls in community-dwelling older adults. *Phys Ther.* 1997:77: 812–819; with permission.

express the odds of the occurrence of a particular outcome between the case group and the control group. Risk and odds ratios are calculated from categorical data cast into a 2×2 table, as in Figure 6.7. The factor that has been identified for association with an outcome measure is plotted against the outcome measure. If the factor and the outcome data are not in a dichotomous form, that is, in two categories, then two categories must be created. The categories created from continuous data such as a test score must be reduced to above or below a certain score. This is the same procedure utilized for diagnostic statistics that are described in detail in Chapter 8.

Risk Ratio

The risk ratio relates the information in the *rows* of the 2×2 table. The following formula is used:

$$\text{Risk ratio} = [a/(a + b)]/[c/(c + d)]$$

From Figure 6.7, the incidence of injury for each group of subjects, the group above the cutoff score and then the group below the cutoff score, are calculated separately. The proportion of subjects below the cutoff score who were injured is compared with the number of subjects below the cutoff score who were injured. These proportions create the risk ratio.

Odds Ratio

The odds ratio relates the information in the *columns* of the 2×2 table. Proportions are not calculated; rather, the data within the table are used directly. Odds ratios are expressed with the following formula:

$$\text{Odds ratio (OR)} = (a/c)/(b/d)$$
$$\text{or}$$
$$OR = ad/bc$$

The difference between the risk ratio and the odds ratio is more obvious if you put values in the 2×2 table in Figure 6.8 and calculate the ratios. There were 34 athletes with lower extremity (LE) injury who also had a positive value on the "risk factor of muscle imbalance." There were 13 athletes with LE injury with a negative "risk factor Z." There were 11 athletes with no LE injury who had a positive "risk factor Z" and 72 athletes without LE injury who had a negative "risk factor Z."

Clinical statements from these ratios:

A. Risk ratio = $[a/(a + b)]/[c/(c + d)]$
"The risk of lower extremity injury for an athlete with a positive risk factor score is five times greater than an athlete without a positive risk factor."

B. Odds ratio = Odds ratio (OR) = $(a/c)/(b/d)$
"The odds of experiencing a lower extremity injury for an athlete with a positive risk score is 17 times greater than the odds of an athlete without a positive risk score experiencing injury."

These statements are clearly similar, although the estimated values are different. Risk ratios are typically calculated with a cohort design study in which the risk status is identified and the cohort is followed to determine who develops the problem. Odds ratios are used with case control studies in which the problem is identified and then risk factors are investigated.

Outcome of Interest

Risk Factor		Positive (yes)	Negative (no)	
	+	a	b	a/a+b
	−	c	d	c/c+d

FIGURE 6.7 A 2×2 table to calculate risk ratio.

Outcome of Interest
(Lower extremity injury)

Risk Factor "muscle imbalance"		Positive (yes)	Negative (no)	
	+	34	11	34/34+11
	−	13	72	13/13+72

FIGURE 6.8 A 2×2 table to calculate risk ratio and odds ratio.

QUESTION 10: *Will this prognostic research make a difference for my recommendations to my patient?*

A prognostic study is helpful to you if it affects the treatment or management decisions for your patient. You must determine if the outcomes are important to your patient and if the factors associated with the outcomes are relevant. In addition, it is important to weigh the magnitude of the predictive statement.

There may be a small but clinically significant prognostic statement from a study or a large and clinically insignificant statement. You and your patient must weigh the value of this literature for clinical decisions.

Some of the most common statistics used in prognostic research are included in Table 6.2. Table 6.3 is a summary of the appraisal questions for prognostic studies.

TABLE 6.2 **Common Statistics for Prognosis**

STATISTIC	DEFINITION	EXPRESSION OF STATISTICAL RESULTS
Correlation	A correlation is a measure of the extent to which two variables are associated; a measure of how these variables change together	r: varies between −1.0 and +1.0 r^2: expresses the percentage of variance that is shared by the two variables; the percentage of the variability within one variable that can be accounted for by the other variable p value: the probability that the coefficient of determination (r^2) occurred by chance; even small correlations might be statistically significant, but this does not mean they are important
Simple linear regression	In simple linear regression, one variable (X) is used to try to *predict* the level of another variable (Y)	r^2: expresses the percentage of variance that is shared by the two variables; one variable can be used to predict the second variable p value: the probability that the coefficient of determination (r^2) occurred by chance Confidence interval (CI): a measure of the accuracy of the prediction; a range of values that includes the possible range of the predicted value; a smaller range indicates a better prediction
Multiple regression	In multiple regression, more than one variable (X, Y . . .) is used to try to *predict* the level of another variable when this variable is continuous	R^2: the correlation among all variables used for prediction and the predicted variable p value: the probability that the R^2 value occurred by chance Confidence interval (CI): a measure of the accuracy of the prediction; a range of values that includes the possible range of the predicted value; a smaller range indicates a better prediction
Logistic regression	In multiple regression, more than one variable (X, Y . . .) is used to try to *predict* the level of another variable when this variable is dichotomous	Same as multiple regression
Risk ratio (RR)	The ratio of the risk in the treated group to the risk in the control group	RR is expressed as numeric values with or without decimals
Odds ratio (OR)	The odds of having an outcome of interest versus the odds of not having the outcome of interest	OR is expressed as numeric values with or without decimals

TABLE 6.3 **Key Questions for Appraising Studies of Prognosis**

QUESTION	YES/NO	WHERE TO FIND THE INFORMATION	COMMENTS AND WHAT TO LOOK FOR
1. Is there a defined, representative sample of patients assembled at a common point that is relevant to the study question?	__ Yes __ No	Methods and Results	The study should report specific details about how the sample of participants was assembled. It is important that participants are at a similar stage in the event of interest (or recovery process) prior to starting the study. Finally, it is important that all participants are measured at study outset on the primary outcome that will be used to detect change in status.
2. Were end points and outcome measures clearly defined?	__ Yes __ No	Methods	The study should describe specific details about how participants' change in status will be measured. Ideally, a standardized outcome measure will be used to determine change in status.
3. Are the factors associated with the outcome well justified in terms of the potential for their contribution to prediction of the outcome?			The factors chosen for association to the outcomes should be justified from previous literature combined with the logic of clinical reasoning in associating the factors with the outcome.
4. Were evaluators blinded to reduce bias?	__ Yes __ No	Methods	Because all outcome measures are subject to bias, when possible, it is ideal for evaluators to be blinded to the primary hypothesis and previous data collected by a given participant.
5. Was the study time frame long enough to capture the outcomes of interest?	__ Yes __ No	Methods and Results	The study should report the anticipated follow-up time in the methods and the actual follow-up time in the results. Ideally, the follow-up time will be sufficient to ensure that the outcome of interest has sufficient time to develop in study participants.
6. Was the monitoring process appropriate?	__ Yes __ No	Methods	The study should report how information was collected over the length of the study. Ideally, the monitoring process results in valid and reliable data and does not cause participants to be substantially different from the general population.
7. Were all participants followed to the end of the study?	__ Yes __ No	Methods and Results	The greater the percentage of participants who have completed a study, the better. Ideally, >80% of participants will have follow-up data and the reason for those without follow-up data will be reported.
8. What statistics were used to determine the prognostic statements? Were the statistics appropriate?	__ Yes __ No	Methods and Results	The statistical analysis should be clearly described and a rationale given for the chosen methods.
9. Were clinically useful statistics included in the analysis?	__ Yes __ No	Methods and Results	Have the authors formed their statistical statement in a way that has an application to your patient?
10. Will this prognostic research make a difference for my recommendations to my patient?	__ Yes __ No	Discussion and Conclusions	How will your recommendations or management of your patient change based on this study?

SUMMARY

The prognostic literature has specific types of designs and statistical analyses. The research designs most typically applied to prognostic questions are observational. These typically include cohort and case control designs. Statistical analyses of prognostic studies are based on measures of association and include correlation, regression, and estimates of relative risk.

Prognostic studies can assist you in making statements about expected outcomes for a patient or patient group and provide estimates of the likelihood of certain outcomes. Just as with all other study types, the clinical usefulness of a study of prognosis depends on both the applicability to your patient and to the rigor of the study.

REVIEW QUESTIONS

1. State your interpretation of the following: correlation coefficient of 0.24 that has a p value of 0.01

2. What is the major difference between a cohort study and case control study?

3. State the difference between a risk ratio and an odds ratio.

REFERENCES

1. Framingham Heart Study. http://www.framinghamheartstudy.org/. Accessed December 26, 2010.
2. Domholdt B. *Physical Therapy Research*. 2nd ed. Philadelphia: Saunders; 2000.
3. Plisky PJ, Rauh MJ, Kaminski TW, et al. Star Excursion Balance Test as a predictor of lower extremity injury in high school basketball players. *J Orthop Sports Phys Ther*. 2006;36:911–919.
4. Stucki G, Ewert T, Cieza A. Value and application of the ICF in rehabilitation medicine. *Disabil Rehabil*. 2003;25:628–634.
5. Munro BH. *Statistical Methods for Health Care Research*. 5th ed. Philadelphia: Lippincott Williams & Wilkins; 2004.
6. Jaeschke R, Guyatt G, Shannon H, et al. Basic statistics for clinicians. 3. Assessing the effects of treatment: measures of association. *CMAJ*. 1995;152:351–357.
7. Shumway-Cook A, Baldwin M, Polissar NL, et al. Predicting the probability for falls in community-dwelling older adults. *Phys Ther*. 1997;77:812–819.

7 Appraising Research Studies of Systematic Reviews

1. Describe the differences between a systematic review and a narrative review.

2. State three differences between systematic reviews and randomized clinical trials.

3. What elements of a systematic review impact applicability to a searchable clinical question?

4. What is the PEDro scale and how can it be used in a systematic review?

5. How are systematic reviews used to inform clinical practice?

CHAPTER-AT-A-GLANCE

This chapter will help you understand the following:

- The difference between systematic and narrative reviews

- The difference between primary and secondary studies

- The nature and value of systematic reviews

- Determining the applicability of a systematic review to your practice

- Appraising the quality of a systematic review

■ Introduction

What is a Systematic Review?

Systematic reviews are a special type of research study characterized as secondary research. **Secondary research studies** are "studies of studies" that summarize information from multiple primary studies. **Primary studies** are "original studies," such as the randomized clinical trials and cohort studies described in previous chapters. Systematic reviews are the principal scientific method for secondary research. Systematic reviews are developed using a documented, systematic approach that minimizes bias.[1] Authors of a systematic review define a specific purpose for the study. Methods that minimize bias are determined prior to the beginning of the study. Unlike a randomized clinical trial, a systematic review does not include recruiting and enrolling participants. Specific inclusion and exclusion criteria are used to select appropriate studies for review. The sample size for a systematic review is the number of studies identified that meet the specific criteria.

Systematic reviews of treatment interventions are most common; however, reviews can also appraise diagnostic tests, outcome measures, and prognostic factors. For example, Dessaur and Magarey[2] conducted a systematic review of diagnostic studies to determine the diagnostic accuracy of clinical tests for superior labral anterior-posterior lesions in the shoulder. In another example, Blum and Korner-Bitensky[3] conducted a systematic review of studies of the Berg Balance Scale to better understand its usefulness in stroke rehabilitation. In

this chapter, we focus on systematic reviews of intervention studies; however, the same principles and appraisal processes can be applied to other types of systematic reviews (Fig. 7.1).

A **meta-analysis** is a statistical method used to summarize outcomes across multiple primary studies, usually as a part of a systematic review. The sample size of a meta-analysis is considered the total number of participants from all studies combined. Not all systematic reviews contain a meta-analysis. This analysis depends on the nature of the data included in the selected primary studies. In a meta-analysis, data are "normalized" across studies and the results are expressed as a quantitative value representing all included studies (e.g., effect size; see Chapter 4).

Narrative reviews provide an overview of literature and are commonly published in peer-reviewed research journals. These reports are sometimes confused with systematic reviews. A narrative review is not a systematic study and analysis of the literature.[4,5] Rather, it is a description of the content of articles selected by an expert with the review expressing the expert's perspective. As such, narrative reviews are subject to the bias associated with personal opinion. Narrative reviews are a useful resource of expert opinion, but they are not research. Hence, narrative reviews are represented at the lowest level of the research evidence pyramid, whereas systematic reviews are at the top of the pyramid. Clinical expertise is, however, one of the three pillars of evidence based practice (EBP). A narrative review is useful as an expression of clinical expertise. Table 7.1 includes a comparison of the methods and results typically included in systematic and narrative reviews.

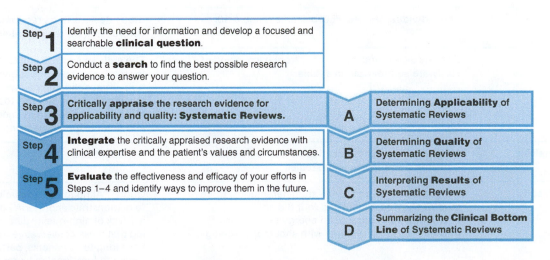

Step 1 Identify the need for information and develop a focused and searchable **clinical question**.

Step 2 Conduct a **search** to find the best possible research evidence to answer your question.

Step 3 Critically **appraise** the research evidence for applicability and quality: **Systematic Reviews**.

A Determining **Applicability** of Systematic Reviews

Step 4 **Integrate** the critically appraised research evidence with clinical expertise and the patient's values and circumstances.

B Determining **Quality** of Systematic Reviews

Step 5 **Evaluate** the effectiveness and efficacy of your efforts in Steps 1–4 and identify ways to improve them in the future.

C Interpreting **Results** of Systematic Reviews

D Summarizing the **Clinical Bottom Line** of Systematic Reviews

FIGURE 7.1 This illustration focuses on appraising a research systematic review.

TABLE 7.1   **Comparing the Design of a Typical Systematic Review and a Narrative Review**

	SYSTEMATIC REVIEW[4]	NARRATIVE REVIEW[5]
Type of review and citation	Alexander LD, Gilman DRD, Brown DR, Brown JL, Houghton PE. Exposure to low amounts of ultrasound energy does not improve soft tissue shoulder pathology: a systematic review. *Phys Ther.* 2010;90:14–25.	Valen PA, Foxworth J. Evidence supporting the use of physical modalities in the treatment of upper extremity musculoskeletal conditions. *Current Opinion in Rheumatology.* 2010;22:194–204.
INTRODUCTION		
Purpose	"The purposes of this study were to identify relevant randomized clinical trials (RCTs) and to evaluate ultrasound treatment protocols to determine whether certain ultrasound treatment parameters were associated with improvements in soft tissue shoulder impairments or function."	"To evaluate recent trials and reviews of physical modalities and conservative treatments for selected upper extremity musculoskeletal conditions for evidence supporting their use."
METHODS		
Literature search	Five electronic databases were searched (database names and years searched are provided). Search terms are provided.	Not reported
Inclusion and exclusion criteria	Detailed criteria are provided describing the nature of primary studies included and excluded from the review.	Not reported
Quality assessment	Three reviewers independently assessed each study using the Physiotherapy Evidence Database (PEDro) scale.	Not reported
Data extraction	A description of how ultrasound parameters were characterized is provided.	Not reported
RESULTS/FINDINGS		
Studies reviewed	The initial search identified 727 studies. Eight studies met the pre-established inclusion and exclusion criteria. Reasons are provided for studies that were excluded.	A total of 120 references are cited. Two studies are cited relating to the shoulder and ultrasound therapy.
Study quality	The individual studies' PEDro scores range 4–10.	Study designs (e.g., randomized controlled trial) are described.
Interventions and outcome measures assessed	Specific ultrasound parameters from each included study are summarized in a table.	The authors address eight interventions for rotator cuff tendinopathy: acupuncture, ultrasound, microwave diathermy, low-energy laser therapy, topical nitroglycerine, corticosteroid injections, tape, and manual therapy, among others.
Statistical analysis	Meta-analysis was not conducted due to inconsistent outcome measures among studies.	Not applicable
Qualitative result	For patients with soft tissue shoulder injuries, three studies showed benefit and four did not. Low amounts of ultrasound energy did not result in improvements for patients with shoulder pathology.	Quote: "Although most studies are able to demonstrate short-term benefits, there is a lack of high-quality data demonstrating that these conservative treatments have long-term benefits, particularly with regard to functional outcomes."
HOW THIS ARTICLE CONTRIBUTES TO CLINICAL PRACTICE		
	A secondary research study that provides a minimally biased analysis of primary literature on the topic of ultrasound for patients with shoulder pathology.	A summary of selected articles illustrating the author's opinion from the literature regarding modalities for patients with upper extremity conditions.

■ SELF-TEST 7.1 Differentiating

Use the abstracts in Table 7.2 to practice differentiating between systematic and narrative reviews.

Patient Case: James Green is a 42-year-old driver for a shipping company. He experienced a lumbar strain while lifting heavy boxes at work. He has improved as a result of your physical therapy intervention and feels ready to return to work. In preparation for discharge, you would like to prescribe a preventive therapeutic exercise program for Mr. Green. However, Mr. Green reports that he has tried starting an exercise program in the past and found that "I just ended up getting hurt." Mr. Green is skeptical about the value of a therapeutic exercise program. You plan to review the best available research evidence with him and arrive at a shared, informed decision about exercise after discharge from physical therapy.

Searchable Clinical Question:

"For a 42-year-old male with history of a low back injury, are therapeutic exercise programs effective for preventing injury recurrence?"

Search: The Systematic Reviews section of the Clinical Queries feature in PubMed[6] was used to identify the following articles that might be applicable to the clinical question.

Activity: Read the abstracts in Table 7.2, and discriminate between systematic reviews and narrative reviews.

Why Are Systematic Reviews at the Top of the Evidence Pyramid?

Systematic reviews are at the top of the Evidence Pyramid because they overcome many of the limitations of individual studies. A single research study rarely provides a definitive answer to a clinical or research question because it represents only one sample from the population. This is particularly true in rehabilitation literature because sample sizes are typically small. A high-quality systematic review combines all of the high-quality studies published on a given topic into one study. Systematic reviews provide a more comprehensive analysis and summary of the research available on a given topic than can be obtained from primary research studies.

Systematic reviews also save time for the evidence based therapist. The number of articles published in peer-reviewed journals increases every year (Fig 7.2). It is unrealistic to expect to read and appraise all of the literature on the broad range of clinical questions encountered in your practice. Systematic reviews provide important literature for addressing this challenge.

In a systematic review, Choi et al[9] identified over 2000 potentially relevant articles that addressed the clinical question in Self-Test 7.1. Through a documented and systematic process, those 2000 articles were narrowed to 13 articles, all of which had high applicability to the specific question and rigorous research quality. The authors applied meta-analytic statistics to four of the studies to quantitatively express the effectiveness of post-treatment exercise programs. By combining four separate primary studies with a total of 407

TABLE 7.2 Abstracts for Self-Test 7.1

	CHECK THE CORRECT BOX
Abstract 7-1	☐ Systematic
	☐ Narrative
Introduction: Low back pain (LBP) is one of the most costly conditions to manage in occupational health. Individuals with chronic or recurring LBP experience difficulties returning to work due to disability. Given the personal and financial cost of LBP, there is a need for effective interventions aimed at preventing LBP in the workplace. The aim of this systematic review was to examine the effectiveness of exercises in decreasing LBP incidence, LBP intensity, and the impact of LBP and disability.	
Methods: A comprehensive literature search of controlled trials published between 1978 and 2007 was conducted, and 15 studies were subsequently reviewed and analyzed.	
Results: There was strong evidence that exercise was effective in reducing the severity and activity interference from LBP. However, due to the poor methodological quality of studies and conflicting results, there was only limited evidence supporting the use of exercise to prevent LBP episodes in the workplace. Other methodological limitations, such as differing combinations of exercise, study populations, participant presentation, workloads, and outcome measures; levels of exercise adherence and a lack of reporting on effect sizes, adverse effects, and types of sub-groups, make it difficult to draw definitive conclusions on the efficacy of workplace exercise in preventing LBP.	
Conclusions: Only 2 out of the 15 studies reviewed were high in methodological quality and showed significant reductions in LBP intensity with exercise. Future research is needed to clarify which exercises are effective and the dose-response relationships regarding exercise and outcomes.	

From: Bell JA, Bornett A. Exercise for the primary, secondary and tertiary prevention of low back pain in the workplace: a systematic review. *J Occup Rehabil.* 2009;19(1):8-24 with permission.

Continued

TABLE 7.2 **Abstracts for Self-Test 7.1—cont'd**

	CHECK THE CORRECT BOX

Abstract 7-2

☐ Systematic
☐ Narrative

We reviewed the literature to clarify the effects of exercise in preventing and treating nonspecific low back pain. We evaluated several characteristics of exercise programs including specificity, individual tailoring, supervision, motivation enhancement, volume, and intensity. The results show that exercise is effective in the primary and secondary prevention of low back pain. When used for curative treatment, exercise diminishes disability and pain severity while improving fitness and occupational status in patients who have subacute, recurrent, or chronic low back pain. Patients with acute low back pain are usually advised to continue their everyday activities to the greatest extent possible rather than to start an exercise program. Supervision is crucial to the efficacy of exercise programs. Whether general or specific exercises are preferable is unclear, and neither is there clear evidence that one-on-one sessions are superior to group sessions. Further studies are needed to determine which patient subsets respond to specific characteristics of exercise programs and which exercise volumes and intensities are optimal.

From: Henchoz Y, So AKL. Exercise and nonspecific low back pain: A literature review. *Joint Bone Spine.* 2008;75:533-539. with permission.

Abstract 7-3

☐ Systematic
☐ Narrative

Background: Back pain is a common disorder that has a tendency to recur. It is unclear if exercises, either as part of treatment or as a post-treatment program, can reduce back pain recurrences.

Objectives: To investigate the effectiveness of exercises for preventing new episodes of low back pain or low back pain–associated disability.

Search Strategy: We searched CENTRAL (The Cochrane Library 2009, issue 3), MEDLINE, EMBASE, and CINAHL up to July 2009.

Selection Criteria: Inclusion criteria were: participants who had experienced back pain before, an intervention that consisted of exercises without additional specific treatment, and outcomes that measured recurrence of back pain or time to recurrence.

Data Collection and Analysis: Two review authors independently judged if references met the inclusion criteria. The same review authors independently extracted data and judged the risk of bias of the studies. Studies were divided into post-treatment intervention programs and treatment studies. Study results were pooled with meta-analyses if participants, interventions, controls, and outcomes were judged to be sufficiently homogenous.

Main Results: We included 13 articles reporting on nine studies with nine interventions. Four studies with 407 participants evaluated post-treatment programs, and five studies with 1113 participants evaluated exercise as a treatment modality. Four studies had a low risk of bias, one study a high risk, and the remainder an unclear risk of bias. We found moderate quality evidence that post-treatment exercises were more effective than no intervention for reducing the rate of recurrences at one year (Rate Ratio 0.50; 95% Confidence Interval 0.34 to 0.73). There was moderate quality evidence that the number of recurrences was significantly reduced in two studies (Mean Difference −0.35; 95% CI −0.60 to −0.10) at one-half to two years follow-up. There was very low quality evidence that the days on sick leave were reduced by post-treatment exercises (Mean Difference −4.37; 95% CI −7.74 to −0.99) at one-half to two years follow-up. We found conflicting evidence for the effectiveness of exercise treatment in reducing the number of recurrences or the recurrence rate.

Author's Conclusions: There is moderate quality evidence that post-treatment exercise programs can prevent recurrences of back pain but conflicting evidence was found for treatment exercise. Studies into the validity of measurement of recurrences and the effectiveness of post-treatment exercise are needed.

From: Choi BKL, Verbeek JH, Tam WWS, Jiang JY. Exercises for prevention of recurrences of low-back pain. *Cochrane Database Syst Rev.* 2010 with permission.

Abstract 7-4

☐ Systematic
☐ Narrative

The principle of core stability has gained wide acceptance in training for the prevention of injury and as a treatment modality for rehabilitation of various musculoskeletal conditions in particular of the lower back. There has been surprisingly little criticism of this approach up to date. This article re-examines the original findings and the principles of core stability/spinal stabilization approaches and how well they fare within the wider knowledge of motor control, prevention of injury, and rehabilitation of neuromuscular and musculoskeletal systems following injury.

From: Lederman E. The myth of core stability. *J Body Mov Ther.* 2010;14(1):84-98 with permission.

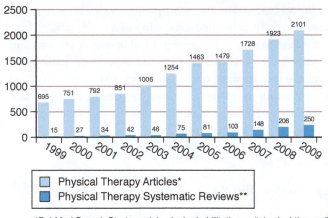

*PubMed Search Strategy: (physical rehabilitation or "physical therapy" treatment or physiotherapy) and ("YYYY"[PDAT]))

**PubMed Search Strategy: (physical rehabilitation or "physical therapy" treatment or physiotherapy) and ("YYYY"[PDAT]) and "systematic review"

FIGURE 7.2 The number of primary articles and systematic reviews in PubMed that include physical therapy over a 10-year period.

participants we learn that injury recurrence decreased by 50% following a post-treatment exercise program for patients with low back pain. If we determine the review to be of high quality, it provides an efficient resource to guide our care for Mr. Green.

Appraising Systematic Reviews

How do You Determine if a Systematic Review is of Sufficient Quality to Inform Clinical Decisions?

The next two sections of this chapter detail the appraisal process for systematic reviews. Just as with intervention, diagnostic, or any other type of research study, the quality of the study must be appraised before it can be appropriately applied in the clinic. The sections that follow are organized into parts A through D to consider when appraising quality of a systematic review. The 12 questions within these parts form the checklist in Table 7.6.

Part A: Determining Applicability of a Systematic Review

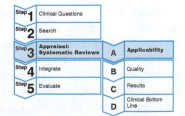

Determining the applicability of a systematic review to your clinical question is similar to the process used for other study types. The questions

about applicability presented in Chapter 3 have been modified for appraising systematic reviews.

*QUESTION 1: **Is the study's purpose relevant to my clinical question?***

As with other study types that we have reviewed, systematic reviews should provide a specific purpose, usually stated at the end of the Introduction. Because a systematic review is intended to appraise a body of literature, the purpose is likely to be broader than your clinical question. You may find that several clinical questions are addressed within one systematic review.

*QUESTION 2: **Are the inclusion and exclusion criteria clearly defined, and are studies that would answer my clinical question likely to be included?***

Systematic reviews should provide specific inclusion and exclusion criteria for studies (not patients) to be considered for the review. It is important to appraise the appropriateness of the criteria used to select studies in the context of your question. Review the inclusion and exclusion criteria to determine if studies that address your patient characteristics and intervention of interest are included in the review. Also consider the study types included in the review. For example, a systematic review of constraint-induced movement therapy (CIMT) for children with hemiplegia due to cerebral palsy[11] included only the three randomized clinical trial (RCT) studies on this topic. Recommendations were weakly supportive of CIMT for children and gave recommendations for future studies. A systematic review by Huang et al[12] included all studies on this topic regardless of design type. This review gave stronger recommendations for CIMT and also gave recommendations for clinical application. You would need to appraise each review to determine which is more appropriate to guide your clinical practice regarding CIMT.

*QUESTION 3: **Are the types of interventions investigated relevant to my clinical question?***

Because primary research studies investigate a broad variety of interventions, authors of a systematic review should clearly identify the specific interventions included in the systematic review. Assess if the included interventions are relevant to your clinical question and clinical practice. A systematic review could assist you in developing a treatment strategy that you have not used before, or it could provide evidence to support interventions that are already a part of your clinical practice.

QUESTION 4: Are the outcome measures relevant to my clinical question?

Consider if the systematic review addresses your outcome of interest (e.g., return to work, walking endurance, shoulder range of motion). The methods section should provide information about the outcome measures included in the review. Ultimately, however, the outcome measures assessed are dependent on the measures provided by the primary studies included in the review. A common challenge for authors conducting a systematic review is to draw conclusions from the diversity of outcome measures often used across primary studies.

QUESTION 5: Is the study population sufficiently similar to my patient to justify the expectation that my patient would respond similarly to the population?

The authors should provide a summary of the demographics of the participants in the primary studies included in the systematic review. Consider differences and similarities between the sample population and your patient. The study sample might be close enough, even if it does not exactly match your patient. Often the population will be broad (e.g., large age range, multiple diagnoses, different severities of disease). Use your clinical expertise to determine the relation of the information to your patient.

Part B: Determining Quality of a Systematic Review

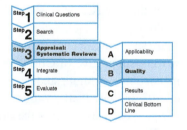

The clinical usefulness of a systematic review is dependent on its applicability to the clinical case and to the rigor (quality) with which the study is conducted. To determine the quality of a systematic review, we appraise many of the same general concepts presented in Chapters 3 and 4. However, there are aspects of quality that are unique to systematic reviews.[1,13] The gold standard method for conducting systematic reviews has been developed and maintained by the Cochrane Collaboration. Digging Deeper 8.1 describes this influential group.

Study Sample

QUESTION 6: Was the literature search comprehensive?

Once a specific purpose has been defined for a systematic review, the next step is for the authors to conduct a comprehensive literature search to identify all articles that may be associated with the topic. You should consider several aspects of the search to determine if it was comprehensive.

- **Did the authors use appropriate search terms to search for articles about the topic of interest?**

  Ideally, a systematic review should provide a detailed list of the terms and search strategies used to conduct the literature search. As you gain skills in searching you will be able to appraise the effectiveness of the authors' strategy. Table 7.3 illustrates the search strategy reported in a systematic review provided by Alexander et al[4] (from Table 7.1).

- **Was a comprehensive number of appropriate databases used?**

  The objective of the search methods described in Chapter 2 was to find the best available research to answer a clinical question. Authors of a systematic review attempt to find all of the available literature on a topic. Given this objective, a systematic review should describe numerous (usually three to seven) databases used to conduct the literature search. Chapter 2

 DIGGING DEEPER 7.1

The Cochrane Collaboration

The Cochrane Collaboration, founded by Archie Cochrane, a British medical researcher and epidemiologist, was formally launched in 1993.[14] The Cochrane Collaboration consists of groups of expert clinicians and scientists that conduct systematic reviews of health-care interventions. The collaboration has been an international leader in establishing methods for conducting systematic reviews. According to its Web site (www.cochrane. org), "Cochrane Reviews are intended to help providers, practitioners and patients make informed decisions about health care. . . ."[14] Within the community of evidence based practitioners, methods established by the Cochrane Collaboration are regarded as a gold standard for the development of systematic reviews.

When searching for the best available evidence, Cochrane Systematic Reviews should be a first stop for high-quality evidence. However, you will find that many Cochrane Reviews of physical therapy interventions report that there is "insufficient evidence" to draw conclusions in support of or against the intervention. Many physical therapy interventions have few studies that meet the rigorous criteria required to be included in a Cochrane Review. This limitation is shrinking as the physical therapy body of literature expands.

TABLE 7.3 **Search Terms Used to Identify Potentially Relevant Studies from Alexander LD, Gilman DRD, Brown DR, Brown JL, et al. Exposure to low amounts of ultrasound energy does not improve soft tissue shoulder pathology: a systematic review. *Phys Ther.* 2010;90:14–25; with permission.**

PART	SEARCH TERMS
A	Ultrasound OR physical therapy OR physiotherapy OR rehabilitation OR pulsed ultrasound OR ultrasonic therapy OR continuous ultrasound OR therapeutic ultrasound OR sonic therapy OR high-frequency sound waves OR MHz OR kHz OR sound wave OR cavitation OR acoustic microstreaming
B	Shoulder tendonitis OR shoulder tendinitis OR shoulder tendinopathy OR shoulder tendinosis OR shoulder strain OR rotator cuff pathology OR rotator cuff tear OR rotator cuff injury OR rotator cuff strain OR rotator cuff tendonitis OR rotator cuff tendinitis OR rotator cuff tendinosis OR shoulder bursitis OR subdeltoid bursitis OR subacromial bursitis OR rotator cuff impingement OR supraspinatus impingement OR shoulder impingement OR calcific tendonitis OR calcific tendinitis OR acromioclavicular sprain OR coracoclavicular sprain OR rotator cuff rupture OR frozen shoulder OR adhesive capsulitis OR biceps tendonitis OR biceps tendinitis OR biceps tendinosis OR bicipital tendonitis OR bicipital tendinitis OR bicipital tendinopathy OR infraspinatus tear OR supraspinatus tear OR infraspinatus tendonitis OR infraspinatus tendinitis OR infraspinatus tendinosis OR infraspinatus tendinopathy OR bicipital strain OR biceps strain OR supraspinatus strain OR infraspinatus strain

TABLE 7.4 **Databases Commonly Used to Conduct Systematic Reviews in Physical Therapy**

TYPE	DATABASE NAME AND COMPANY/ORGANIZATION
General databases	PubMed, U.S. Government National Library of Medicine Ovid, Ovid Technologies EMBASE (Excerpta Medica Database), Elsevier B.V. Cochrane Central Register of Controlled Trials, Cochrane Collaboration
Special collections	CINAHL (Cumulative Index to Nursing and Allied Health Literature), EBSCO Industries Sports Discus, EBSCO Industries AMED (Allied and Complementary Medicine), British Library PEDro (Physiotherapy Evidence Database), Centre of Evidence-Based Physiotherapy

emphasizes freely available databases (e.g., MEDLINE via PubMed; TRIP database; and PEDro). Table 7.4 illustrates a list (not exhaustive) of databases commonly used in systematic reviews of physical therapy literature.

■ **Were articles from a wide range of languages included in the literature review?**

Although the English language is predominant in physical therapy literature, it not the only language used for publication. Including articles in multiple languages may require the resources of a translator; as a consequence, language inclusion is commonly limited in systematic reviews. **Language bias** results when important study results are excluded from a systematic review because of language.

■ **Were efforts made to identify unpublished data relevant to the topic?**

Authors of systematic reviews should make an effort to identify studies about the topic of interest that were conducted but have not been published. **Publication bias** is the tendency for studies with positive results to be published more often than studies with nonsignificant results. Clinical trial registries list clinical trials at their initiation and provide a method to monitor studies that are conducted but the results not yet published. Unpublished data are usually obtained by personally contacting the researcher who conducted the study.

Primary Study Appraisal

QUESTION 7: Was an objective, reproducible, and reliable method used to judge the quality of the studies in the systematic review?

Once the authors have identified studies that meet the pre-established inclusion and exclusion criteria, each primary research article included in the systematic review should be systematically appraised for quality. Ideally, two or more independent reviewers use a standardized study appraisal tool. Each reviewer conducts the appraisal independently and without knowledge of the other reviewer's appraisal. After the appraisals are complete, discrepancies are addressed by discussion between the reviewers and, if needed, a third reviewer is consulted to resolve the discrepancy. Ideally, the authors should use a study appraisal tool with established reliability and validity in addition to reporting their own raters' reliability.

There are several standardized appraisal tools used for appraisal. These tools assign a corresponding score for quality. The most commonly used tool in the physical therapy literature is the Physiotherapy Evidence Database (PEDro) scale.[15] The PEDro scale ranges from 0 to 10, with 10 representing the highest score for quality. Figure 7.3 illustrates the PEDro scale

and the use of the scale to appraise the quality of primary studies included in a systematic review.

Data Reduction and Analysis

QUESTION 8: *Was a standardized method used to extract data from studies included in the systematic review?*

Extraction of data from each primary study must be done carefully to prevent errors and omissions. For some studies, the authors of the primary studies must be contacted to obtain details beyond those in the published paper. Systematic reviews should provide an explicit description of data extraction. For

A.   PEDro scale

	no	yes
1. eligibility criteria were specified	☐	☐
2. subjects were randomly allocated to groups in a crossover study, subjects were randomly allocated in order in which treatments were received	☐	☐
3. allocation was concealed	☐	☐
4. the groups were similar at baseline regarding the most important prognostic indicators	☐	☐
5. there was blinding of all subjects	☐	☐
6. there was blinding of all therapists who administered the therapy	☐	☐
7. there was blinding of all assessors who measured at least one key outcome	☐	☐
8. measures of at least one key outcome were obtained from more than 85% of the subjects initially allocated to the groups	☐	☐
9. all subjects for when outcome measures were available received the treatment or control condition as allocated or, where this was not the case, data for at least one key outcome were analysed by "intention to treat"	☐	·yes ☐
10. the results of between-group statistical comparisons are reported for at least one key outcome	☐	☐
11. the study provides both point measure and measures of variability for at least one key outcome	☐	☐

B.   Table 1. Breakdown of PEDro scores.

Author	2	3	4	5	6	7	8	9	10	11	PEDro scores
González-Iglesias et al[18]	Y	Y	Y	Y	N	Y	Y	Y	Y	Y	9
González-Iglesias et al[17]	Y	Y	Y	Y	N	Y	Y	Y	Y	Y	9
Bergman et al[4]	Y	Y	Y	N	N	Y	Y	Y	Y	Y	8
Cleland et al[13]	Y	Y	Y	N	N	Y	Y	Y	Y	Y	8
Cleland et al[10]	Y	Y	Y	N	N	Y	Y	Y	Y	Y	8
Cleland et al[6]	Y	Y	Y	N	N	Y	Y	Y	Y	Y	8
Fernández-de-las-Peñas et al[16]	Y	Y	Y	N	N	Y	Y	Y	Y	Y	8
Fernández-de-las-Peñas et al[14]	Y	N	Y	N	N	N	Y	Y	Y	Y	6
Krauss et al[19]	Y	Y	Y	N	N	Y	N	N	Y	Y	6
Winters et al[46]	Y	Y	N	N	N	Y	N	Y	Y	Y	6
Savolainen et al[21]	Y	N	N	N	N	Y	Y	N	Y	Y	5
Parkin-Smith and Penter[47]	Y	N	Y	N	N	N	N	N	Y	Y	4
Strunk and Hondras[22]	Y	Y	N	N	N	N	Y	Y	N	N	4
Total "yes" scores and percentage (%) of "yes" scores in each criterion	**13 (100)**	**10 (77)**	**10 (77)**	**2 (15)**	**0 (0)**	**10 (77)**	**10 (77)**	**10 (77)**	**12 (92)**	**12 (92)**	

Y = Criterion was satisfied; N = Criterion was not satisfied

FIGURE 7.3 A. The 11-item PEDro scale (www.pedro.org.au; upper half) is one tool used to appraise validity of primary studies in systematic reviews. Item 1 does not contribute to the final 10-point PEDro score. B. Performance on the scale for 13 studies in Walser et al's systematic review, "The Effectiveness of Thoracic Spine Manipulation for the Management Of musculoskeletal conditions." *From: Walser RF, Meserve BB, Boucher TR. The effectiveness of thoracic spine manipulation for the management of musculoskeletal conditions: a systematic review and meta-analysis of randomized clinical trials. J Man Manip Ther. 2009;17:237–246, Table 1; with permission.*

example, the review by Alexander et al[4] provides specific details of the extraction procedures used for the ultrasound parameters from eight primary studies.

QUESTION 9: *Was clinical heterogeneity assessed to determine whether a meta-analysis was justified?*

One of the most challenging elements of a systematic review, particularly in physical therapy literature, is determining if the data from multiple studies can be combined in a meta-analysis.[16] A meta-analysis is useful because it allows data from several studies to be combined. However, to produce valid results, combined studies must be similar in study population, intervention, and outcome measures. When authors conduct a qualitative analysis of these variables among the included studies, it is called an assessment of clinical heterogeneity. Meta-analyses should only be used to pool study results when the studies can be justified as having clinical homogeneity in patient characteristics, interventions, and outcomes.

In the systematic review of motor control exercises for patients with nonspecific low back pain by Macedo et al,[17] 14 RCTs met the inclusion and exclusion criteria. However, those studies varied widely with regard to the interventions studied and the outcomes measured. Therefore, several different meta-analyses were conducted on subsets of studies within the systematic review. For example, seven studies were included in a meta-analyses contrasting motor control exercise with minimal intervention. Among those studies, three studies were pooled to assess the impact of motor control exercises on short-term (<3 mo) pain relief. A fourth study was added to the meta-analysis to assess the impact of disability on intermediate-term (>3 and <12 mo) disability. You should appraise the process used for qualitative analysis of heterogeneity prior to pooling data for meta-analyses.

QUESTION 10: *If a meta-analysis was conducted, was statistical heterogeneity assessed?*

When a meta-analysis is conducted it should be paired with a test of statistical heterogeneity (also called a test of statistical homogeneity). Tests of statistical heterogeneity assess the likelihood that the variability between studies is due to chance. If the result indicates that differences are unlikely to be due to chance (i.e., $p < 0.05$), the meta-analysis result is called into question and the authors are expected to explore explanations for the differences by further analyzing subgroups of studies.

Different statistical methods are used for meta-analysis depending on the result of heterogeneity testing. For example, in the systematic review by Macedo et al,[17] groups of studies with a positive test for heterogeneity were analyzed differently compared with those with a negative test. If the statistical

TABLE 7.5	Statistical Tests Used to Assess Heterogeneity and Their Symbols
NAME	**SYMBOL**
Between study variance	τ^2
Cochran's Q	χ^2
Index of variability	I^2

heterogeneity test is positive, a random effects model might be used for the meta-analysis. If the statistical heterogeneity test is negative, a fixed effects model may be more appropriate. As a consumer of systematic reviews, it is important for you to recognize whether or not a test of statistical heterogeneity was conducted. Statistical tests commonly used to assess heterogeneity are described in Table 7.5.[1] Interpretation of these tests (beyond their presence or absence) is complex, controversial, and exceeds the scope of this text. For more information we recommend the text by Egger et al.[1]

Part C: Interpreting Results of a Systematic Review Study

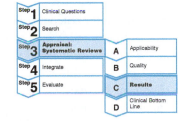

QUESTION 11: *What methods were used to report the results of the systematic review?*

Interpretation of Qualitative Results

At this point in your appraisal, you have already determined if a meta-analysis was conducted as part of the systematic review and if heterogeneity was considered as part of the analysis. If a meta-analysis was not conducted, the systematic review should provide a qualitative summary of the included studies. In addition, a "vote counting" analysis can also be included.[1] Using vote counting, the authors count the number of studies favoring one intervention compared to the number of studies favoring an alternative intervention (or control). Your appraisal of a qualitative summary should include your assessment of the studies given the details provided by the authors. Figure 7.4 illustrates a qualitative summary of the eight studies included in the systematic review by Alexander et al[4] regarding ultrasound therapy and soft tissue shoulder pathology.

Interpretation of Quantitative Results

If a meta-analysis was conducted, the results will include a statistical result that allows multiple studies to be expressed in the

Table 5.
Comparison of Studies in Which Ultrasound Was Reported to Be Beneficial and Studies in Which
No Statistical Difference Was Found Between Treatment and Control Groups

Parameter	Ultrasound Found Beneficial	Ultrasound Found Equivalent to Control
No. of studies	3	5
Total no. of participants	121	465
Energy density, J/cm^2, $\overline{X}$ (range)[a]	768 (432–1,422)	413 (27–900)
Total energy per session, J, X (range)[a]	4,228 (2,250–6,114)	2,019 (181–4,095)
Total exposure, h, $\overline{X}$ (range)[a]	5.3 (1.2–10.3)	1.3 (0.5–2.5)
Total energy over study duration, J, (range)[a]	107,289 (51,840–216,028)	20,394 (1,085–67,500)

"Vote counting" the number of studies that found ultrasound to be equivalent to a control.

[a] Values for studies in which a benefit of ultrasound was seen or in which no benefit was seen in the ultrasound group compared with the control group. Studies were considered "beneficial" when a statistically significant improvement in 1 or more of the chosen outcome measures was reported.

Equations were as follows:
Energy density = spatial average − temporal average × treatment time
Total energy/per session = spatial average − temporal average × transducer head size × treatment time
Total exposure = treatment time per session × number of sessions
Total energy over study duration = total energy per session × number of sessions

The treatment area sizes were considered to be the same for all of the studies because only the shoulder area was included in these studies.

FIGURE 7.4 A table summarizing the characteristics of studies in the systematic review that did and did not demonstrate benefit from ultrasound. *From: Alexander LD, Gilman DRD, Brown DR, et al. Exposure to low amounts of ultrasound energy does not improve soft tissue shoulder pathology: a systematic review. Phys Ther. 2010;90:14–25; with permission.*

same units. If the outcome of interest is dichotomous, relative risks and odds ratios can be used to represent each study and the results compared. If the outcome of interest is continuous, the mean difference or effect size (weighted mean difference) between treatment and control groups is most commonly reported.[1]

Forest plots are a graphical representation of the studies included in a systematic review. When a meta-analysis is included in the review, the forest plot is often used to illustrate individual studies and pooled results from the meta-analysis. Consider the forest plot in Figure 7.5 that illustrates three meta-analyses comparing motor control exercises to minimal intervention for long-term impact on disability for persons with nonspecific low back pain.[17]

In the top third of the graph, results from five studies were pooled in a meta-analysis to determine the cumulative effect of motor control exercises versus minimal intervention on short-term disability. The effect size (boxes) and 95% confidence interval (lines) for each comparison are represented. Data to the left of the vertical line, termed "Line of No effect," favor motor control exercises. Data to the right of the Line of No Effect favor control interventions. The "Pooled" line represents the results of a meta-analysis, which indicates that overall there was a large effect size (9.6) in favor of motor control exercises. However, because the 95% confidence interval crosses zero (Line of No Effect), there is a greater than 5% chance that the difference in level of disability between patients who received motor control exercises and minimal intervention was due to chance. In

contrast, the meta-analysis for long-term recovery (>12 mo) demonstrates a statistically significant difference between groups. The effect size is −10.8 (the negative sign indicates that the difference favors motor control exercises) and the 95% confidence interval ranges from −18.7 to −2.8. We can determine that there was a statistically significant difference in the pooled effect because the confidence interval is to the left of the Line of No effect.

Within the top box (outlined in blue) in Figure 7.5, the study authors illustrate the result of a meta-analysis for the impact of motor control exercise compared to minimal intervention in the short-term (<3 mo).

1. Each of six studies included in the analysis are listed, followed by "Pooled," which represents the result of the meta-analysis.
2. The small squares represent the mean effect size for each individual study. The squares on one side (left, in this case) represent results that favor motor control exercises; squares on the other side (right, in this case) represent results that favor minimal intervention.
3. The horizontal lines represent the confidence interval for each study's effect sizes.
4. The diamond represents the mean effect size from the meta-analysis.
5. The vertical line is called the Line of No Effect and represents the point on the scale at which neither treatment is favored over the other. If the horizontal Confidence Interval lines (C) cross the Line of No Effect

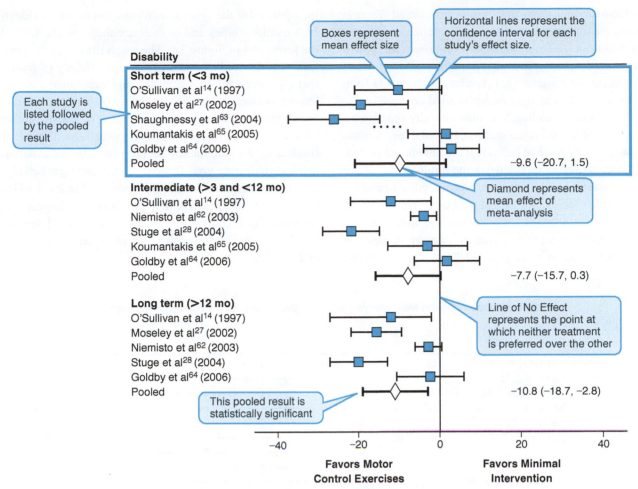

FIGURE 7.5 Forest plots illustrating three meta-analyses comparing motor control exercises to minimal intervention for long-term impact on disability for patients with low back pain over three time periods. *Redrawn from: Macedo LG, Maher CG, Latimer J, et al. Motor control exercise for persistent, nonspecific low back pain: a systematic review.* Phys Ther. *2009;89:9–25; with permission.*

we know that there was not a statistically significant difference between groups.

6. We identify that the result is statistically significant because the 95% Confidence Interval line does not cross the Line of No Effect.

■ SELF-TEST 7.2 Interpreting Forest Plots

Use Figure 7.5 to answer the following questions:

1. Which studies did not find a statistically significant benefit for motor control compared to minimal intervention at the intermediate time point?
2. What was the mean effect size identified by the meta-analysis at the intermediate time point? Is this a large effect size (see Chapter 4)? Was this a statistically significant result?
3. Review the long-term time period. Which primary study had the greatest benefit of motor control exercises compared to minimal intervention?

4. Does this graph support that motor control exercises are preferable to minimal intervention in the Intermediate recovery period? Was this a statistically significant result?

Part D: Summarizing the Clinical Bottom Line of a Systematic Review

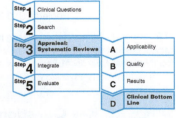

QUESTION 12: Does the systematic review inform clinical practice related to my clinical question?

A high-quality, clinically applicable systematic review provides a comprehensive literature review, appraisal, and synthesis of study results in one document. The culmination of many studies can be more powerful for informing practice than single primary studies. However, because systematic reviews combine studies, there are limitations that must be considered. There is wide variation in intervention and outcome measurements. Pooling data from studies in which interventions were applied with disparate frequency, intensity, duration, and methods of application can be misleading. Likewise, pooling data from studies in which the outcome measures used are widely disparate can also be misleading. You must carefully appraise the characteristics of the individual studies included in a systematic review (a summary table of individual studies should be provided) before accepting and applying the results.

Many systematic reviews do not provide the necessary details to guide specifics for patient treatment. These reviews can be used to gain insight into the body of literature that relates to your question and to identify primary studies that provide more detail to guide practice. The literature review incorporated in the systematic review can be used to identify high-quality studies and to compare their results. Consider the forest plot in Figure 7.6. The graph illustrates the pooled results of 15 studies that assessed the efficacy of physical therapy interventions on motor and functional outcomes among persons with chronic stroke.[18] The pooled result favors physical therapy. However, most of the studies have 95% Confidence Intervals that cross the Line of No Effect (indicating no statistically significant difference between groups). To inform your clinical practice, it might be helpful to read the article by Yang et al,[19] published in 2006, to learn more about the methods that produced the largest effect favoring physical therapy over a control. The 12 questions that inform Parts A through D are included in the checklist in Table 7.6.

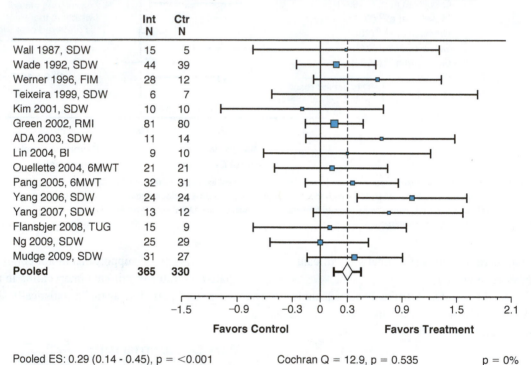

Plot of Random Effects Meta-analysis of Effect Size for All the Outcomes Considered.

	Int N	Ctr N
Wall 1987, SDW	15	5
Wade 1992, SDW	44	39
Werner 1996, FIM	28	12
Teixeira 1999, SDW	6	7
Kim 2001, SDW	10	10
Green 2002, RMI	81	80
ADA 2003, SDW	11	14
Lin 2004, BI	9	10
Ouellette 2004, 6MWT	21	21
Pang 2005, 6MWT	32	31
Yang 2006, SDW	24	24
Yang 2007, SDW	13	12
Flansbjer 2008, TUG	15	9
Ng 2009, SDW	25	29
Mudge 2009, SDW	31	27
Pooled	**365**	**330**

−1.5   −0.9   −0.3   0   0.3   0.9   1.5   2.1

Favors Control   **Favors Treatment**

Pooled ES: 0.29 (0.14 - 0.45), p = <0.001   Cochran Q = 12.9, p = 0.535   p = 0%

FIGURE 7.6 Forest plot illustrating individual studies and the pooled effect size for a comparison of the efficacy of physical therapy interventions on motor and functional outcomes among persons with chronic stroke. *From: Ferrarello F, Baccini M, Rinaldi LA, et al. Efficacy of physiotherapy interventions late after stroke: a meta-analysis.* J Neurol Neurosurg Psychiatry. 2010; with permission.

TABLE 7.6 **Key Questions for Appraising Systematic Reviews**

QUESTION	YES/NO	EXPLAIN
1. Is the study's purpose relevant to my clinical question?	__ Yes __ No	
2. Are the inclusion and exclusion criteria clearly defined and are studies that would answer my clinical question likely to be included?	__ Yes __ No	
3. Are the types of interventions investigated relevant to my clinical question?	__ Yes __ No	

TABLE 7.6 **Key Questions for Appraising Systematic Reviews—cont'd**

QUESTION	YES/NO	EXPLAIN
4. Are the outcome measures relevant to my clinical question?	__ Yes __ No	
5. Is the study population (sample) sufficiently similar to my patient to justify expectation that my patient would respond similarly to the population?	__ Yes __ No	
6. Was the literature search comprehensive?	__ Yes __ No	
7. Was an objective, reproducible, and reliable method used to judge the quality of the studies in the systematic review.	__ Yes __ No	
8. Was a standardized method used to extract data from studies included in the systematic review?	__ Yes __ No	
9. Was clinical heterogeneity assessed to determine whether a meta-analysis was justified?	__ Yes __ No	
10. If a meta-analysis was conducted, was statistical heterogeneity assessed?	__ Yes __ No	
11. What methods were used to report the results of the systematic review?		
12. How does the systematic review inform clinical practice related to my clinical question?		

SUMMARY

Systematic reviews are the principal scientific method for secondary research. There is a difference between narrative reviews and systematic reviews. Narrative reviews are not research studies and provide a nonsystematic summary of research that is at risk for author bias. A systematic review uses a documented and systematic approach to obtain and analyze studies that meet set criteria for answering a clinical question. High-quality systematic reviews provide a transparent and reproducible process for identifying studies, judging their quality, extracting data, and conducting qualitative or quantitative analyses. Systematic reviews reduce the risk of bias inherent in informing practice based on single primary studies. However, as with any study, systematic reviews must be appraised for applicability and quality before they can be used to inform clinical practice.

REVIEW QUESTIONS

1. Conduct a PubMed search using a searchable clinical question of your choosing. Identify at least one narrative and one systematic review applicable to your question.

2. Answer the 12 questions in Table 7.6 using the systematic review from question 1.

3. Why is the quality of the search conducted by the authors of a systematic review important?

4. What is the PEDro scale and how is used in systematic reviews?

5. What is the difference between clinical and statistical heterogeneity?

6. Draw a hypothetical forest plot that compares the impact of mechanical and manual traction for the lumbar spine on pain-free range of motion. Include the following:
   a. a study with a statistically significant benefit for mechanical traction with a narrow confidence interval
   b. a study with a nonsignificant benefit for manual traction with a large confidence interval
   c. three more studies with mean effect size and confidence intervals of your choosing
   d. based on what you have drawn, estimate the pooled effect size for the five studies.

7. Using the systematic review that you found for question 1, identify a primary study used in the systematic review that you expect would provide useful details about the intervention or diagnostic test.

REFERENCES

1. Egger M, Smith GD, Altman DG. *Systematic Reviews in Health Care: Meta-Analysis in Context*. 2nd ed. London, England: BMJ Books; 2001.
2. Dessaur WA, Magarey ME. Diagnostic accuracy of clinical tests for superior labral anterior posterior lesions: a systematic review. *J Orthop Sports Phys Ther.* 2008;38:341–352.
3. Blum L, Korner-Bitensky N. Usefulness of the Berg Balance Scale in stroke rehabilitation: a systematic review. *Phys Ther.* 2008.88:559–566
4. Alexander LD, Gilman DRD, Brown DR, et al. Exposure to low amounts of ultrasound energy does not improve soft tissue shoulder pathology: a systematic review. *Phys.Ther.* 2010;90:14–25.
5. Valen PA, Foxworth J. Evidence supporting the use of physical modalities in the treatment of upper extremity musculoskeletal conditions. *Curr Opinion Rheumatol.* 2010;22:194–204.
6. www.ncbi.nlm.nih.gov/sites/entrez/ Accessed October 21, 2011.
7. Bell JA, Bornett A. Exercise for the primary, secondary and tertiary prevention of low back pain in the workplace: a systematic review. *J Occup Rehabil.* 2009;19(1):8–24 wth permission.
8. Henchoz Y, So AKL. Exercise and nonspecific low back pain: a literature review. *Joint Bone Spine.* 2008;75:533–539.
9. Choi BKL, Verbeek JH, Tam WWS, et al. Exercises for prevention of recurrences of low-back pain. *Cochrane Database Syst Rev.* 2010.
10. Lederman E. The myth of core stability. *J Bodyw Mov Ther.* 2010;14:84–98.
11. Hoare BJ, Wasiak J, Imms C, et al. Constraint-induced movement therapy in the treatment of the upper limb in children with hemiplegic cerebral palsy. *Cochrane Database Syst Rev.* 2007:CD004149.
12. Huang HH, Fetters L, Hale J, et al. Bound for success: a systematic review of constraint-induced movement therapy in children with cerebral palsy supports improved arm and hand use. *Phys Ther.* 2009;89:1126–1141.
13. Moher D, Liberati A, Tetzlaff J, et al; the PG. Preferred reporting items for systematic reviews and meta-analyses: the PRISMA statement [reprint]. *Phys Ther.* 2009;89:873–880.
14. The Cochrane Collaboration. *Cochrane Reviews.* www.cochrane.org/reviews/ Accessed April 10, 2008.
15. Criteria for inclusion on PEDro: PEDro scale. www.pedro.fhs.usyd.edu.au/scale_item.html Accessed May 2, 2008.
16. Walser RF, Meserve BB, Boucher TR. The effectiveness of thoracic spine manipulation for the management of musculoskeletal conditions: a systematic review and meta-analysis of randomized clinical trials. *J Man Manip Ther.* 2009;17:237–246.
17. Macedo LG, Maher CG, Latimer J, et al. Motor control exercise for persistent, nonspecific low back pain: a systematic review. *Phys Ther.* 2009;89:9–25.
18. Ferrarello F, Baccini M, Rinaldi LA, et al. Efficacy of physiotherapy interventions late after stroke: a meta-analysis. *J Neurol Neurosurg Psychiatry.* 2010; 82:136-43.
19. Yang YR, Wang RY, Lin KH, et al. Task-oriented progressive resistance strength training improves muscle strength and functional performance in individuals with stroke. *Clin Rehabil.* 2006;20:860–870.

8 Appraising Clinical Practice Guidelines

PRE-TEST

1. What is the difference between clinical practice guidelines and systematic reviews?

2. Which U.S. government database can be used to search for clinical practice guidelines?

3. List two characteristics to assess when searching for clinical practice guidelines.

4. List two important appraisal questions for assessing a guideline's applicability, quality, and clinical utility.

5. What is a grade of recommendation?

6. Why do clinical practice guideline recommendations tend to be vague?

CHAPTER-AT-A-GLANCE

This chapter will help you understand the following:

- The purpose of clinical practice guidelines (CPGs)

- Special search considerations for CPGs

- Appraisal of CPGs for applicability, quality, and clinical utility

■ Introduction

What Are Clinical Practice Guidelines?

Clinical practice guidelines (CPGs) are systematically developed statements designed to facilitate evidence based decision making for the management of specific health conditions, such as knee osteoarthritis or stroke.[1] CPGs incorporate evidence from research, clinical expertise, and, ideally, patient perspectives. They can be developed to meet the needs of various stakeholders including clinicians (from a single discipline or interdisciplinary teams), patients, payers, legislators, public health authorities, and the general public (Fig. 8.1).

Government health-care agencies and professional associations fund the development of most CPGs. For example, the

Agency for Healthcare Research and Quality (AHRQ), a U.S. government agency, produces CPGs targeted at American health-care providers and the public.[2] Special interest sections of the American Physical Therapy Association (APTA) create guidelines for physical therapy, targeted at physical therapists, policy makers, and insurance companies in the United States.[3]

If you are not familiar with CPGs, it may be difficult to discern the difference between a systematic review (see Chapter 7) and a CPG. A high-quality CPG includes both a systematic review of research evidence and explicit recommendations regarding clinical decisions. CPGs also tend to be broader than systematic reviews, addressing multiple aspects of care (i.e., diagnosis, prognosis, and interventions) associated with a particular health condition. Table 8.1 illustrates the similarities and differences between CPGs and systematic reviews.

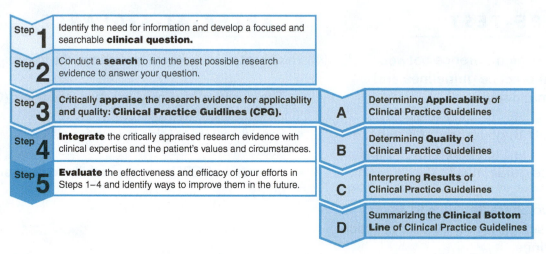

FIGURE 8.1 Clinical practice guidelines should be appraised for applicability and quality.

TABLE 8.1 Comparison of CPGs and Systematic Reviews

	HIGH-QUALITY CLINICAL PRACTICE GUIDELINES	HIGH-QUALITY SYSTEMATIC REVIEWS
Purpose	To make recommendations for best clinical practice based on the best available research evidence, clinical expertise, and patient perspectives for a relatively broad set of clinical questions associated with a specific health condition.	To summarize the research on a specific question, or specific set of questions, by systematically reviewing and summarizing existing research evidence.
Literature search	Comprehensive search of numerous databases with pre-set inclusion and exclusion criteria.	Comprehensive search of numerous databases with pre-set inclusion and exclusion criteria.
Research appraisal	Conducted using a standardized method by >1 independent reviewer.	Conducted using a standardized method by >1 independent reviewer.
Research analysis	Includes meta-analysis as possible.	Includes a meta-analysis as possible.
Clinical expertise	Experts are consulted to facilitate interpretation of research evidence and to provide recommendations when research evidence is lacking.	Not a component of methods.

TABLE 8.1 **Comparison of CPGs and Systematic Reviews—cont'd**

	HIGH-QUALITY CLINICAL PRACTICE GUIDELINES	HIGH-QUALITY SYSTEMATIC REVIEWS
Patient perspective	Patients are consulted to facilitate appropriate prioritization of patient concerns and needs	Not a component of methods
Results	Evidence quality and results are summarized. Specific recommendations for practice are made	Meta-, quantitative, and/or qualitative analyses are reported
Implications for clinical practice	Clinicians are provided with specific recommendations for practice	Clinicians identify what clinical action to take based on the results of the study
Document location	Published on the Internet or in book format; may be a special item in a peer-reviewed journal	Peer-reviewed journals
Document size	Large documents often 30–100+ pages	Average article length (~5–15 pages)

What Search Strategies are Best for CPGs?

Clinical practice guidelines are often published in documents other than peer-reviewed journals. They may be located on a Web site (usually free to access) or in book or pamphlet form for purchase. Thus, although search engines such as PubMed may identify CPGs, they are unlikely to produce a comprehensive list. The AHRQ maintains a searchable database of author-submitted CPGs at the National Guidelines Clearinghouse (NGC) Web site (www.guidelines.gov; Fig. 8.2). In addition, the PEDro database[4] includes physical therapy–specific CPGs. Finally, individual organizations may maintain a list of CPGs

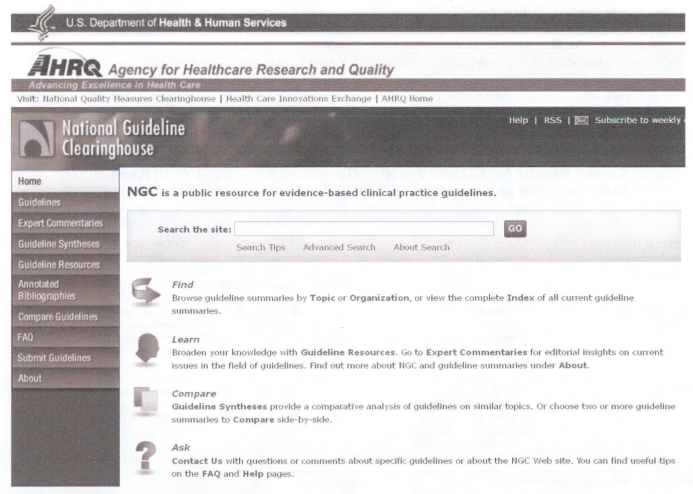

FIGURE 8.2 Screenshot from the National Guidelines Clearinghouse Web site.

targeted to their users. In the text that follows, we introduce a new patient case, Mrs. White, and describe where to search for CPGs to guide her physical therapy care.

 CASE STUDY 8.1 Bernice White

Bernice White is a 72-year-old retired woman who lives alone. She is widowed with three grown children who live nearby. Bernice enjoys gardening, "power walks" with friends, and volunteering for her church. Over the years, she has experienced a gradual increase in knee pain secondary to osteoarthritis. She reports that lately, her knee pain is really slowing her down. Mrs. White has difficulty climbing stairs, completing her normal 3-mile walk, and gardening as a result of her knee pain. Her co-morbidities include bilateral hip and hand osteoarthritis, obesity (body mass index [BMI] = 31), coronary artery disease, hypertension, hypercholesterolemia, and occasional bouts of gout. Mrs. White likes to exercise and would like to know what exercises would help to control her knee pain.

Mrs. White's presentation is consistent with the complex array of issues that we often encounter in practice. It can be overwhelming to think about how to search for information about the best exercises for someone with her number and complexity of co-morbidities. It is helpful to focus on the most immediate problem. We want to know what exercises will be most effective for Mrs. White given her primary problem of knee pain secondary to osteoarthritis. Therefore, our searchable clinical question could be, "For a 72-year-old female with knee osteoarthritis, what exercise regimens are most effective for reducing pain and improving function?"

When we find research evidence to answer this question, we can use our own expertise and Mrs. White's values and circumstances (including her co-morbidities) to come to a shared informed decision about the most appropriate exercise program for her.

Our search for CPGs in three sources (NGC, PEDro, and PubMed) identified three [5–7] potential guidelines to inform care for Mrs. White (Table 8.2). We recommend that you start searches for CPGs using the NGC. However, CPGs have to be submitted to the NGC by the authors, and as a consequence not all CPGs can be located at the NGC Web site. Therefore, we followed our search of NGC by searching with PEDro and PubMed. We located two additional CPGs, including one sponsored by the American Academy of Orthopedic Surgeons (AAOS).[7] Professional association guidelines often address multiple aspects of care for a condition; this CPG may provide recommendations relevant to the physical therapist. Further appraisal of the CPG is required to determine if it is appropriate to guide physical therapy care. In addition, in recent years, the Orthopedic Section of the APTA has published numerous CPGs in the *Journal of Orthopaedic and Sports Physical Therapy*. Although a CPG relevant to Mrs. White did not emerge in our search at this site, the associated Web site (www.jospt.org) and other APTA sections are valuable to monitor.

You will need to do a cursory screening process when searching for CPGs. Note the sponsoring organization, purpose, overall clarity, and depth of the CPG. Table 8.3 describes the relevance of this information and where to locate it within the CPG. When you identify a CPG of interest, you will need to appraise it for applicability and quality before proceeding to use it to inform you practice.

TABLE 8.2 **Search Results for Clinical Practice Guidelines Associated With Knee Osteoarthritis and Exercises to Reduce Pain and Improve Function***

SOURCE	SEARCH STRATEGY	SAMPLE RESULTS
National Guidelines Clearinghouse www.guideline.gov	Search box: • "Knee osteoarthritis" and "Exercise"	National Collaborating Centre for Chronic Conditions. Osteoarthritis. The care and management of osteoarthritis in adults. London, England: National Institute for Health and Clinical Excellence (NICE); 2008:22. Clinical Guideline, no. 59.[5]
PEDro database www.pedro.org.au	• Abstract and title: knee osteoarthritis and exercise • Method: practice guideline • Date: since 2005	Zhang W, Moskowitz RW, Nuki G, et al. OARSI recommendations for the management of hip and knee osteoarthritis, Part II: OARSI evidence-based, expert consensus guidelines. *Osteoarthritis and Cartilage*. 2008;16:137–162. [6]
PubMed www.pubmed.gov	Keywords: • "Knee osteoarthritis" • "Exercise" Limits: • "Practice Guidelines" • "Last 5 years"	Richmond J, Hunter D, Irrgang J, et al. Treatment of osteoarthritis of the knee (nonarthroplasty). *J Am Acad Orthop Surg*. Sep 2009;17:591–600.[7]

*Searches were conducted in September 2010.

TABLE 8.3 **Characteristics to Consider When Reviewing CPG Search Results**

CHARACTERISTIC	WHERE TO LOOK	RELEVANCE
Age *Is the CPG <5 years old?*	Title page	CPGs are out of date as soon as substantial new data emerge on the topic. CPGs must be revised at least every 5 years to be considered current.
Sponsoring organization *Is the sponsoring organization likely to produce an objective summary of the evidence?*	First page	Because CPGs involve interpretation of evidence, they are at risk of bias. Knowledge of the sponsoring organization gives you insight into potential conflicts of interest for the CPG developer. Knowledge of the sponsoring organization provides insight into the intended audience.
Topic *Is the topic relevant to your clinical question?*	Opening text	The purpose or aim defines the intended audience and objectives. A rapid review of this information facilitates your understanding of the CPG's applicability to your clinical question.
Clarity of information *Is the information efficient to access?*	Scan document	Guidelines should organize a large amount of information for efficient use and the guideline should be easy to navigate.
Depth *Does the depth of information correspond to your needs?*	Scan document	Some guidelines contain substantial depth (100+ pages), wheras others are short (a few pages). The depth of the required information effects comprehensiveness.
Availability of full text *Is the full-text easily accessible?*	PDF link on Web site	CPGs that are not freely available require additional time and expense to access. Weigh the value of instant access to an online CPG versus the time or money associated with obtaining a well-developed, but more difficult to access, CPG.

■ SELF-TEST 8.1

Use Self-Test 8.1 to practice your CPG search skills and record them in the table provided in the Answers to Self-Test section at the end of this chapter.

New and updated CPGs are published on a regular basis. Practice reproducing the searches presented in Table 8.2. Screen the result of each search using the list from Table 8.3 and record your findings. Identify the CPG that is most relevant to Mrs. White.

■ Appraising Clinical Practice Guidelines

The next sections of this chapter detail the appraisal process for clinical practice guidelines (see Fig. 8.1). Just as with intervention, diagnostic, or systematic reviews, or any other type of research study, the quality of the study must be appraised before it can be appropriately applied in practice.

We use the Appraisal of Guidelines Research and Evaluation II (AGREE II)[8] as we describe the appraisal process. AGREE II is one established tool for CPG appraisal (Fig. 8.3). AGREE II is the product of the AGREE Collaboration (http://www.agreecollaboration.org), an international collaboration of researchers and policy makers. AGREE II consists of

23 items to consider in the appraisal process organized into six domains:

1. Scope and purpose
2. Stakeholder involvement
3. Rigor of development
4. Clarity of presentation
5. Applicability
6. Editorial independence

We have modified these appraisal items into questions that we include in parts A through D of the appraisal process used throughout this book. The 23 questions modified from AGREE II form the checklist in Table 8.6.

Part A: Determining Applicability of a CPG

Like any source of evidence, it is important to determine if a CPG is relevant to your clinical practice. Because recommendations from CPGs are written broadly you want to determine if the objective and clinical question for the guideline is informative for your practice.

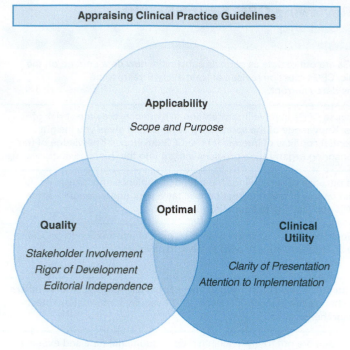

Appraising Clinical Practice Guidelines

FIGURE 8.3 CPG appraisal requires consideration of the CPG's applicability, quality, and clinical utility.

QUESTION 1: Is the overall objective(s) of the guideline described?

QUESTION 2: Is your clinical question(s) addressed by the guideline?

QUESTION 3: Are the patients to whom the guideline is meant to apply specifically described, and do they match your clinical question?

Determine if answers to these three questions are well described, and if the objectives, clinical questions, and patients addressed in the CPG are relevant to your clinical question.

Part B: Determining Quality of a CPG

Part C: Interpreting the Results of a CPG

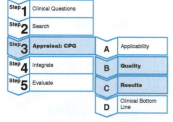

CPGs are designed to make recommendations for clinical practice. As a consumer of CPGs, you trust others to appraise and interpret primary sources of evidence for you; however, you should appraise the quality of a CPG before you follow its recommendations. Based on the AGREE II, the following domains include items that address quality of the CPG and assist you in interpreting the results: stakeholder involvement, rigor of development, and

editorial independence. We include the questions from Table 8.6 under these domain headings from AGREE II.

Stakeholder Involvement

There is risk for bias when CPG authors translate objective data into recommendations. One method of reducing bias is to ensure that authors from a broad range of interest groups are represented in the development process. When diverse biases are represented, there is less risk that one particular bias will skew a CPG's recommendations.

QUESTION 4: Were individuals from all relevant professional groups included?

QUESTION 5: Were patients' views and preferences sought?

QUESTION 6: Are target users of the guideline clearly defined?

Determine which professional groups provide a balanced assessment of evidence for a given CPG. For example, a CPG about rehabilitation after shoulder arthroplasty might include physical therapists, occupational therapists, orthopedic surgeons, payers (representatives from insurance companies), and pharmacists. Each professional group brings opinions and possible bias. Working together, they are more likely to produce recommendations that balance their biases in the best interest of patients.

Patients' views and preferences are critical to evidence based practice (EPB). This most important stakeholder group can influence recommendations for clinical practice and should be included in CPG development. Patients have too often been omitted from the CPG process; however, this is changing with the increased emphasis on patient perspectives in clinical decisions.

Rigor of Development

Developing CPGs is a resource intensive process. The authors should conduct a systematic review for each clinical question addressed by the CPG and then determine recommendations for practice through a consensus process among the diverse stakeholders. If resources are limited, the rigor of CPG development might be compromised. The impact of possible compromises should be weighed when appraising the validity of a CPG's development.

QUESTION 7: Were systematic methods used to search for evidence?

QUESTION 8: Are criteria for selecting the evidence clearly described?

The authors should provide detailed information about the databases searched, including terms and limits. Inclusion and exclusion criteria for included studies should also be provided. Many CPGs do not provide this level of detail; in these cases, you must decide if sufficient information is provided for an adequate appraisal of the validity of the CPG's recommendations.

QUESTION 9: Were the strengths and limitations of the body of evidence clearly described?

Authors of a CPG should provide readers with a clear and concise summary of the strengths and limitations of the body of evidence. This information allows you to quickly assess the quality of research evidence available for making clinical practice recommendations.

QUESTION 10: Are the methods for formulating recommendations clearly described?

QUESTION 11: Were health benefits, side effects, and risks considered in formulating the recommendations?

QUESTION 12: Is there an explicit link between recommendations and the supporting evidence?

The purpose of CPGs is to provide recommendations for practice. A transparent method for formulating recommendations must be provided to determine the clinical usefulness of the CPG. Integrating the three sources of evidence—research, patient perspective, and clinician expertise—into CPG recommendations for practice is a complex process and methods for formulating recommendations vary among guidelines. Authors should express their level of confidence in the clinical recommendations from the CPG. An important mechanism for confirming the validity of recommendations is to link the summarized evidence to the recommendations. You should be able to identify the specific sources of evidence used to make each recommendation. If the recommendations appear to be independent of the evidence synthesis, there is reason to suspect that the recommendations are more heavily influenced by informal opinion rather than research evidence, systematically collected clinical expertise, or patient perspective.

QUESTION 13: Was the guideline externally reviewed by experts?

CPGs should be peer reviewed, just as with primary and secondary research. CPGs may be published in peer-reviewed journals. Other CPGs may report a peer-review process as a part of the methods even if they are not published in a peer-reviewed journal.

QUESTION 14: Was a procedure for updating the guideline provided?

Finally, CPGs can rapidly become out of date. New research evidence may influence or contradict outdated CPG recommendations. In addition, changes in the health-care environment can influence patient perspective and clinical expertise. CPGs should be published with a specific plan for revision. A commonly accepted plan is that a CPG is updated when either important new research is published *or* every 5 years, whichever occurs first.

Editorial Independence

If CPGs are developed in conjunction with an external funding agency, then it is important that the authors develop the CPG without undue influence from the funding agency. For example, if a funding agency has a bias toward specific clinical interventions, then the authors must have editorial independence to recommend for or against use of those interventions based on the best available evidence.

QUESTION 15: Was the guideline developed independently of the views of the funding body?

QUESTION 16: Were competing interests of guideline development members recorded and addressed?

A CPG should have a statement that defines the source of funding and explicitly states that the views and interests of the funding body have not influenced the CPG recommendations. Any conflict of interest for individual authors should be stated. For example, consider an orthotist who is an author of a CPG about use of orthotics and prosthetics. If the orthotist owns a company that fabricates orthotics, that conflict of interest should be reported in the CPG.

Part D: Summarizing the Clinical Bottom Line of a CPG

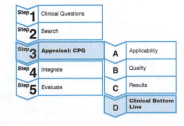

The final step in appraising a CPG is to determine if the recommendations can be utilized in clinical practice. You have already scanned the CPG for helpful, clear recommendations during the search process. Now, examine the recommendations more closely for clarity and presentation, consideration of barriers, and implementation resources.

Clarity of Presentation

QUESTION 17: Are the recommendations specific and unambiguous?

QUESTION 18: Are different options for management of the condition clearly presented?

QUESTION 19: Are key recommendations easily identified?

The best CPGs provide well-supported, specific recommendations based on systematically collected, appraised, and integrated evidence. The most useful recommendations are supported by strong evidence and have a direct impact on patient care.

Attention to Implementation

QUESTION 20: Does the CPG address facilitators and barriers to its application?

QUESTION 21: Are advice and/or tools provided on how the CPG can be put into practice?

QUESTION 22: Does the CPG address potential resource implications of applying the recommendations?

QUESTION 23: Does the CPG provide monitoring and/or auditing criteria?

Changing health-care practice as new evidence emerges is challenging. The authors of CPGs are in an excellent position to provide methods to successfully implement their recommendations. For example, educational tools and user-friendly summaries for both clinicians and patients may facilitate implementation of CPG recommendations. Implications for financial, personnel, and other costs should be addressed. Consider a CPG that recommends that patients who undergo a certain surgical procedure should receive 1 week of inpatient physical therapy. The CPG should address the impact that an increased (or decreased) length of stay might have on hospital services. It might also address the implications of the costs to provide this service in comparison to home care physical therapy.

CPGs are increasingly used to monitor quality of care.[9] CPGs should provide review criteria that could be used to monitor or audit adherence to the guideline. For example, a CPG about fall prevention in the elderly should provide a list of "best" practice criteria that could be assessed through chart review in a multi-disciplinary setting.

Using Clinical Practice Guidelines in Clinical Practice

You may be disappointed at the lack of detail provided in recommendations from CPGs. For example, the AAOS[7] recommendations do not tell us how *much* aerobic exercise Mrs. White should do, what she should do if the exercises cause increased pain, or whether quadriceps strengthening exercises should be done under weight-bearing or non–weight-bearing conditions.

This lack of specificity can be partially explained by three main issues:

1. Guideline recommendations are not meant to be prescriptive. Rather, they are designed to summarize a large body of evidence and distill that information into general recommendations that can be applied to most patients with a particular condition.
2. Guideline recommendations can be overly general or limited because of the lack of research evidence. Students and clinicians are often surprised at the relatively small amount of research available to inform common clinical questions. Physical therapy's body of research evidence is growing; however, there will always be gaps between the questions we have and the available evidence.
3. The consensus nature of CPGs, by design, reduces the detail contained in recommendations. Large groups of diverse stakeholders can agree to general recommendations but often have difficulty agreeing on highly detailed directions for clinical practice.

Given the general nature of most CPG recommendations, you may find that they are particularly helpful to answer clinical questions about populations of patients. For example, you could update your knowledge and practice for patients with knee meniscus injuries using the Orthopedic Section of the APTA's CPG, "Knee Pain and Mobility Impairments: Meniscal and Articular Cartilage Lesions."[10] This CPG provides excellent insight into the best available research and clinical expert evidence for many important clinical questions for this population.

Finally, CPGs are an important resource for identifying primary research articles that provide more specific details to inform practice. For example, the CPG by Logerstedt et al[10] gives a grade B recommendation that "Neuromuscular electrical stimulation can be used with patients following meniscal injuries to increase quadriceps muscle strength." Specific articles associated with that recommendation would be helpful to obtain more detailed information about the neuromuscular electrical stimulation protocols that were most effective.

DIGGING DEEPER 8.1

Turning evidence into recommendations

Appraising a large body of research evidence and translating that evidence into a cohesive set of CPG recommendations are complex processes. Research studies included in the CPG may vary in design (type and quality), outcome measures, participant characteristics, and results. Recommendations for clinical practice emerge from a multi-step process that includes conducting a systematic review of the literature, characterizing the strengths and limitations of the literature, and developing consensus-based recommendations. As a consumer of CPGs, it is important to have insight into the diversity of systems used to convert evidence into recommendations.

Typically, CPGs present findings in two parts: (1) a summary of the quality of available research evidence and (2) a recommendation that includes the strength of that recommendation. Commonly, numeric levels of evidence are used to characterize the quality of available research. Alphabetical grades of recommendation are used to characterize recommendations for practice. The details, however, of how this important process is conducted can vary significantly between CPGs. Table 8.4 illustrates a side-by-side comparison of this two-step process for two CPGs, one previously identified in our search regarding Mrs. White (Table 8.2)[7] and one from the Orthopedic Section of the APTA.[10]

The processes illustrated in Table 8.4 are the most commonly observed in rehabilitation-associated CPGs. However, another system termed GRADE (Grading of Recommendations Assessment, Development, and Evaluation, Table 8.5) has emerged as a popular alternative for characterizing the quality of a body of literature and communicating the strength of recommendations.[11] The GRADE method is similar to the systems in Table 8.5 in that it is composed of a two-step process. GRADE uses a description rather than a numerical or alphabetical ranking.

TABLE 8.4 **Comparison of the Process Used by Two CPGs for Summarizing the Quality of Research Evidence (Part 1) and Making Explicit Recommendations for Practice (Part 2)**

Clinical practice guidelines illustrated:
* Logerstedt DS, Snyder-Mackler L, Ritter RC, Axe MJ. Knee pain and mobility impairments: meniscal and articular cartilage lesions. *J Orthop Sports Phys Ther.* 2010;40(6):A1–A35.
* Richmond J, Hunter D, Irrgang J, et al. Treatment of osteoarthritis of the knee (nonarthroplasty). *J Am Acad Orthop Surg.* 2009;17(9):591–600.

PART 1: LEVEL OF EVIDENCE

Both guidelines used similar criteria to define level of evidence for the body of literature:

Level	Description
I	Evidence obtained from high-quality diagnostic, prospective studies, or randomized controlled trials
II	Evidence obtained from lesser-quality diagnostic studies, prospective studies, or randomized controlled trials (e.g., weaker diagnostic criteria and reference standards, improper randomization, no blinding, <80% follow-up)
III	Case-controlled studies or retrospective studies
IV	Case series
V	Expert opinion

Continued

TABLE 8.4 **Comparison of the Process Used by Two CPGs for Summarizing the Quality of Research Evidence (Part 1) and Making Explicit Recommendations for Practice (Part 2)—cont'd**

PART 2: GRADE OF RECOMMENDATION			
The CPGs used different grading systems Logerstedt et al 2010[10] Authors assign a grade to each recommendation based on the cumulative body of evidence:		Richmond et al 2009[7] Recommendations and their grades were voted on using a standard technique:	
Grade	**Recommendation is supported by**	**Grade/Recommendation**	**Recommendation is supported by**
A Strong evidence	A preponderance of level I and/or level II studies support the recommendation. Must include at least 1 level I study	A *We Recommend*	Level I evidence
B Moderate evidence	A single high-quality randomized controlled trial or a preponderance of level II studies	B *We suggest*	Level II or III evidence
C Weak evidence	A single level II study or a preponderance of level II and IV studies including statements of consensus by content experts	C *Option*	Level IV or V evidence
D Conflicting evidence	Higher-quality studies that disagree with respect to their conclusions	I *We are unable to recommend for or against*	None or conflicting evidence
E Theoretical/ foundational evidence	A preponderance of evidence from animal or cadaver studies, from conceptual models/principles or from basic sciences/bench research		
F Expert opinion	Best practice based on the clinical experience of the guidelines development team		

TABLE 8.5 **The GRADE System for Developing CPG Recommendations**[11]

Part 1: Quality of the body of research evidence is defined as:

DESCRIPTION	DEFINITION
High quality*	Further research is very unlikely to change confidence in the estimate of effect
Moderate quality†	Further research is likely to have an important impact on confidence in the estimate of effect and may change the estimate
Low quality	Further research is very likely to have an important impact on our confidence in the estimate of effect and is likely to change the estimate
Very low quality	Any estimate of effect is very uncertain

*Randomized controlled trials are initially considered high quality but are downgraded based on study limitations and inconsistencies between trials.
†Observational studies are initially considered low quality but are upgraded based on magnitude of effect size and other elements of the results.

TABLE 8.5 **The GRADE System for Developing CPG Recommendations[11]—cont'd**

Part 2: A recommendation is graded as either strong or weak based on a balance of the following four criteria:

CRITERIA THAT INFLUENCE RECOMMENDATIONS	STRONG	WEAK
1. Quality of evidence	High	Low
2. Balance between benefits and risks	Large difference between desirable and undesirable effects	Small difference between desirable and undesirable effects
3. Values and preferences	Low variability or uncertainty in clinician/patient preferences	High variability or uncertainty in clinician/patient preferences
4. Costs (resource allocation)	Low cost/resource demand	High cost/resource demand

SUMMARY

High-quality CPGs provide clinicians with a summary of research evidence with consideration from multiple stakeholders, ideally including patient perspectives. CPGs are not research evidence, but are based on a systematic review of the research literature. CPGs are developed by experts to facilitate EBP by developing a plan of care for specific clinical questions. A rigorously developed CPG reduces the need to appraise each primary research study associated with a patient population. Because CPGs are published through a variety of methods, different search strategies are required. Valuable resources include the National Guidelines Clearinghouse and the PEDro database in addition to PubMed. Table 8.6, "Key Questions for the Appraisal of Clinical Practice Guidelines," follows.

TABLE 8.6 **Key Questions for Appraising Clinical Practice Guidelines (Modified From the AGREE II Tool)[8]**

DOMAIN	STATEMENT	
Part A: Applicability		
Scope and purpose	1. The overall objective(s) of the guideline is (are) specifically described and addresses my clinical question.	__Yes __No
	2. The clinical question(s) addressed by the guideline is (are) specifically described and addresses my clinical question.	__Yes __No
	3. The patients to whom the guideline is meant to apply are specifically described and match my clinical question.	__Yes __No
Part B: Quality **Part C: Interpreting Results**		
Stakeholder involvement	4. The guideline development group includes individuals from all the relevant professional groups.	__Yes __No
	5. The patients' views and preferences have been sought.	__Yes __No
	6. Target users of the guideline are clearly defined.	__Yes __No
Rigor of development	7. Systematic methods were used to search for evidence.	__Yes __No
	8. The criteria for selecting the evidence are clearly described.	__Yes __No
	9. The strengths and limitations of the body of evidence are clearly described.	__Yes __No
	10. The methods used for formulating the recommendations are clearly described.	__Yes __No
	11. The health benefits, side effects, and risks have been considered in formulating the recommendations.	__Yes __No

Continued

TABLE 8.6   **Key Questions for Appraising Clinical Practice Guidelines (Modified From the AGREE II Tool)[8]—cont'd**

DOMAIN	STATEMENT	
	12. There is an explicit link between the recommendations and the supporting evidence.	__Yes __No
	13. The guideline has been externally reviewed by experts prior to its publication.	__Yes __No
	14. A procedure for updating the guideline is provided.	__Yes __No
Editorial independence	15. The views of the funding body have not influenced the content of the guideline.	__Yes __No
	16. Competing interests of guideline development members have been recorded and addressed.	__Yes __No
Part D: Clinical Bottom Line		
Clarity of presentation	17. The recommendations are specific and unambiguous.	__Yes __No
	18. The different options for management of the condition are clearly presented.	__Yes __No
	19. Key recommendations are easily identifiable.	__Yes __No
Attention to implementation	20. The guideline describes facilitators and barriers to its application.	__Yes __No
	21. The guideline provides advice and/or tools on how the recommendations can be put into practice.	__Yes __No
	22. The potential cost implications of applying the recommendations have been considered.	__Yes __No
	23. The guideline presents key review criteria for monitoring and/or audit purposes.	__Yes __No

REVIEW QUESTIONS

1. Use the National Guidelines Clearinghouse (www.guideline.gov) to search for a CPG about a diagnosis and treatment of interest to you. Limit the search time to 20 minutes at the Web site. What did you find?

2. Conduct searches for the same diagnosis and treatment in the PEDro (www.pedro.org.au) and PubMed (www.pubmed.org) databases. How do the searches compare?

3. Use the characteristics listed in Table 8.3 to choose one CPG to appraise. Use the checklist in Table 8.6 to appraise the quality of the CPG. Summarize the CPG's strengths and weaknesses.

4. Describe the system used to summarize the quality of the research evidence used in the CPG you chose.

5. Describe the system used to grade the strength of the recommendations provided by the CPG.

6. Use the CPG you found (if it is high quality) or retrieve the Logerstedt et al[10] CPG cited in this chapter. How could you improve your clinical care for patients using recommendations from the CPG?

7. Identify a recommendation from the CPG that you would apply in practice. Then identify and obtain an individual article that was used to support that recommendation. Does this article provide important details for applying the CPG recommendation?

ANSWERS TO SELF-TEST

■ SELF-TEST 8.1

Source	Search Strategy	Your Results
National Guidelines Clearinghouse www.guideline.gov **PEDro database** www.pedro.org.au **PubMed** www.pubmed.gov	Search box: • "knee osteoarthritis" and "exercise" • Abstract and title: knee osteoarthritis and exercise • Method: practice guideline • Date: since 2005 Keywords: • "Knee osteoarthritis" • "Exercise" Limits: • "Practice guidelines" • "Last 5 years"	

REFERENCES

1. Appraisal of Guidelines for Research and Evaluation (AGREE) Instrument. www.agreecollaboration.org Published 2001. Accessed September 3, 2010.
2. Agency for Healthcare Research. Clinical practice guidelines archive Web site. www.ahrq.gov/clinic/cpgarchv.htm
3. Orthopaedic Section of the American Physical Therapy Association. ICF project. www.orthopt.org/ICF.php
4. PEDro Web site. www.pedro.fhs.usyd.edu.au/ Accessed March 26, 2008.
5. National Collaborating Centre for Chronic Conditions. Osteoarthritis. The care and management of osteoarthritis in adults. London, England: National Institute for Health and Clinical Excellence (NICE); 2008:22 p. Clinical Guideline no. 59.
6. Zhang W, Moskowitz RW, Nuki G, et al. OARSI recommendations for the management of hip and knee osteoarthritis. Part II: OARSI evidence-based, expert consensus guidelines. *Osteoarthritis and Cartilage.* 2008;16:137–162.
7. Richmond J, Hunter D, Irrgang J, et al. Treatment of osteoarthritis of the knee (nonarthroplasty). *J Am Acad Orthop Surg.* 2009;17:591–600.
8. AGREE Next Steps Consortium. *The AGREE II Instrument* [Electronic version]. http://www.agreetrust.org. Published 2009. Accessed Septermber 3, 2010.
9. Brouwers M, Kho ME, Browman GP, et al; AGREE Next Steps Consortium. AGREE II: advancing guideline development, reporting and evaluation in healthcare. *Can Med Assoc J.* 2010. doi:10.1503/cmaj.090449.
10. Logerstedt DS, Snyder-Mackler L, Ritter RC, et al. Knee pain and mobility impairments: meniscal and articular cartilage lesions. *J Orthop Sports Phys Ther.* 40:A1–A35.
11. Atkins D, Eccles M, Flottorp S, et al. Systems for grading the quality of evidence and the strength of recommendations I: critical appraisal of existing approaches the GRADE Working Group. *BMC Health Serv Res.* 2004;4:38.

9 Appraising Studies With Alternative Designs

PRE-TEST

Use Figure 9.1 to answer questions 1 and 2 of the Pre-Test.

1. What is the meaning of the letters A and B in the graph in Figure 9.1?

2. What conclusions could you draw from the graph of data?

3. What characteristic(s) of single-subject studies are different from a randomized clinical trial?

4. What are the primary differences between qualitative and quantitative research designs?

5. What types of clinical questions are best addressed with a qualitative research study?

CHAPTER-AT-A-GLANCE

This chapter will help you understand the following:

- Advantages and disadvantages of single-subject research designs

- Appraising the applicability, quality, and results of single-subject research designs

- The purposes of qualitative research versus quantitative research

- Appraising the applicability, quality, and results of qualitative research

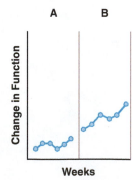

FIGURE 9.1 Example of an SSR design with one baseline phase (A), one treatment phase (B), and one withdraw of treatment phase.

■ Introduction

We include single-subject and qualitative research in this chapter. These two types of research are not common in the physical therapy literature, but both types are useful for clinical decisions (Fig. 9.2). Many of the appraisal concepts described in depth in previous chapters can be applied to single-subject research;[1] therefore, they are mentioned but not repeated in depth in this chapter. The different concepts used in the appraisal of qualitative research are described in more depth.

■ Single-Subject Research

Understanding single-case experimental designs, analyses, and applications improves your ability to evaluate the evidence based literature and eventually to answer your clinical questions. Rigorous research with single participants can be applied to your patients, sometimes more directly than the results of group randomized clinical trials (RCTs). In a typical single-subject design (SSD) one participant is followed intensely. During a baseline period, before intervention begins, the variables of interest are repeatedly measured. This may occur over successive days or weeks. The baseline period establishes what is typical for each of the variables for the participant. For example, during a baseline period, the gait characteristics of a participant walking on a treadmill might be measured every day for a week. The intervention period begins after baseline and then data are collected periodically on the single subject during the intervention. There might then be a period after intervention, during which the participant is measured, but no treatment is given. The change in the variables during the treatment period is then compared to the variables during baseline and post-treatment periods. An SSD typically creates abundant data, but on only one participant.

In contrast to an SSD, case studies are typically written retrospectively and detail the characteristics of one case and the course of intervention for that case. A case study is *not* a controlled single-case experimental design and the two terms should not be interchanged. A case study is a systematically reported single-patient example that does not include a controlled manipulation of intervention or the other experimental controls that are implemented in an SSD. Case studies may be helpful to our clinical decisions but they lack systematic control, implementation, and evaluation of treatment.

Example Designs and Notation

Research notation is a shorthand method to describe the overall design of a study. Research notation for SSDs is different from notation for other intervention designs (see Chapter 3 for research notation for group designs). Examples of SSDs are included in Figures 9.3 through 9.6. The following letters are used to designate phases of a single-subject research (SSR) study:

A = Phase of observation with measurement; A designates baseline or treatment withdrawal phases
B = Intervention
C, D, etc. = comparison interventions

Combining Multiple SSR Studies

RCTs

RCTs can be implemented using SSDs.[2] The key here is that multiple single-subject studies are grouped together. The participants in the multiple SSR studies should have characteristics that are as similar as possible. For an RCT with single subjects, one subject is randomly assigned to treatment condition A and the next subject is assigned to an alternative (comparison) treatment B. The treatment protocol is standardized across subjects, just as in a group design. The benefit of this type of design is that multiple measures are obtained on each subject. These repeated measures document the natural fluctuations of the outcome of interest during phases of no treatment and also give insight into the trend and variability of responses to treatment.

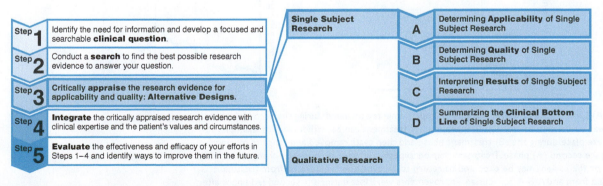

Step **1**	Identify the need for information and develop a focused and searchable **clinical question**.
Step **2**	Conduct a **search** to find the best possible research evidence to answer your question.
Step **3**	Critically **appraise** the research evidence for applicability and quality: **Alternative Designs**.
Step **4**	**Integrate** the critically appraised research evidence with clinical expertise and the patient's values and circumstances.
Step **5**	**Evaluate** the effectiveness and efficacy of your efforts in Steps 1–4 and identify ways to improve them in the future.

Single Subject Research

A — Determining **Applicability** of Single Subject Research
B — Determining **Quality** of Single Subject Research
C — Interpreting **Results** of Single Subject Research
D — Summarizing the **Clinical Bottom Line** of Single Subject Research

Qualitative Research

FIGURE 9.2 Both SSR and qualitative research are useful for clinical decisions.

Design Example 1:

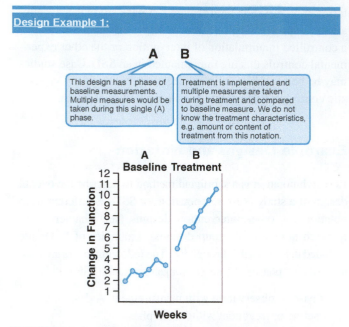

FIGURE 9.3 Data from an A-B SSR design. This design would be appropriate if other "events" were not expected during the (A) baseline phase that might affect the (B) treatment outcome. For example, this design might be used prior to treatment initiation. Measures are taken before treatment is initiated and compared to the measures taken during the treatment phase. This type of design is also appropriate if change is not expected to occur as a result of spontaneous recovery or with maturation during the intervention phase.

RCT With Crossover

A crossover design can also be used with a group of single-subject studies. A subject is randomly assigned to treatment A, the outcome is measured and this is followed by the same subject receiving treatment B with measurements taken after the second treatment. Kluzik et al[3] used this design to detail each subject's responses to two treatments and the aggregate responses of the group of 10 subjects to each treatment and to the treatments combined. There were no significant differences between treatments but there were significant differences when both treatments were combined. They determined that 9 of the 10 subjects benefited from the combined treatments, but one subject became progressively worse during the study. The specific characteristics that might have contributed to poor outcome were analyzed for future treatment recommendations and research.

The explanatory sections that follow are organized by questions to consider when appraising the quality of a single-subject study. We have included these questions in Table 9.1.

Romeiser-Logan et al[1] have also published a set of key questions for the appraisal of SSR. These questions are similar to the questions for group designs (Chapters 3 and 4) with specific questions modified for SSR.

Design Example 2:

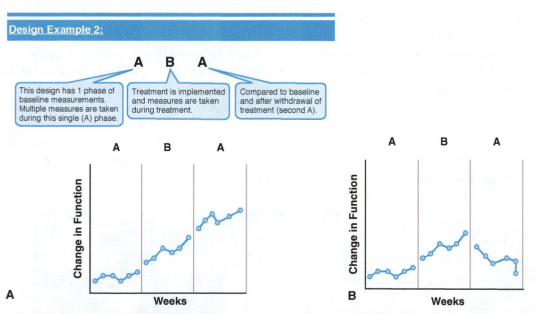

FIGURE 9.4 (A) Data from and A-B-A SSR design. Improvements continued during the second A phase after treatment was withdrawn. This design is appropriate if treatment can be withdrawn. For example, serial casting may take place during the (B) treatment phase and then casts removed and range of motion measured during the second (A) phase. Treatment may be expected to have permanently changed the condition (Fig. 9.4A) or the patient may be expected to return to baseline after withdrawal from treatment (Fig. 9.4B). (B) Data from and A-B-A SSR design. Improvements were lost during the second (A) phase after treatment was withdrawn.

Design Example 3:

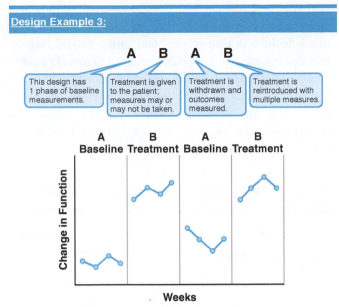

FIGURE 9.5 Data from an A-B-A-B SSR design. Losses may be observed after treatment withdrawal, but may recur when treatment is reintroduced (second A phase). This design is appropriate to more fully determine the effects of treatment. By reintroducing treatment following a phase of withdrawal, it is expected that the treatment effects will again be apparent.

Design Example 4:

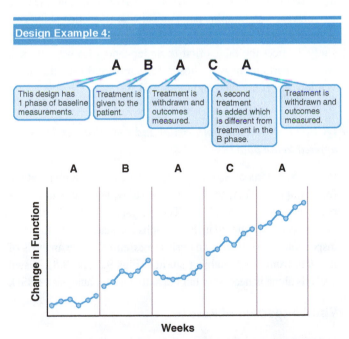

FIGURE 9.6 Data from an A-B-A-C-A SSR design. The effects of a second treatment in combination with the first treatment are measured. This design is appropriate if a combination of treatments offered in a series rather than together might be expected to be beneficial to the patient. For example, the first treatment might be manual therapy treatment given by a physical therapist and the second treatment might be a home exercise program.

■ Appraising SSR Designs

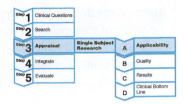

Part A: Determining Applicability of SSR

QUESTION 1: **Is the study's purpose relevant to my clinical question?**

QUESTION 2: **Is the study subject sufficiently similar to my patient to justify the expectation that my patient would respond similarly to the population?**

QUESTION 3: **Are the inclusion and exclusion criteria clearly defined and would my patient qualify for the study?**

The development of evidence based practice (EBP) is largely based on intervention studies that include a large number of individuals. The major advantage of having a large number of subjects in a clinical trial is that it is more likely that differences between treatment effects will be detected when they actually exist. In a group design, at least some of the participants, if not all, will benefit from treatment. However, the disadvantage of this design is the inter-subject variability introduced with a large sample. This in itself may reduce the likelihood of finding a significant difference between the effects of different interventions when they actually exist. In an SSD, the subject acts as his own control, and the participant's baseline and intervention periods are compared to detect possible treatment effects.

Another challenge of RCT designs is the application of study findings from a group to a single patient. We may find that participants in a group study are less like our patient than a participant in a single-subject study. The challenges of applicability for large group studies are described in Chapter 3. A group of patients may have characteristics that are close to those of our patient, but still leave us questioning if the study is truly helpful for the clinical decisions for our specific patient. The trade-off between SSDs and group designs is that the treatment responses of a single participant are not as powerful as the treatment responses from a group of participants.

Part B: Determining the Quality of SSR

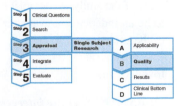

The same systematic appraisal of quality and many of the same quality criteria used to appraise research with group designs are used in the appraisal of SSR. Just as with other experimental designs, measurement must be valid and reliable and other factors that might affect outcomes must be controlled during the study. For example, intervention protocols are specified prior to the study initiation and adhered to as rigorously as in an RCT design.

Rigorous controls in SSR ensure that the study outcomes are the result of treatment and reduce the likelihood that factors other than the intervention under study affected the subject's outcomes. Control of the experimental procedures is a characteristic of all quality research, regardless of design.

Measurement

QUESTION 4: Are the outcome measures relevant to the clinical question and are they conducted in a clinically realistic manner?

As mentioned previously, in SSR measures are taken repeatedly on a single participant over the course of several days or even weeks before intervention is initiated. This allows the investigators to measure natural fluctuations in the outcomes of interest. For example, if strength is a primary outcome of the study, it may be measured every day for a week and the natural fluctuations in strength can be established for the individual participant. With group designs, participants' measurements are typically taken only once at baseline. This single measurement of each participant assumes that the variable being measured is stable and that the measure accurately represents the variable of interest. In our strength example, if an individual tests unusually weak on a given day, this will be considered baseline for that participant in the group. Group study designs accommodate for this by having a large number of individuals; those who measure unusually weak are balanced by those who measure as unusually strong on a given day. Again, the trade-off is a single measurement of many subjects versus multiple measures of a single person.

An important consideration for SSR is the possible impact of multiple measures on the outcome of interest. Practicing a measure may alter a subject's performance on that measure, either positively or negatively. For example, repeatedly measuring a subject's balance may improve performance on that balance measure.

QUESTION 5: Was blinding/masking optimized in the study design (evaluators)?

Therapists must be reliable in their measurements, and the treating therapist should not measure the subject during the study. This blinding is often challenging in an SSD, but it is critical to the rigor of the study. A therapist from another clinic may be asked to be an independent evaluator of the subject at the completion of the study.

Intervention

QUESTION 6: Is the intervention clinically realistic?

QUESTION 7: Are the outcome measures relevant to the clinical question and are they conducted in a clinically realistic manner?

In SSD, the intervention is specific to the participant. Subject characteristics and the specific intervention are typically more fully described, often making it easier to determine if the study outcomes are appropriate for your patient and if the intervention is feasible in your clinic. Many group designs include a standard treatment that is given to each participant in a similar "dose." Alternative group designs create individual treatment for participants in the group and systematically measure the progress of each participant.[2] These studies are more costly and typically take longer to complete, but they do address the issue that no one treatment fits all.

QUESTION 8: Aside from the planned intervention, could other events have contributed to my patient's outcome?

SSDs should be rigorously controlled. This should include monitoring the patient for all possible contributions to outcomes during the study period.

Part C: Interpreting Results of a Single-Subject Research Study

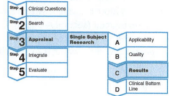

The same process of appraisal of results that we used from group studies can be applied to the results of SSD. The tables in an SSD research article have the relevant demographic and clinical characteristics of the participant as well as the results of the outcomes measured in the study. Inspect the tables first to understand who was studied, why the participant was chosen for study, and how the intervention was conducted and measured.

QUESTION 9: Were both visual and statistical analyses applied to the data?

Published reports of SSR typically include the research notation, for example, A-B-A, to describe the study, and the data are reported according to the phases. The analysis of the results of a single-subject study should include graphs and statistics. Both visual inspection and statistical analysis are *essential* in the analysis of the data from single-subject studies (Figs 9.7 and 9.8). Visual analysis alone is necessary but not sufficient for analysis of SSD.

Visual Inspection of Results

Determining and describing the trend in data are supported with the use of trend line analysis (Fig. 9.8). One common procedure to quantify trends is the celeration line. The *celeration line* is a "best fit" line through the data beginning in the first phase and extending through each phase in the study.[4,5] This technique assumes that the data can be fit with a linear function. Celeration lines assist in describing increasing and decreasing trends in the data. A celeration line is created by computing the median value for each phase of the study beginning with the baseline (A) phase. The median value is marked on the vertical line dividing A and B phases as in Figure 9.8. A line is then drawn from the Y-axis value of the first data point to the horizontal line representing the median value. The celeration line is then extended into the treatment phase (B). This assists in the visual interpretation of the data in the treatment phase in comparison to the data in the baseline phase.

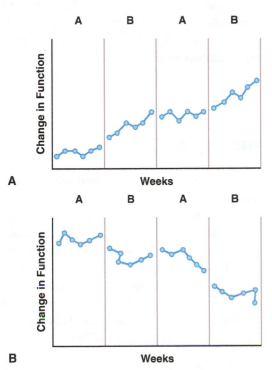

A

B

FIGURE 9.7 Graphs present variable data with an increasing trend (A) and a decreasing trend (B). The data in each phase should be visually inspected for *variability and trend*. The data in Figure 9.7A have considerable variability in each phase of the data, but there is also a somewhat linear increasing trend from the first (A) phase through the second (B) phase. Figure 9.7B graphs variable data with a decreasing trend.

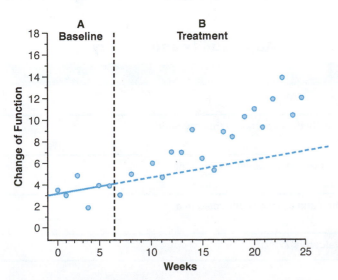

FIGURE 9.8 Celeration line assists in the visual interpretation of the data in the treatment phase in comparison to the data in the baseline phase.

The slope of the celeration line is also a part of the visual interpretation of the data. The direction and pitch of the slope convey the amount and rate of increase or decrease in the data, again assuming a linear trend. The data values at one point, for example, day 1, in the baseline phase (A) is divided into the data value at day 6 of the baseline. In this example, day 1 value is 2 and day 7 value is 4. Thus, the slope can be represented as 0.5. This slope value represents the rate of change during the baseline week, that is, before treatment begins. Slopes for all phases in the study and the slope from the beginning of the study to the end visually capture the nature of change in the outcomes.

Statistical Analysis of Results

QUESTION 10: Were data trends in the baseline removed from the intervention data?

Detrending Data and Serial Dependency

As mentioned, one of the strengths of an SSD is the repeated measures that are taken of each subject during baseline and treatment withdrawal phases and, in some designs, during the treatment phase. Repeated measures provide a description of the natural variation of the variables of interest during the baseline phase, before treatment initiation. Because this natural trend would be expected throughout the study, it must then be removed from the subsequent treatment phase. The trend(s) that remains is then considered the result of the treatment with the natural fluctuation removed. There are a variety of methods to "detrend" the data,[6,7] but the important point in the appraisal of SSD is that this issue has been addressed in the analysis of the results of the study.

As mentioned previously, repeated measurement of an individual has potential drawbacks. Performance may improve or be degraded through the repetition of measurement. The problem for statistical analysis is that repeated measures on the same person create dependency in the data, termed *serial dependency*. Data points from the same person are positively correlated, also termed *autocorrelation*. Autocorrelation can be computed on a data set. As with detrending data, there are a variety of methods to appropriately analyze serial dependency prior to further statistical analysis. Autocorrelation should be analyzed in terms of statistical significance. If autocorrelation values remain significant, then further statistical analysis will be problematic.

Two-Standard Deviation Band

The two-standard deviation band method is a statistic used in combination with celeration line.[4,8] Data must be normally distributed (see Chapter 4) and not have a significant autocorrelation coefficient.[4] Figure 9.9 graphs the two-standard deviation band method. The mean and standard deviation for the baseline data are computed and parallel lines representing +2SD and -2SD are drawn through the baseline and treatment phase data graphs. By convention, if two data points are above or below the 2SD bands in the treatment phase, the change is considered statistically significant.

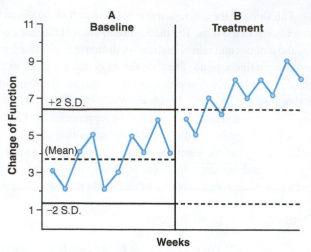

FIGURE 9.9 Two-standard deviation band method. More than two data points fall outside of the +2sd and thus the change would be considered statistically significant.

There are other statistical tests that can be used with single-subject data including computing the statistical significance of a celeration line (in addition to the two-standard deviation band method) and the C statistic.[4,9] Again, the important point for the appraisal of SSR is that the appropriate statistical analyses are included with a visual analysis of the data.

Part D: Summarizing the Clinical Bottom Line

QUESTION 11: Were outcome measures clinically important and meaningful to my patient?

Just as with the outcome of all research, the relevance of the outcomes of SSR is based on what constitutes a successful

intervention from the patient's perspective. Research outcomes may be statistically significant, as we have discussed in previous chapters of this book, but that significant difference may not be clinically relevant. Clinical meaningfulness of the outcomes of research, regardless of design, is relative to each patient. SSR could provide a framework for your clinical practice. Controlled single-case experimental design offers an efficient and clinically valid method for identifying differences in efficacy between treatment forms. Successful implementation of SSR requires the same rigor as implementation of an RCT design, but it is a convenient and effective design to measure the effects of your treatment with your specific patient. Although requiring additional clinical treatment time, an SSR project can be designed and implemented in your clinic to provide systematic data for your practice.

■ Summary of SSR

SSR is an alternative to group design research that can contribute to your clinical decisions. Appraising the applicability and validity of SSR follows the same guidelines as the appraisal process for group designs, with the specific questions modified to fit the reduced number of participants, design alternatives, and statistics for analysis of SSR. Rigorous control of the research process is essential in SSR, just as it is with all research regardless of design. Although SSR requires additional clinic time, it can be conducted in most clinical settings. We have included appraisal questions in Table 9.1.

■ Qualitative Research

Qualitative research focuses on questions of experience, culture, and social/emotional health. Study designs used in qualitative research facilitate understanding of the *processes* that

TABLE 9.1 **Key Questions to Determine an SSR Study's Applicability and Quality**

	YES/NO
Question 1: Is the study's purpose relevant to my clinical question?	
Question 2: Is the study subject sufficiently similar to my patient to justify the expectation that my patient would respond similarly to the population?	
Question 3: Are the inclusion and exclusion criteria clearly defined and would my patient qualify for the study?	
Question 4: Are the outcome measures relevant to the clinical question and are they conducted in a clinically realistic manner?	
Question 5: Was blinding/masking optimized in the study design (evaluators)?	
Question 6: Is the intervention clinically realistic?	

TABLE 9.1 **Key Questions to Determine an SSR Study's Applicability and Quality—cont'd**

	YES/NO
Question 7: Are the outcome measures relevant to the clinical question, and are they conducted in a clinically realistic manner?	
Question 8: Aside from the planned intervention, could other events have contributed to my patient's outcome?	
Question 9: Were both visual and statistical analyses applied to the data?	
Question 10: Were data trends in the baseline removed from the intervention data?	
Question 11: Were outcome measures clinically important and meaningful to my patient?	

are experienced by an individual, group of individuals, or an entire culture of people during everyday life. The design and results of qualitative research are distinctly different from those used in quantitative research, and each type of research is best used based on the nature of the question for study. In a poignant editorial on research in neurodisability, Rosenbaum[10] states, "I hope people will resist the siren call of the RCT simply because it is there—and use the best designs for the 'big' questions we need to answer."

One purpose of qualitative research is to generate hypotheses.[11] This is in contrast to quantitative research in which stated hypotheses are tested. Table 9.2 includes a comparison of qualitative and quantitative research. In quantitative research, tests of statistical inference are used for hypothesis testing. But there are topics of importance to physical therapy that may not have sufficient theoretical development to generate hypotheses. For example, Tyson and De Souza[12] described the lack of a model to adequately define and describe the rehabilitation process. They used a qualitative design that included focus groups of physical therapists to generate themes to define the rehabilitation

process. The themes that emerged could then be developed into a testable model of a generalizable rehabilitation process.

The sections that follow are organized by questions to consider when appraising a study using a qualitative design. Parts A through D have not been applied to these sections because of the different characteristics of qualitative designs and the different types of questions that are posed in the appraisal process. We have included questions in Table 9.3.

■ Appraising Qualitative Research

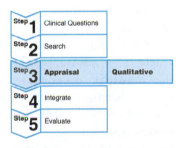

QUESTION 1: Is the study's purpose relevant to my clinical question?

Just as with any study design, the purpose of the study should relate to your question of interest. You may be developing your

TABLE 9.2 **Comparison of Qualitative and Quantitative Research**

QUALITATIVE	QUANTITATIVE
Hypothesis generating; understanding life experiences	Hypothesis testing; establishing causal relations
Example designs: ethnographic, phenomenology, grounded theory, biography	Example designs: RCT, case control, cohort, single subject
Sampling: participants are chosen for a specific purpose; sample size is small and determined by the question and processes under study	Sampling: participants are randomly selected; sample size is critical and can be determined prior to conducting the study
Methods: interviews, focus groups, participant observation, review of documents; all methods are fully described, but control of factors is not primary	Methods: includes a range of procedures but all experimental procedures are highly controlled
Types of data: in-depth descriptions of personal experiences, field notes, records, and documents; no statistical analysis	Types of data: quantifiable and appropriate for statistical analysis; predetermined and controlled

clinical ideas about a patient or population of patients, and qualitative research may assist your clinical reasoning in this process.

Qualitative Research Designs

QUESTION 2: *Was a qualitative approach appropriate?*

There are five general designs used in qualitative research: ethnology, phenomenology, grounded theory, biography, and case study. As in quantitative research, the design is chosen based on the best fit between the research question and research design. The three most common designs, phenomenology, ethnology, and grounded theory, are detailed in the text that follows and include examples.

Phenomenology

Phenomenology is useful to study experiences in life. Bendez[13] studied the life experience of having a stroke. She interviewed 15 patients during the first year post-stroke and reviewed the documentation of their health-care professionals. Themes were identified through patient interviews and included loss of control, fatigue, and fear of relapse. Although health-care professionals also identified these themes, they ignored these aspects in their documentation of the rehabilitation process. The phenomenological design was used to understand and interpret lived experiences and provide information from the people as they were living the experience. From these personal perspectives, it is often possible to generate insights into themes that may not be revealed with quantitative research or through clinical treatment.

Ethnology

Ethnology study design is typically used to study questions in anthropology. Questions of group behavior including daily life patterns, attitudes, and beliefs during rehabilitation could be studied with this design. Kirk-Sanchez[14] studied the factors related to activity limitations in a group of Cuban Americans recovering from hip fractures. They used extensive interviews as well as questionnaires to understand the psychosocial determinants of activity limitations in this group during the process of recovery from fracture.

Grounded Theory

Grounded theory design is used to construct or validate a theory. Researchers focus on core processes in a given life experience and develop a theoretical model to represent the processes. Again, these models might generate a hypothesis that could then be tested with a quantitative design. Gustafsson et al[15] used the grounded theory design to study chronic pain. The study provided validation for the theory that the rehabilitation process begins the process of change from shame to respect for women with chronic pain. They conducted semistructured interviews of 16 females who were experiencing chronic pain. They grounded their theoretical perspective in the real world of people with chronic pain experiencing the rehabilitation process.

QUESTION 3: *Was the sampling strategy clearly defined and justified?*

Qualitative research includes an in-depth study of a specific topic, typically with a small and select group of participants. Random selection of participants is not a part of qualitative study sampling; rather, participants are selected specifically because they can contribute to the understanding of a topic. Petursdottir et al[16] studied the experience of exercising for patients with osteoarthritis (OA). They conducted purposive sampling and chose 12 participants who they believed would have sufficient experience with OA and exercise to inform their research question. All participants had a diagnosis of OA for at least 5 years, and they were all over age 50, capable of a dialogue with the researcher, and willing to share their experiences. Lyons and Tickle-Degnen[17] also purposively sampled and chose four participants, two males and two females with varying amounts of experience with their diagnosis of Parkinson's disease (PD). The goal of their research was to explore the social challenges experienced by people with PD. These researchers anticipated that different issues would emerge with disease progression. The samples in both of these examples were *selected* based on the particular population, culture, and experiences that could inform the specific goals of the research.

QUESTION 4: *What methods did the researcher use for collecting data?*

Valid qualitative research is rigorously conducted and reported. The methods used for collecting and analyzing data must be thoroughly reported so that a complete understanding of the processes used in the qualitative study is achieved and the context for the study is detailed. Various data collection methods, including triangulation, add to the rigor of the study.

Triangulation is the use of different perspectives to study the identified process.[18] For example individuals from three different professions might serve as interviewers, or multiple methods such as interviews, focus groups, and records review might be used within a single study. The triangulation method strengthens a qualitative study's results by investigating the process under study from different perspectives.

QUESTION 5: What methods did the researcher use to analyze the data, and what quality control measures were implemented?

Member checking is a method to verify that the investigator has adequately represented the participant's contributions to the question under study.[18] The investigator may share preliminary drafts of the interpretation of the participant's interview and then revise the draft with further comment from the participant.

QUESTION 6: What are the results, and do they address the research question? Are the results credible?

QUESTION 7: What conclusions were drawn and are they justified by the results? In particular, have alternative explanations for the results been explored?

The results of a qualitative study should be reviewed in light of the overall purpose of the study. Data may be expressed in terms of a narrative from subjects around specific themes that were identified and that occurred across subjects. Because qualitative research often generates hypotheses to be explored, you may search for follow-up quantitative research that may have tested these hypotheses.

■ Summary of Qualitative Research

Qualitative research focuses on questions of experience, culture, and social/emotional health. The designs used in qualitative research emphasize the *processes* that are experienced by an individual, group of individuals, or an entire culture of people during everyday life. Both qualitative and quantitative research are used to address important questions in physical therapist practice. There is no hierarchy of best type of research design. The design features must fit the nature of the research question under consideration. Qualitative research has yielded rich insights into rehabilitation processes that emerge from individuals and group experiences of daily life events. We have included questions in Table 9.3.

TABLE 9.3 **Key Questions for Appraisal of Qualitative Research**

	YES	NO
1. Is the study's purpose relevant to my clinical question?		
2. Was a qualitative approach appropriate? Consider: Does the research seek to understand or illuminate the experiences and/or views of those taking part?		
3. Was the sampling strategy clearly defined and justified? Consider: • Has the method of sampling (subjects and setting) been adequately described? • Have the investigators studied the most useful or productive range of individuals and settings relevant to their question? • Have the characteristics of the subjects been defined? • Is it clear why some participants chose not to take part?		
4. What methods did the researcher use for collecting data? Consider: • Have appropriate data sources been studied? • Have the methods used for data collection been described in enough detail to allow the reader to determine the presence of any bias? • Was more than one method of data collection used (e.g., triangulation)? • Were the methods used reliable and independently verifiable (e.g., audiotape, videotape, field notes)? • Were observations taken in a range of circumstances (e.g., at different times)?		
5. What methods did the researcher use to analyze the data, and what quality control measures were implemented? Consider: • How were themes and concepts derived from the data? • Did more than one researcher perform the analysis, and what method was used to resolve differences of interpretation? • Were negative or discrepant results fully addressed, or just ignored?		

Continued

TABLE 9.3 **Key Questions for Appraisal of Qualitative Research—cont'd**

	YES	NO
6. What are the results, and do they address the research question? Are the results credible?		
7. What conclusions were drawn, and are they justified by the results? In particular, have alternative explanations for the results been explored?		

Data from: Critical Appraisal Skills Programme (CASP), Public Health Resource Unit, Institute of Health Science, Oxford.
Greenhalgh T. Papers that go beyond numbers (qualitative research). In: Dept. of General Practice, University of Glasgow.
How to Read a Paper. The Basics of Evidence Based Medicine. London, England: BMJ Publishing Group; 1997.

REVIEW QUESTIONS

1. State one advantage of an SSD over a group design.

2. State one advantage of a group design over an SSD.

3. Why is visual inspection necessary but not sufficient for the reporting of an SSR?

4. How is the choice made between a using a quantitative versus qualitative research design?

REFERENCES

1. Romeiser-Logan LR, Hickman RR, Harris SR, et al. Single-subject research design: recommendations for levels of evidence and quality rating. *Dev Med Child Neurol.* 2008;50:99–103.
2. Størvold GV, Jahnsen R. Intensive motor skills training program combining group and individual sessions for children with cerebral palsy. *Pediatr Phys Ther.* 2010;22:150–159
3. Kluzik J, Fetters L, Coryell J. Quantification of control: a preliminary study of effects of neurodevelopmental treatment on reaching in children with spastic cerebral palsy. *Phys Ther.* 1990;70:65–68.
4. Ottenbacher KJ. *Evaluating Clinical Change. Strategies for Occupational and Physical Therapists.* Baltimore, MD: Williams & Wilkins; 1986.
5. White OR, Haring NG. *Exceptional Teaching.* 2nd ed. Columbus, OH: Charles E. Merrill; 1980.
6. Campbell JM. Statistical comparison of four effect sizes for single-subject designs. *Behav Modif.* 2004;28:234–246.
7. Allison DB, Faith MS, Franklin RD. Antecedent exercise in the treatment of disruptive behavior: a meta-analytic review. *Clin Psychol.* 1995;2:279–303.
8. Miller EW, Combs SA, Fish C, et al. Running training after stroke: a single-subject report. *Phys Ther.* 2008;88:511–522.
9. Tryon WW. A simplified time-series analysis for evaluating treatment interventions. *J Appl Behav Anal.* 1995;15:423–429.
10. Rosenbaum P. The randomized controlled trial: an excellent design, but can it address the big questions in neurodisability? *Dev Med Child Neurol.* 2010;52:111.
11. Giacomini MK, Cook DJ. Users' guides to the medical literature: XXIII. Qualitative research in health care A. Are the results of the study valid? Evidence-Based Medicine Working Group. *JAMA.* 2000;284:357–362.
12. Tyson SF, DeSouza LH. A clinical model for the assessment of posture and balance in people with stroke. *Disabil Rehabil.* 2003;25:120–126.
13. Bendz M. The first year of rehabilitation after a stroke—from two perspectives. *Scand J Caring Sci.* 2003;17:215–222.
14. Kirk-Sanchez NJ. Factors related to activity limitations in a group of Cuban Americans before and after hip fracture. *Phys Ther.* 2004;84: 408–418.
15. Gustafsson M, Ekholm J, Ohman A. From shame to respect: musculoskeletal pain patients' experience of a rehabilitation programme, a qualitative study. *J Rehabil Med.* 2004;36:97–103.
16. Petursdottir U, Arnadottir SA, Halldorsdottir S. Facilitators and barriers to exercising among people with osteoarthritis: a phenomenological study. *Phys Ther.* 2010;90:1014–1025.
17. Lyons KD, Tickle-Degnen L. Dramaturgical challenges of Parkinson's disease. *Occup Ther J Res.* 2003;23:27–34.
18. Giacomini MK, Cook DJ. Users' guides to the medical literature: XXIII. Qualitative research in health care B. What are the results and how do they help me care for my patients? Evidence-Based Medicine Working Group. *JAMA.* 2000;284:478–482.

10 | Appraising Research Studies of Outcome Measures

PRE-TEST

1. State three or more psychometric properties that are commonly reported in studies of outcome measures.

2. State two important characteristics to consider when appraising the applicability of a study of an outcome measure.

3. State two types of outcome measure reliability that are studied.

4. Describe two important design features you consider when appraising the quality of a reliability study.

5. State two types of outcome measure validity that are studied.

6. State important design features to consider when appraising the quality of a criterion-related study of outcome measure validity.

CHAPTER-AT-A-GLANCE

This chapter will help you understand the following:

- The different psychometric properties of clinical outcome measures that are studied

- The types of studies used to assess outcome measure psychometric properties

- Appraisal of studies that assess outcome measure reliability, quality, and clinical meaningfulness

- Interpretation of the results of studies of outcome measure reliability, validity, and clinical meaningfulness

Introduction

This chapter addresses the appraisal of studies of outcome measures. Outcome measures provide information about patients and their progress. Choosing appropriate outcome measures for your patients is critical to understanding their status and progress over time. Ideally, the psychometric properties of an outcome measure used in practice have been developed and tested through a series of research studies. **Psychometric properties** are the intrinsic properties of an outcome measure and include reliability, validity, and clinical meaningfulness (Fig. 10.1). Understanding the research used to develop and assess outcome measure psychometric properties empowers you to select and use outcome measures effectively in your practice.

We begin this chapter by defining common features of outcome measures and describing the different categories of outcome measures that you are likely to encounter in clinical practice, that is, questionnaires and performance-based measures. This chapter does not focus on the appropriate use of outcome measures in a particular research study; rather, we focus on how you can use the appraisal process to determine whether a study of an outcome measure is applicable, valid, and clinically useful. We review the appraisal of studies of reliability, validity, and clinical meaningfulness of outcome studies and provide corresponding checklists of appraisal with key questions in Tables 10.6, 10.8, and 10.9.

Types and Utility of Outcome Measures

What Is an Outcome Measure?

An outcome measure is any characteristic or quality measured to assess a patient's status. Outcome measures are commonly collected at the beginning, middle, and end of a course of physical therapy care. Outcome measures that you are likely to encounter in clinical practice can be divided into two categories: (1) questionnaires and (2) performance-based measures. Questionnaires require that either a therapist interviews a patient or the patient independently completes the questionnaire. Questionnaires are typically scored by applying a pre-set point system to the patient's answers. Performance-based measures require the patient to perform a set of movements or tasks. Scores for performance-based measures can be based on either an objective measurement (e.g., time to complete a task) or a

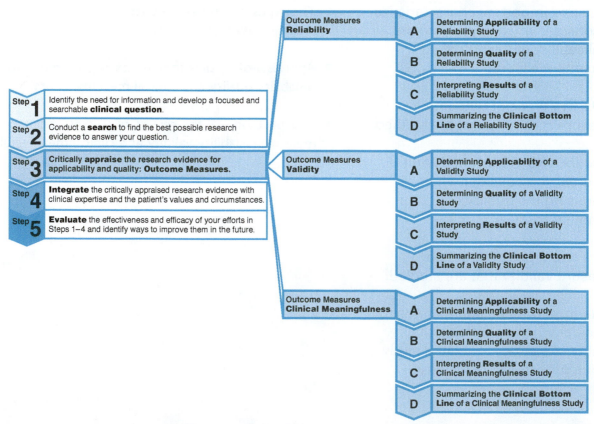

FIGURE 10.1 The appraisal process for studies of reliability, validity, and clinical meaningfulness of outcome measures.

qualitative assessment that is assigned a score (e.g., normal or abnormal mechanics for a given task).

Two commonly used outcome measures are shown in Figure 10.2. The modified Oswestry Disability Questionnaire[1] (Fig. 10.2A) uses a series of questions to measure disability associated with low back pain. The Berg Balance Scale[2] (Fig. 10.2B) is a performance-based measure of balance. Note that the Oswestry Disability Questionnaire is a series of

questions answered by the patient, whereas the Berg Balance Scale requires the patient to physically perform a series of tasks that are then characterized by the therapist.

Outcome measures can also be classified according to one or more components of the International Classification of Functioning, Disability and Health (ICF):[3] body structures and functions, activity, and/or participation (see Chapter 2). Table 10.1 categorizes example outcome measures used

Modified Low Back Pain Disability Questionnaire

This questionnaire has been designed to give your therapist information as to how your back pain has affected your ability to manage in everyday life. Please answer every question by placing a mark in the **one** box that best describes your condition today. We realize you may feel that two of the statements may describe your condition, but **please mark only the box that most closely describes your current condition**.

Pain Intensity
- ❑ I can tolerate the pain I have without having to use pain medication.
- ❑ The pain is bad, but I can manage without having to take pain medication.
- ❑ Pain medication provides me with complete relief from pain.
- ❑ Pain medication provides me with moderate relief from pain.
- ❑ Pain medication provides me with little relief from pain.
- ❑ Pain medication has no effect on my pain.

Personal Care (e.g. Washing, Dressing)
- ❑ I can take care of myself normally without causing increased pain.
- ❑ I can take care of myself normally, but it increases my pain.
- ❑ It is painful to take care of myself, and I am slow and careful.
- ❑ I need help, but I am able to manage most of my personal care.
- ❑ I need help every day in most aspects of my care.
- ❑ I do not get dressed, I wash with difficulty, and I stay in bed.

Lifting
- ❑ I can lift heavy weights without increased pain.
- ❑ I can lift heavy weights, but it causes increased pain.
- ❑ Pain prevents me from lifting heavy weights off the floor, but I can manage if the weights are conveniently positioned (e.g., on a table).
- ❑ Pain prevents me from lifting heavy weights, but I can manage light to medium weights if they are conveniently positioned.
- ❑ I can lift only very light weights.
- ❑ I cannot lift or carry anything at all.

Walking
- ❑ Pain does not prevent me from walking any distance.
- ❑ Pain prevents me from walking more than 1 mile.
- ❑ Pain prevents me from walking more than 1/2 mile.
- ❑ Pain prevents me from walking more than 1/4 mile.
- ❑ I can walk only with crutches or a cane.
- ❑ I am in bed most of the time and have to crawl to the toilet.

Sitting
- ❑ I can sit in any chair as long as I like.
- ❑ I can only sit in my favorite chair as long as I like.
- ❑ Pain prevents me from sitting for more than 1 hour.
- ❑ Pain prevents me from sitting for more than 1/2 hour.
- ❑ Pain prevents me from sitting for more than 10 minutes.
- ❑ Pain prevents me from sitting at all.

Standing
- ❑ I can stand as long as I want without increased pain.
- ❑ I can stand as long as I want, but it increases my pain.
- ❑ Pain prevents me from standing for more than 1 hour.
- ❑ Pain prevents me from standing for more than 1/2 hour.
- ❑ Pain prevents me from standing for more than 10 minutes.
- ❑ Pain prevents me from standing at all.

Sleeping
- ❑ Pain does not prevent me from sleeping well.
- ❑ I can sleep well only by using pain medication.
- ❑ Even when I take medication, I sleep less than 6 hours.
- ❑ Even when I take medication, I sleep less than 4 hours.
- ❑ Even when I take medication, I sleep less than 2 hours.
- ❑ Pain prevents me from sleeping at all.

Social Life
- ❑ My social life is normal and does not increase my pain.
- ❑ My social life is normal, but it increases my level of pain.
- ❑ Pain prevents me from participating in more energetic activities (e.g., sports, dancing).
- ❑ Pain prevents me from going out very often.
- ❑ Pain has restricted my social life to my home.
- ❑ I have hardly any social life because of my pain.

Traveling
- ❑ I can travel anywhere without increased pain.
- ❑ I can travel anywhere, but it increases my pain.
- ❑ My pain restricts my travel over 2 hours.
- ❑ My pain restricts my travel over 1 hour.
- ❑ My pain restricts my travel to short necessary journeys under 1/2 hour.
- ❑ My pain prevents all travel except for visits to the physician/therapist or hospital.

Employment/Homemaking
- ❑ My normal homemaking/job activities do not cause pain.
- ❑ My normal homemaking/job activities increase my pain, but I can still perform all that is required of me.
- ❑ I can perform most of my homemaking/job duties, but pain prevents me from performing more physically stressful activities (e.g., lifting, vacuuming).
- ❑ Pain prevents me from doing anything but light duties.
- ❑ Pain prevents me from doing even light duties.
- ❑ Pain prevents me from performing any job or homemaking chores.

FIGURE 10.2 (A) Modified Oswestry Disability Questionnaire. *Modified by: Fritz & Irrgang. The Chartered Society of Physiotherapy, from Fairbanks JCT, Couper J, Davies JB, et al. The Oswestry Low Back Pain Disability Questionnaire. Physiotherapy. 1980;66:271–273; with permission.*

Continued

Berg Balance Test

INSTRUCTIONS: Demonstrate each task and/or give instructions as written. When scoring, record the lowest response category for each item. Patient cannot use an assistive device for this test.

1. Sitting to Standing: Please stand up
Instructions: Try not to use your hands for support.
- ❏ 4 Able to stand independently, does not use hands and is stable
- ❏ 3 Able to stand independently using hands
- ❏ 2 Able to stand using hands after several tries
- ❏ 1 Needs min assistance to stand or stabilize
- ❏ 0 Needs mod-max assistance to stabilize

2. Standing Unsupported
Instructions: Stand for 2 minutes without holding onto anything.
- ❏ 4 Stands safely for 2 minutes
- ❏ 3 Stands for 2 minutes with supervision
- ❏ 2 Stands unsupported for < 2 minutes
- ❏ 1 Needs several tries to stand 30 seconds
- ❏ 0 Unable to stand 30 seconds unassisted

3. Standing to Sitting: Please sit down
Instructions: Try to use your hands as little as possible.
- ❏ 4 Sits with minimal use of hands
- ❏ 3 Controls descent with hands
- ❏ 2 Uses back of legs against chair to control descent
- ❏ 1 Sits independently but has uncontrolled descent
- ❏ 0 Needs assistance to sit

4. Sitting Unsupported with Feet on Floor
Instructions: Sit with your arms folded across chest for 2 minutes.
- ❏ 4 Sits safely for 2 minutes
- ❏ 3 Sits 2 minutes with supervision
- ❏ 2 Sits 30 seconds
- ❏ 1 Sits 10 seconds
- ❏ 0 Unable to sit for 10 seconds unsupervised

5. Transfers
Instructions: Please move from the chair you are sitting in to the other chair (place chairs at 45° angle, one chair with arm rests, one without).
- ❏ 4 Transfers safely with minimal use of hands
- ❏ 3 Transfers safely with definite need of hands
- ❏ 2 Transfers with verbal cues or supervision
- ❏ 1 Needs 1 person assist or supervision for safety
- ❏ 0 Needs 2 person assist

6. Standing Unsupported with Eyes Closed
Instructions: Stand with feet shoulder-width apart. Close your eyes and stand still for 10 seconds.
- ❏ 4 Stands for 10 seconds safely
- ❏ 3 Stands for 10 seconds with supervision
- ❏ 2 Stands 3 seconds
- ❏ 1 Unable to keep eyes closed for 3 seconds but stays steady
- ❏ 0 Needs help to keep from falling

7. Standing Unsupported with Feet Together
Instructions: Place your feet together and stand without holding. Hold for 1 minute.
- ❏ 4 Able to place feet together independently and stand 1 minute safely
- ❏ 3 Places feet together independently and stands for 1 min with supervision
- ❏ 2 Places feet together independently but unable to hold for 30 seconds
- ❏ 1 Needs help to attain position but able to stand for 15 seconds
- ❏ 0 Needs help to attain position and unable to hold for 15 seconds

8. Reaching Forward with Outstretched Arm
Instructions: Raise your arm to shoulder height and reach forward with your fist as far as you can.
- ❏ 4 Greater than 10 inches
- ❏ 3 Greater than 5 inches
- ❏ 2 Greater than 2 inches
- ❏ 1 Reaches forward but needs supervision
- ❏ 0 Needs help to keep from falling

9. Pick Up Object from Floor
Instructions: Please pick up plastic cup. (Place on floor 6-12 inches in front of feet.)
- ❏ 4 Able to pick up safely and easily
- ❏ 3 Able to pick up but needs supervision
- ❏ 2 Unable to pick up but reaches 1-2 inches from object and keeps balance independently
- ❏ 1 Unable to pick up and needs supervision while trying
- ❏ 0 Unable to try or tries and needs assist to keep from falling

10. Turn to Look Behind over Left and Right Shoulders
Instructions: Turn to look behind you over toward the left shoulder without moving your feet. Repeat with the right.
- ❏ 4 Looks behind from both sides and weight shifts well
- ❏ 3 Looks behind one side only, other side shows less weight shift
- ❏ 2 Turns sideways only but maintains balance
- ❏ 1 Needs supervision while turning
- ❏ 0 Needs assistance to keep from falling

11. Turning 360°
Turn completely around in full circle. Pause. Now turn in the other direction.
- ❏ 4 Turns full circle in < 4 seconds each side.
- ❏ 3 Turns safely to only one side in < 4 seconds
- ❏ 2 Turns safely but slowly
- ❏ 1 Needs close supervision or verbal cuing
- ❏ 0 Needs assist while turning

12. Dynamic Weight Shifting while Standing Unsupported
Instructions: Place each foot alternately on the stool for a count of 8 (demonstrate with foot flat; count touches).
- ❏ 4 Completes 8 steps in 20 seconds safely
- ❏ 3 Completes 8 steps in > 20 seconds
- ❏ 2 Completes 4 steps without aid and with supervision
- ❏ 1 Able to complete > 2 steps, needs min assist
- ❏ 0 Needs assist to keep from falling/unable to try

13. Standing Unsupported One Foot in Front
Instructions: Place one foot directly in front of other as close as possible and hold for 30 sec.
- ❏ 4 Places foot in tandem independently and holds 30 seconds
- ❏ 3 Places one foot in front of other independently and holds for 30 seconds
- ❏ 2 Takes small step independently and holds for 30 seconds
- ❏ 1 Needs help to place foot, holds 15 seconds
- ❏ 0 Loses balance while stepping or standing

14. Standing on One Leg
Instructions: Stand on one leg for as long as you can without holding.
- ❏ 4 Lifts leg independently and holds > 10 seconds
- ❏ 3 Lifts leg independently and holds 5-10 seconds
- ❏ 2 Lifts leg independently and holds ≥ 3 seconds
- ❏ 1 Tries to lift leg, unable to hold 3s but remains standing independently
- ❏ 0 Unable to try or needs assist to prevent fall

Total Score: _____ **(maximum = 56)**

FIGURE 10.2 cont'd (B) The Berg Balance Scale. *From: Berg KO, Wood-Dauphinee SL, Williams JI, et al. Measuring balance in the elderly: validation of an instrument. Can J Public Health. 1992;83(suppl 2):7–11; with permission.*

TABLE 10.1 **Types of Outcome Measures**

OUTCOME MEASURE	QUESTIONNAIRE OR PERFORMANCE BASED	WHAT IT MEASURES	ICF LEVEL MEASURED
Geriatric Depression Scale[8]	Questionnaire	Screens for depression in older adults	Body function
Mini-Mental State Exam[26]	Performance-based	Cognitive function	Body function
Activities-Specific Balance Confidence Scale (ABC Scale)[27]	Questionnaire	Balance confidence	Activity
10-Meter Walk Test[28]	Performance-based	Walking speed	Activity
Pediatric Evaluation of Disability Inventory (PEDI)[29]	Questionnaire	Children's functional capabilities	Activity
Neck Disability Index[4]	Questionnaire	Impact of neck pain on life participation	Participation
Oswestry Disability Questionnaire[14]	Questionnaire	Impact of low back pain on life participation	Participation

ICF = International Classification of Functioning, Disability and Health.

in physical therapy practice by type (questionnaire or performance-based) and the ICF characteristic measured.

What Makes an Outcome Measure Useful in the Clinic?

To be clinically useful, an outcome measure must be applicable to your patient population and demonstrate high-quality psychometric properties. A general definition and example of reliability, validity, and clinical meaningfulness are as follows:

- **Reliability refers to an outcome measure's consistency in score production.** For example, if you and a colleague use the Berg Balance Scale for the same patient on the same day, you should get a similar score. This is an example of **inter-tester reliability** as described in Chapter 4. We explore several types of outcome measure reliability studies in the next section of this chapter.
- **Validity refers to an outcome measure's ability to measure the characteristic or feature that it is intended to measure.** For example, if you choose the Neck Disability Index[4] to measure the impact of neck pain on a patient's ability to participate in life roles, it is important to know whether the Neck Disability Index actually measures the impact of neck pain on participation in life roles. This is an example of **content validity.** We explore several types of validity later in this chapter.
- **Clinical meaningfulness refers to an outcome measure's ability to provide the clinician and the patient with consequential information.** For example, if you used the 10-meter walk to measure a patient's walking speed before and after therapy, you might question the relationship

between improvement in walking speed and your patient's ability to function in daily life. This is an example of a measure's meaningfulness. We explore several measures of clinical meaningfulness later in this chapter.

These three psychometric properties of outcome measures are typically studied separately. Therefore, in this chapter we describe the appraisal process for studies of reliability, validity, and clinical meaningfulness separately.

■ Studies That Assess Outcome Measure Reliability

Types of Reliability and Terms Associated With Reliability Studies

A variety of study designs are used to explore outcome measure reliability. We explore four different types of reliability and the study designs used to assess them. The first two types of reliability, **internal consistency** and **test-retest reliability,** quantify the consistency of the measure itself, whereas the second two, **intra-rater** and **inter-rater** reliability, quantify the consistency of the raters who conduct the test.[5] Ideally, an outcome measure will have published research studies that address all four types of reliability.

Internal Consistency

Internal consistency establishes the extent to which multiple items within an outcome measure (e.g., the 14 items of the Berg Balance Scale) reflect the same construct. For example, the Berg Balance Scale is intended to measure one construct, balance. To determine internal consistency of the scale, inter-item correlation is commonly assessed using the Cronbach alpha statistical test. Cronbach alpha scores range from 0 to 1. Scores close to 0 indicate that individual items of the measure do not correlate with each other. Scores close to 1 indicate that the individual items have strong correlation. Although somewhat arbitrary, a general rule of thumb is that Cronbach alpha scores should be greater than 0.70 and less than 0.90. Values greater than 0.90 suggest repetition (excessive correlation) between items in an outcome measure.[6]

Continuing with our example, the Berg Balance Scale has demonstrated high internal consistency among older adults with a Cronbach alpha score of 0.83 and for persons with stroke with a Cronbach alpha score of 0.97.[7] These scores indicate that the 14 items are all measuring a very similar construct, in this case, balance for the two populations. In fact, based on the score of 0.97, there may be items that are too similar for persons with stroke—measuring essentially the same balance skill. This finding could present the opportunity for researchers to study the psychometric properties of a shorter version of the test for persons with stroke.

Table 10.2 includes two hypothetical measures of cognitive function, one with low internal consistency and the other with high internal consistency. Scores on the items for Cognitive Test 1 are not consistently high or low for patient A or patient B, illustrating low internal consistency. Scores on the items for Cognitive Test 2 are more consistent. Patient A tends to score high (4s and 5s) on all three items and patient B tends to score low (0–2); hence, the test illustrates high internal consistency.

Test-Retest Reliability

Test-retest reliability establishes the extent to which an outcome measure produces the same result when repeatedly applied to a patient who has not experienced change in the characteristic being measured. For example, if a patient's balance has not changed between Monday and Friday of the same week, the patient's score on a balance measure should be essentially the same on Monday and again on Friday. In a test-retest study, one rater measures the same participants two or more times, usually over several days. Participants chosen for the study should be expected to remain the same or similar in the characteristic being measured. For performance-based tests the rater is usually a clinician (e.g., physical therapist). For questionnaires, the participant (e.g., patient) may self-administer the test and therefore serve a self-rater. Consistency of scores is analyzed to quantify test-retest reliability.

Table 10.3 includes two hypothetical measures of balance confidence. Balance Confidence Test 1 illustrates low test-retest reliability because scores for participants vary substantially from day to day. Balance Confidence Test 2 illustrates high test-retest reliability because scores, although not exactly the same, are similar from day to day for each patient.

Intra-Rater Reliability

Intra-rater reliability refers to the consistency with which an outcome measure produces the same score when used by the same therapist on the same patient. Intra-rater reliability is important in clinical practice to compare outcomes taken by the same rater over time, for example, at the beginning and end of a course of therapy.

Studies of intra-rater reliability involve raters (e.g., physical therapists) who are asked to conduct an outcome measure two or more times on the same individual(s), usually over several days. The consistency of each individual rater's scores is assessed to determine intra-rater reliability. Some studies establish test-retest reliability and intra-rater reliability concurrently. The difference between the two psychometric properties is that test-retest reliability refers only to the outcome measure itself, whereas intra-rater reliability specifically addresses the skills of the raters conducting the test. For this reason, a high-quality

TABLE 10.2 **Hypothetical Outcome Measures With High and Low Internal Consistency**

COGNITIVE TEST 1 LOW INTERNAL CONSISTENCY		COGNITIVE TEST 2 HIGH INTERNAL CONSISTENCY	
Patient A	Patient B	Patient A	Patient B
Item scores from 0 (low) – 5 (high) function		Item scores from 0 (low) – 5 (high) function	
Item 1	5	0	Item 1	5	0
Item 2	1	5	Item 2	5	1
Item 3	4	2	Item 3	4	2

TABLE 10.3 **Hypothetical Outcome Measures With High and Low Test-Retest Reliability**

Two measures of balance confidence
(0 = No confidence, 100 = perfect confidence)

	MONDAY	WEDNESDAY	FRIDAY
Balance Confidence Test 1: Low Test-retest Reliability			
Participant 1	80	92	75
Participant 2	25	45	65
Balance Confidence Test 2: High Internal Consistency			
Participant 1	85	87	83
Participant 2	34	34	31

intra-rater reliability study will investigate the intra-rater reliability of several different raters. In contrast, test-retest reliability can be established with just one rater.

Table 10.4 illustrates the results of a hypothetical study of intra-rater reliability for two therapists. Between the two therapists, therapist 1 has lower intra-rater reliability, with large differences in scores from day 1 to day 2 for each patient. In contrast, therapist 2 demonstrates higher intra-rater reliability, with smaller differences in scores from day 1 to day 2 for each patient.

Inter-Rater Reliability

Inter-rater reliability refers to the consistency with which different raters produce the same score for the same patient. This psychometric property is important in clinical practice. If you know that a certain outcome measure has high inter-rater reliability, you can have more confidence comparing your measurements with those of a colleague. For example, consider a situation in which your patients with total knee arthroplasty typically achieve knee flexion range of motion of 90 degrees after 1 week of therapy. However, when your colleague measures the same patients, they achieve 100 degrees of flexion. To determine why this is occurring, it would be helpful to know the inter-rater reliability of knee flexion range-of-motion measurement after total knee arthroplasty. In addition to reviewing studies of goniometry inter-rater reliability, you and your colleague would want to compare personal measurement techniques to improve inter-rater reliability within your clinic.

Studies of inter-rater reliability ask two or more raters to rate the same patients. The study should include patients with scores that span the range of possible scores for the measure. The consistency of scores between different raters is computed to determine the reliability between raters. When inter-rater reliability is low, there is wide variability in the scores. When inter-rater reliability is high, there is little variability.

Table 10.5 illustrates hypothetical athletic ability scores recorded by two therapists (A and B) for three soccer players. Comparing the two measures, therapists using the Athletic Ability Measure 1 demonstrate lower inter-rater reliability—the differences in scores between therapists A and B are 15 to 30 points. In contrast, the same therapists using the Athletic Ability Measure 2 demonstrate higher inter-rater reliability—the differences in scores between therapists A and B are relatively small, 0 to 4 points.

Appraising the Quality of Studies of an Outcome Measure's Reliability

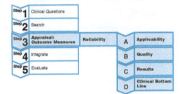

As we have described in previous chapters, appraisal is the third step in the five-step evidence based practice (EBP) process. In this section of the chapter, we describe the process of appraising the literature about the reliability of outcome measures, completing all four parts of appraisal: Part A: Determining Applicability of a Reliability Study, Part B: Determining the Quality of a Reliability Study, Part C: Interpreting Results of a Reliability Study, and Part D: Summarizing the Clinical Bottom Line.

Part A: Determining Applicability of a Reliability Study

Determining the applicability of a reliability study is similar to this determination for other study types. Four questions you should answer when appraising the applicability of studies of reliability (Questions 1–4) are provided and discussed in Table 10.6.

Part B: Determining the Quality of a Reliability Study

The important questions to ask about quality for a reliability study are different from those discussed in Chapter 4 for intervention studies. Table 10.6 describes important questions (questions 5–10) to ask about the quality of studies of outcome measure reliability and why they matter.

TABLE 10.4 Outcome Measures With High and Low Intra-Rater Reliability

Outcome Measure: 10-meter walk test of gait speed
Time elapsed to walk 10 meters was measured on two consecutive days by each therapist. Participants were not expected to experience a change in gait speed.

	THERAPIST 1 LOW INTRA-RATER RELIABILITY			THERAPIST 2 HIGH INTRA-RATER RELIABILITY		
	Day 1	Day 2	Difference	Day 1	Day 2	Difference
Patient 1	15 sec.	10 sec.	−5	15 sec.	13 sec.	−2 sec.
Patient 2	20 sec.	25 sec.	+5	25 sec.	27 sec.	+2 sec.
Patient 3	30 sec.	20 sec.	−10	31 sec.	29 sec.	−2 sec.

TABLE 10.5 **Outcome Measures With High and Low Inter-Rater Reliability**

Outcome Measure: Two hypothetical measures of athletic ability in soccer players
Scores range from 0 (very low athletic ability) to 100 (very high athletic ability)
- Each test is conducted by Therapist A and is video taped.
- Therapist B watches the video tape and scores each test.

	ATHLETIC ABILITY MEASURE 1 LOW INTER-RATER RELIABILITY			ATHLETIC ABILITY MEASURE 2 HIGH INTER-RATER RELIABILITY		
	Therapist A	Therapist B	Difference	Therapist A	Therapist B	Difference
Patient 1	50	70	20	60	64	4
Patient 2	80	65	15	70	69	1
Patient 3	20	50	30	50	50	0

TABLE 10.6 **Key Questions for Appraising Studies of Outcome Measure Reliability**

QUESTION	ANSWER	WHY IT MATTERS
1. Is the study's purpose relevant to my clinical question?	Yes____ No____	If the purpose of the study is not relevant to your question, it is unlikely to be applicable.
2. Are the inclusion and exclusion criteria clearly defined and would my patient qualify for the study?	Yes____ No____	Ideally, the study inclusion and exclusion criteria for both study participants (e.g., patients) and testers (e.g., therapists) should be similar to your clinical environment. If they are not, you need to take this into consideration when integrating the study findings into your practice.
3. Are the outcome measures relevant to my clinical question and are they conducted in a clinically realistic manner?	Yes____ No____	Consider if the outcome measure was applied in a clinically replicable manner. This includes consideration of the amount of training provided to testers.
4. Is the study population (sample) sufficiently similar to my patient and to my clinical setting to justify the expectation that I would experience similar results?	Yes____ No____	Beyond the inclusion and exclusion criteria (question 2), it is important to consider the similarity of the study participants and therapists to your clinical environment.
5. Consider the number of participants being rated and the number of raters. Does the study have sufficient sample size?	Yes____ No____	Sufficient sample size is required to reduce the chance for random error to affect the results. A study that reports the method used to determine the minimum sample size (i.e., sample size calculation) has higher quality.
6. Do participants have sufficient diversity to assess the full range of the outcome measure?	Yes____ No____	A study of reliability should include the full spectrum of people that the outcome measure was designed to test. For example, consider a measure designed to assess a child's ability to engage in elementary school activities. Study participants should include all ages of elementary school children and children with a full range of participation abilities.
7. Are study participants stable in the characteristic of interest?	Yes____ No____	If the participants in a reliability study change substantially in the characteristic of interest, the reliability result will not be accurate. For example, in the case of an outcome measure designed to assess urinary incontinence, it is important that the participants not change any medication regimen that could change the severity of their incontinence between study assessments. Such a change would produce erroneous results for a study of reliability.

TABLE 10.6 **Key Questions for Appraising Studies of Outcome Measure Reliability—cont'd**

QUESTION	ANSWER	WHY IT MATTERS
8. Is there evidence that the outcome measure was conducted in a reasonably consistent manner between assessments?	Yes____ No____	If it is conducted differently between assessments, the reliability of the outcome measure will be inaccurate. Consider a questionnaire completed by patients regarding their satisfaction with therapy services. If the first assessment is conducted in a quiet, private room and the second assessment is conducted over the phone and without privacy, patients might be prone to give different answers. This scenario would give inaccurate estimates of the measure's test-retest reliability.
9. Were raters blinded to previous participant scores?	Yes____ No____	Raters should not have knowledge of previously collected scores. For example, for a study of PT students' inter-rater reliability in taking manual blood pressure measurements, students must be blinded to the measures collected by other students. Lack of blinding is likely to produce inaccurate results.
10. Is the time between assessments appropriate?		If assessments are conducted within too short a time interval, the reliability may be inaccurate because raters (or participants) are influenced by the initial test. Consider a study of the intra-rater reliability of manual muscle testing. If assessments are taken with only a minute between tests, the raters are likely to remember the strength scores from one test to another and participants may have fatigue that causes a decrease in their strength. In this case, rater recall could *overestimate* intra-rater reliability and participant fatigue could *underestimate* intra-rater reliability, making the results difficult to interpret.

Part C: Interpreting the Results of a Reliability Study

There are several common statistical methods that can be used for making comparisons of test-retest, intra-rater, and inter-rater reliability (e.g., intraclass correlation coefficient [ICC], Spearman's rho [r], kappa [κ]). Table 4.1 summarizes these methods and provides a quick guide to their interpretation.

Part D: Summarizing the Clinical Bottom Line

Ultimately, the bottom line from a study of an outcome measure's reliability will inform whether the measure is sufficiently reliable to use in clinical practice. In addition, research studies about outcome measures should provide details about the methods used to conduct the measure. Replicating the protocol used in a high-quality study may improve your reliability with the measure. It may not be possible to exactly duplicate the study protocol in clinical practice. You should expect that the measure's reliability may decrease as a result of any modifications implemented.

■ Studies That Assess Outcome Measure Validity

Throughout this book, we describe the process of appraisal using the word *quality* in place of the word *validity*. We believe that the word *quality* is clearer for the reader. In the following section, the word *validity* refers to a psychometric property of outcome measures.

Types of Validity

As we described in the introduction to this chapter, the validity of an outcome measure refers to the measure's relevance to the underlying construct it is intended to measure. For example, if you are selecting an outcome measure to screen for depression in older adults, you might identify the Geriatric Depression Scale.[8] Before using this measure to determine if your geriatric patients are at risk for depression, you need to know if this measure is a valid measure of depression. Does it actually identify depression in older adults? A validation study of the Geriatric Depression Scale would help you answer this question. There are different types of validity: **content validity, criterion validity,** and **construct validity.**[9–11]

Consequently, different study designs are used to evaluate different aspects of what is collectively referred to as *outcome measure validity*. Table 10.7 includes study designs for specific types of validity.

Content Validity

Content validity establishes that an outcome measure includes all the characteristics that it purports to measure. For example, if an outcome measure assesses activity limitations associated with low back pain, a study of content validity would attempt to establish that all aspects of activity that might be affected by low back pain are included. A panel of experts subjectively establishes content validity. Each expert determines whether the outcome measure includes all aspects of the characteristics

TABLE 10.7 **Types of Validity and Study Designs**

TYPE	STUDY DESIGN	QUESTION ANSWERED
Content Validity	Expert panel	Does the measure include all important components of the construct?
Subtype: Face	Informal expert input	Does the measure appear to measure what it is intended to measure?
Criterion Validity	Compare measure to an established measure of the same characteristic or construct ■ Gold standard: Virtually irrefutable measure ■ Reference standard: Best available comparison when gold standard is not available	How does the measure compare to other more established measures?
Subtypes: Concurrent	Compare measure to a gold or reference standard at the same point in time.	Does the measure being tested correlate with the gold or reference standard when the two are administered concurrently?
Predictive	Compare measure to a gold or reference standard after time has passed.	Does the measure being tested correlate with a gold or reference standard administered after time has passed?
Construct Validity	Test the measure under conditions that establish that it measures the theoretical construct that it is designed to measure.	Does the measure demonstrate that it represents the theoretical construct that it is designed to measure?
Subtypes: Known groups	Compare performance on the measure from groups with known differences in the characteristic of interest.	Does the outcome measure distinguish between the different known groups?
Convergent	Assess the similarity in scores between the measure of interest and another measure or variable that should correlate with the characteristic of interest.	Does performance on the measure converge with other measures, characteristics, or variables that represent the same characteristic or construct?
Discriminant	Assess the similarity in scores between the measure of interest and another measure or variable that should not correlate with the characteristic of interest.	Does performance on the measure diverge from measures, characteristics, or variables that do not represent the same characteristic or construct?

that it is intended to measure. The experts also look for elements of the measure that are extraneous to the characteristic of interest. This information is then used to modify the measure until the panel and developers believe that satisfactory content validity has been achieved.

A less formal evaluation of content validity is referred to as face validity. **Face validity** is based on informal evaluation by experts that a measure *appears* to measure what it is intended to measure. If you decide to measure patient satisfaction in your clinic, you might develop a questionnaire that asks patients about their satisfaction with therapy. If you and others who work in your clinic believe that the survey addresses patient satisfaction, you could consider the survey to have face validity. You could, however, enhance its face validity by asking current and former patients if they believe that the questionnaire sufficiently explores patient satisfaction.

■ **SELF-TEST 10.1**

Understanding Content Validity

You have been invited to serve on an expert panel to assess the content validity of a new measure designed to assess activity limitations associated with low back pain. List five activities that the measure should assess for each of the following patient groups.

Ambulatory Adults	Ambulatory Children	Adults Using Wheelchairs
1.	1.	1.
2.	2.	2.
3.	3.	3.
4.	4.	4.
5.	5.	5.

Now, compare and contrast your lists. Do you think that one outcome measure could be developed with content validity for each of these populations or would separate measures be needed? Compare your answers to the answers at the end of the chapter.

Criterion Validity

Criterion validity establishes the validity of an outcome measure by comparing it to another, more established measure. The measure used for comparison, the criterion measure, can be designated as either a gold standard or a reference standard. A **gold standard** criterion measure has virtually irrefutable validity for measuring the characteristic of interest. For example, arthroscopic visualization of the knee would be considered a gold standard criterion for assessment for anterior cruciate ligament (ACL) tears. Likewise, the Berg Balance Scale has been studied so extensively as a measure of balance that it has served as a gold standard criterion for balance.[12]

When a gold standard criterion does not exist for a given characteristic, a reference standard criterion is used. A **reference standard** is less irrefutable than a gold standard but is considered a reasonable comparison for the outcome measure of interest. It is the burden of researchers conducting a criterion-related validity study to justify the gold standard or reference standard chosen for their study. For example, George et al.[13] validated a new questionnaire to measure fear of daily activities among persons with low back pain. The previously validated Oswestry Disability Questionnaire (ODS)[14] was one of six scales used as a reference standard for the new scale. The authors justify the use of the ODS by citing two previous studies[15,16] that recommend the ODS as an appropriate outcome measure of self-report for disability among persons with low back pain.

Criterion validity studies can be divided into two main types—concurrent and predictive. **Concurrent validity** is established when researchers demonstrate that an outcome measure has a high correlation with the criterion measure taken at the same point in time. **Predictive validity** is established when researchers demonstrate that an outcome measure has a high correlation with a future criterion measure. For example, if a new measure of balance has a high correlation with falls experienced by individuals over a period of 1 year, the measure would be considered to have predictive validity for falls.

Construct Validity

Construct validity establishes the ability of an outcome measure to assess an abstract characteristic or concept. It is the most complex form of validity to establish. To establish construct validity, outcome measure developers must first provide a theoretical model that describes the constructs being assessed. After that, a series of studies are conducted to establish whether the measure actually assesses those constructs. Three common methods for establishing construct validity are known-groups, convergent, and discriminant validity.

Known-groups validity establishes that an outcome measure produces different scores for groups with known differences on the characteristic being measured. For example, an outcome measure established to assess knee stability would be expected to produce distinctly different scores for persons with and without an ACL injury. Known-groups validity would be established if the measure clearly delineated between knees with and without ACL injury. **Convergent validity** establishes that a new measure correlates with another thought to measure similar a characteristic or concept. In contrast, **discriminant validity** establishes that a measure does not correlate with a measure thought to assess a distinctly different characteristic or concept. For example, a measure of physical strength would not be expected to have a high correlation with a measure of physical endurance. Discriminant validity would be established if a new measure of physical strength established low correlation with a measure of physical endurance.

Appraising the Applicability of Studies of an Outcome Measure's Validity

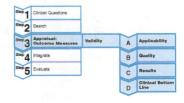

In this section of the chapter, we describe the process of appraising studies on the validity of outcome measures, completing all four parts of appraisal: Part A: Determining Applicability of a Validity Study, Part B: Determining the Quality of a Validity Study, Part C: Interpreting the Results of a Validity Study, and Part D: Summarizing the Clinical Bottom Line.

Part A: Determining Applicability of a Validity Study

This includes the same questions described previously for studies of reliability. These are the first four questions in Table 10.8. You determine that the study's purpose, participants (both persons being measured and raters), and method of conducting the outcome measure(s) are similar enough to your clinical question to justify reading the article.

TABLE 10.8 **Key Questions for Appraising Quality of Studies of Outcome Measure Validity**

QUESTION	EXPLANATION
Applicability is similar across all outcome measure study types.	
1. Is the study's purpose relevant to my clinical question?	If the purpose of the study is not relevant to your question, it is unlikely to be applicable.
2. Are the inclusion and exclusion criteria clearly defined and would my patient qualify for the study?	Ideally, the study inclusion and exclusion criteria for both study participants (e.g., patients) and testers (e.g., therapists) should be similar to your clinical environment. If not, you need to take this into consideration when integrating the study findings into your practice.
3. Are the outcome measures relevant to my clinical question and are they conducted in a clinically realistic manner?	Consider if the outcome measure was applied in a clinically replicable manner. This includes consideration of the amount of training provided to testers.
4. Is the study population (sample) sufficiently similar to my patient and to my clinical setting to justify the expectation that I would experience similar results?	Beyond the inclusion and exclusion criteria (question 2), it is important to consider the similarity of the actual participants enrolled in the study to your clinical environment.
CONTENT VALIDITY	
Content validity is the appraisal of a study that assesses face validity and involves assessment of the quality of the expert panel.	
5. Did the experts have diverse expertise to allow the outcome measure to be assessed from different perspectives?	The purpose of the expert panel is to ensure that the measure addresses all aspects of the characteristics of the construct. A diverse panel helps to ensure the panel's success.
6. Did the researchers systematically collect and respond to the experts' feedback?	Researchers should report their process for collection and analysis to ensure full transparency for the face validity process.
CRITERION AND CONSTRUCT VALIDITY	
Criterion validity establishes the validity of an outcome measure by comparing it to another, more established measure. **Construct validity** establishes the ability of an outcome measure to assess an abstract characteristic or concept.	
7. Have the authors made a satisfactory argument for the credibility of the gold standard or reference criterion measure?	The internal validity of the study is suspect if the gold standard or reference measures were not strong criteria for assessing the validity of the measure of interest.
8. Were raters blinded to the results of the outcome measure of interest and the criterion measure?	It is important to minimize the impact of the outcome measures on each other.
9. Did all participants complete the outcome measure of interest and the gold standard or reference criterion measure?	All participants should be have completed both measures. There is bias if only a subset of subjects had both measures.
10. Was the time between assessments appropriate?	The measures should be conducted either concurrently (concurrent, convergent, and discriminant validity) or with an intervening time period (predictive validity). The appropriate amount of time depends on the purpose of the study. In the former situation it is important that the assessments be done close together but not so close as to have one assessment affect the other. In the case of predictive validity, it is important for enough time to elapse for the characteristic the researchers are trying to predict (e.g., falls) to occur.
11. For known-groups construct validity studies: Are the groups established as being distinctly different on the characteristic of interest?	The groups must be known to be different. If not, the study validity is in question. The authors must provide evidence that they can establish the difference between groups prior to starting the study.

Part B: Determining the Quality of a Validity Study

The most important questions to ask about quality depend on the type of validity under investigation and the method used. In Table 10.8 we have separated important questions by validity type.

Part C: Interpreting the Results of a Validity Study

One of the most common statistical methods used in studies of outcome measure validity is Spearman's rho correlation (r). Table 4.1 summarizes how to interpret Spearman's rho correlation. For studies of criterion validity, the authors report the correlation between the outcome measure of interest and the gold or reference standard. For predictive validity, correlation with the criterion measure is assessed after time has passed.

Convergent and discriminant validity studies, subtypes of construct validity, also produce results that assess the correlation between the outcome measure of interest and another established measure. For convergent validity you would expect to see a positive correlation; for discriminant validity you would expect to see a negative correlation between the two measures. Finally, the known-groups study subtype of construct validity uses inferential statistics, most often analysis of variance to assess the difference in scores between known

groups. For example, researchers could use a known-groups study design to establish that an assessment of respiratory function produces distinctly different scores for persons who are bedridden, wheelchair bound, or ambulatory. If the study result indicated that there was a statistically significant difference (often $p < 0.05$) between the three groups it would support the establishment of construct validity.

Part D: Summarizing the Clinical Bottom Line

Ultimately, the bottom line from a study of an outcome measure's reliability informs whether the measure is sufficiently valid to use in clinical practice. In other words, the study tells us whether we should have confidence that a measure actually measures what it is intended to measure. Before we can base our interpretation of a patient's status or progress on the result of an outcome measure, we need to have confidence in the measure itself.

■ SELF-TEST 10.2 Practice Identifying Studies of Outcome Measure Validity

Read the two abstracts that follow and determine the type of validity under study.

Abstract 1

Objectives: To determine the convergent validity of the 12-item Short-Form Health Survey, version 2 (SF-12v2), with 36-Item Short-Form Health Survey, version 2 (SF-36v2), in patients with spinal disorders, and to determine other key factors that might further explain the variances between the 2 surveys.

Design: Cross-sectional study.

Setting: Orthopedic ambulatory care.

Participants: Eligible participants (N=98; 24 with cervical, 74 with lumbosacral disorders) who were aged 18 years and older, scheduled to undergo spinal surgery, and completed the SF-36v2.

Interventions: Not applicable.

Main Outcome Measures: SF-36v2 and SF-12v2 (extracted from the SF-36v2).

Results: The 2 summary scores, physical and mental component scores (r range, .88-.97), and most of the scale scores (r range, .81-.99) correlated strongly between the SF-12v2 and SF36-v2, except for the general health score (cervical group, r=.69; lumbosacral group, r=.76). Stepwise linear regression analyses showed the SF-12v2 general health scores (cervical: beta=.61, P<.001; lumbosacral: beta=.68, P<.001) and the level of comorbidities (cervical: beta=−.37, P=.014; lumbosacral: beta=−.18, P=.039) were significant predictors of the SF-36v2 general health score in both groups, whereas age (beta=.32, P<.001) and smoking history (beta=−.22, P=.005) were additional predictors in the lumboscacral group.

Conclusions: SF-12v2 is a practical and valid alternative for the SF-36v2 in measuring health of patients with cervical or lumbosacral spinal disorders. The validity of the SF-12v2 general health score interpretation is further improved when the level of comorbidities, age, and smoking history are taken into consideration.

Type of Validity Studied and Why: Abstract 1 describes a study that measures construct validity. The authors report that convergent validity was assessed by determining if the new test (SF-12v2) measures the same construct as the established test (SF-36v2).

Lee CE, Browell LM, Jones DL. Measuring health in patients with cervical and lumbosacral spinal disorders: is the 12-item short-form health survey a valid alternative for the 36-item short-form health survey? *Arch Phys Med Rehabil*. 2008 May;89(5):829-33.

Abstract 2

In the era of life-prolonging antiretroviral therapy, chronic fatigue is one of the most prevalent and disabling symptoms of people living with HIV/AIDS, yet its measurement remains challenging. No instruments have been developed specifically to describe HIV-related fatigue. We assessed the reliability and construct validity of the HIV-Related Fatigue Scale (HRFS), a 56-item self-report instrument developed through formative qualitative research and designed to measure the intensity and consequences of fatigue as well as the circumstances surrounding fatigue in people living with HIV. The HRFS has three main scales, which measure fatigue intensity, the responsiveness of fatigue to circumstances and fatigue-related impairment of functioning. The functioning scale can be further divided into subscales measuring impairment of activities of daily living, impairment of mental functioning and impairment of social functioning. Each scale demonstrated high internal consistency (Cronbach's alpha=0.93, 0.91 and 0.97 for the intensity, responsiveness and functioning scales, respectively). The HRFS scales also demonstrated satisfactory convergent validity when compared to other fatigue measures. HIV-Related Fatigue Scales were moderately correlated with quality of nighttime sleep (rho=0.46, 0.47 and 0.35) but showed only weak correlations with daytime sleepiness (rho=0.20, 0.33 and 0.18). The scales were also moderately correlated with general mental and physical health as measured by the SF-36 Health Survey (rho ranged from 0.30 to 0.68 across the 8 SF-36 subscales with most >0.40). The HRFS is a promising tool to help facilitate research on the prevalence, etiology and consequences of fatigue in people living with HIV.

Pence BW, Barroso J, Leserman J, Harmon JL, Salahuddin N. Measuring fatigue in people living with HIV/AIDS: psychometric characteristics of the HIV-related fatigue scale. *AIDS Care*. 2008;20, 829-37.

◼ Studies That Assess an Outcome Measure's Clinical Meaningfulness

Types of Clinical Meaningfulness

Outcome measures must be valid and reliable and assist us in interpreting change in our patients to have clinical meaning. In this section, we describe concepts related to clinical meaningfulness including floor and ceiling effects, minimal detectible change, responsiveness, and minimal clinically important difference.

Floor and Ceiling Effects

Floor and ceiling effects reflect a lack of sufficient range in the measure to fully characterize a group of patients. For example, consider an outcome measure designed to measure adults' fine motor control. Possible scores on this hypothetical measure range from 0 to 10, with higher scores indicating better performance. Figure 10.3 illustrates scores on this measure from three groups:

1. Persons with stroke
2. Construction workers
3. Musicians

Scores for persons with stroke are clustered at the bottom of the scale, with many earning the minimum score (0). This is an example of floor effect. Scores for musicians are clustered at the top of the scale, with many earning the maximum score (10). This is an example of ceiling effect. The scores for the construction workers are spread across the range, and very few earned the maximum (10) or minimum (0) score. For the construction worker population, this measure does not have a

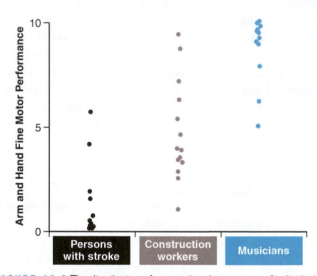

FIGURE 10.3 The distribution of scores that three groups of individuals achieved on a hypothetical measure of adult fine motor control. The measure has a floor effect among patients with stroke and a ceiling effect among musicians.

ceiling or floor effect. Hence, the measure is appropriate for use among construction workers but would have limited meaning for persons with stroke and for musicians.

It is unusual to see a study specifically designed to study ceiling and floor effects, but it is common to encounter studies that discover these effects as part of a larger study. Check for a ceiling or floor effect when appraising studies by visually inspecting the distribution of participants' scores on an outcome measure. The usefulness of a measure is diminished by the presence of a ceiling or floor effect.

Minimal Detectible Change

Minimal detectible change (MDC) is the minimum amount of change required on an outcome measure to exceed anticipated measurement error and variability.[17] For example, if you measured a patient's walking endurance using the Six-Minute Walk Test[18] every day for 5 days, you would expect some variability in the distance that the patient walked each day (e.g., Day 1 = 149 meters (m), Day 2 = 160 m, Day 3 = 155 m, Day 4 = 149 m, Day 5 = 152 m). You need to know the MDC for the Six-Minute Walk Test to determine how much change is needed to exceed this natural variation and represent a true change in the patient's status.

Minimal detectible change is derived using an outcome measure's test-retest reliability and within-subject standard deviation for repeated measurements. The foundation for deriving MDC is a high-quality test-retest reliability study. Because test-retest reliability and variability are different for different patient populations, MDC for an outcome measure must be determined for different populations. For example, the MDC for the Six-Minute Walk Test has been reported as 36 m for persons with Alzheimer's disease,[19] 27 m for persons with Parkinson's disease,[20] and 53 m for persons with chronic obstructive pulmonary disease (COPD).[21] Therefore, if a patient with Parkinson's disease experienced a 40-m improvement in Six-Minute Walk Test distance, the change would be considered beyond the natural variability (27 m) for the population. In contrast, if a patient with COPD experienced the same 40-m improvement, the change fails to exceed the MDC (53 m) for this population and would be considered natural variation rather than true change.

Responsiveness and Minimal Clinically Important Difference

Responsiveness reflects an outcome measure's ability to detect change over time. If your patient improves in a particular characteristic, you want to know that the measure you are using will detect, or respond, to that change. Studies of responsiveness are longitudinal and measure participants who are expected to change over time. One measure of responsiveness is the **minimal clinically important difference (MCID),** also referred to as the minimal important difference (MID). MCID represents the minimum amount of change on an outcome measure that patients perceive as beneficial and that would justify a change in care.[22] MCID answers the question, "How much change on an outcome measure is enough to be meaningful?"

Studies investigating MCID compare the measure of interest to a gold standard, much like studies of validity. For MCID studies, the gold standard is a measure known to detect meaningful change, whenever possible, from the perspective of the patient. A common method is to ask patients how much they have changed (e.g., over a course of

therapy) and have them rate their response from -7 (much worse) to +7 (much better). Those who rate themselves between +3 and +7 are generally considered to have experienced a meaningful improvement (those between -3 and -7 are considered to have experienced a meaningful decline).[23] Statistical methods are used to determine what change on the outcome measure of interest best correlates with the patients' perspective (see Digging Deeper 10.1). Sometimes patient perspective cannot be collected for a MCID study. In these cases, it is appropriate, but less ideal, to use a gold standard comparison that is based on the perspectives of clinicians, family members, or caregivers.

Much like MDC, studies of MCID need to be considered in context. Applicability is an important component of appraisal for studies reporting MCID. For a given outcome measure, the MCID is specific to a particular patient population, taking into consideration, for example, diagnosis, age, or severity of condition.

Finally, when interpreting studies of MCID it is important to consider MDC. MDC is based on anticipated error and variability, and an MCID that is smaller than the MDC has little use. For example, MCID for the Six-Minute Walk Test has been reported as 54 m for people with COPD.[24] People who improved at least 54 m were more likely to rate themselves as being at least a little better. It is important that this value (54 m) be larger than the MDC value of 53 m derived from the work by Brooks et al.[21] If MCID is not larger than the MDC, the natural variability of the measure (53 m) would obscure the ability to detect clinically meaningful change (54 m). Figure 10.4 illustrates the difference between these two properties and their interpretation in clinical practice.

A statistically significant difference is different from the concept of MCID. Remember from Chapter 4 that a statistically significant difference is identified by inferential statistics that compare two or more groups. Statistical significance is influenced by the size and variability (e.g., standard deviation) of the samples being compared. In contrast, MCID addresses whether change experienced by an individual or a group is clinically important. Consider a hypothetical study that reports a statistically significant difference in 6-minute walk distance for persons with COPD who received therapy three times per week compared to a group who received therapy four times per week. If the difference in Six-Minute Walk Test distance between the two groups is only 5 m (much less than the MCID of 54 m), then the clinical meaningfulness of the finding would questionable even though there is a statistically significant difference between groups. In other words, although there was a statistical difference between the groups, the difference is unlikely to be meaningful to patients and might not justify therapy four times per week as opposed to three.

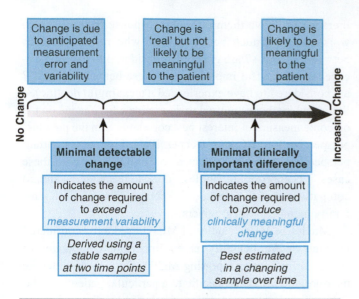

FIGURE 10.4 The relation among commonly reported values associated with clinical meaningfulness.

Appraising Studies That Assess an Outcome Measure's Clinical Meaningfulness

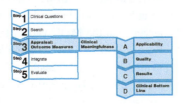

Table 10.9 includes questions regarding appraisal of applicability (questions 1–4) and then additional questions that are specific to concepts of clinical meaningfulness. Parts A through D are included, but they are brief. A full appraisal of each type of study of clinical meaningfulness is beyond the scope of this text. References are included for further in-depth study.[17,23,25]

Part A: Determining Applicability of a Clinical Meaningfulness Study

Applicability for a study of clinical meaningfulness requires a strong similarity between the patient population studied and the patient to whom you wish to apply the result. Meaningfulness is best defined from the patient's perspective. More similar patients will have more similar perspectives. The questions for applicability in Table 10.9 are not different for studies of clinical meaningfulness, but they should be considered with high level of scrutiny.

Part B: Determining the Quality of a Clinical Meaningfulness Study

Because the study design (other than statistical analysis) is the same for studies of test-retest reliability and studies of MDC, the questions for studies of reliability (see Table 10.6) can be used to appraise the quality of studies of MDC. Questions to consider for studies of MCID and for portions of studies that assess ceiling and floor effects are provided in Table 10.9. In addition, Digging Deeper 10.1 describes MCID study methods in more detail to better inform your appraisal of these types of studies.

Part C: Interpreting the Results of a Clinical Meaningfulness Study

Results from studies that include assessment of ceiling and floor effect will provide a proportion (percentage) of individuals who experienced a floor effect (lowest possible score) and ceiling effect (highest possible score). Studies that assess MDC will report a change value that represents the MDC and should also include a confidence interval for the MDC. For example, a study might report that the MDC on an outcome measure is 4 out of 100 points with a 95% confidence interval of 2 to 7. This would tell you that only changes of 4 or greater on the outcome measure (for a given patient) should be considered true change. Change less than 4 would be considered within the natural variation of the measure. The confidence interval tells us that we are 95% confident that the true MDC value for the general population lies between 2 and 7.

Studies of MCID will also report a change value for the outcome measure of interest. In contrast to MDC, this change value represents the minimum amount of change on an outcome measure that is likely to represent a meaningful change for a patient. Interpretation of the MCID value should include consideration of the gold standard used to define meaningful change in the population. MCID results should include a confidence interval as well.

Part D: Summarizing the Clinical Bottom Line of a Clinical Meaningfulness Study

The clinical bottom line for studies of clinical meaningfulness relates to whether a particular outcome measure provides useful information in the clinical environment. With respect to ceiling and floor effects, we learn whether the outcome measure has sufficient range to capture change in patients in the extreme ends of the characteristic being measured. Studies of MDC tell us when to consider change on an outcome measure beyond natural variation.

TABLE 10.9 **Key Questions for Appraising Quality of Studies of Outcome Measure Clinical Meaningfulness**

QUESTION	EXPLANATION
Applicability is similar across all outcome measure study types.	
1. Is the study's purpose relevant to my clinical question?	If the purpose of the study is not relevant to your question, it is unlikely to be applicable.
2. Are the inclusion and exclusion criteria clearly defined and would my patient qualify for the study?	Ideally, the study inclusion and exclusion criteria for both study participants (e.g., patients) and testers (e.g., therapists) should be similar to your clinical environment. If not, you need to take this into consideration when integrating the study findings into your clinic.
3. Are the outcome measures relevant to my clinical question and are they conducted in a clinically realistic manner?	Consider if the outcome measure was applied in a clinically replicable manner. This includes consideration of the amount of training provided to testers.
4. Is the study population (sample) sufficiently similar to my patient and to my clinical setting to justify the expectation that I would experience similar results?	Beyond the inclusion and exclusion criteria (question 2), it is important to consider the similarity of the study participants and therapists to your clinical environment.
FLOOR AND CEILING EFFECTS	
Floor and ceiling effects reflect a lack of sufficient range in the measure to fully characterize a group of patients.	
1. Does the study sample represent individuals who are likely to score across the full range of the outcome measure of interest?	To determine if an outcome measure has a floor and/or ceiling effect, individuals who are likely to perform very poorly (to assess for presence of floor effect) and very well (to assess for presence of ceiling affect) are required.
MINIMAL DETECTABLE CHANGE (MDC)	
The **MDC** is the minimum amount of change required on an outcome measure to exceed anticipated measurement error and variability.[17] Use questions for assessing quality of studies of test-retest reliability.	
MINIMAL CLINICALLY IMPORTANT DIFFERENCE (MCID)	
MCID represents the minimum amount of change on an outcome measure that patients perceive as beneficial and that would justify a change in care.[22]	
1. Is the sampling procedure (recruitment strategy) likely to minimize bias?	The study should describe how and from where participants were recruited. Consecutive recruitment, in which any participant that meets eligibility criteria is invited to join the study, is the strongest design. To understand what change is meaningful to patients as a whole, it is important to have a diverse and unbiased sample.
2. Were the participants recruited likely to experience change during the course of the study?	In the case of studies of MCID (unlike studies of reliability and MDC) it is important that some participants are likely to experience change in the outcome of interest. If no participants experience meaningful change, then a useful result cannot be generated.
3. Were sufficient time and circumstance afforded for participants to experience a meaningful change?	A useful result cannot be generated without sufficient time for meaningful change to occur among participants.
4. Does the study have sufficient sample size?	Sufficient sample size is required to reduce the chance that random error will affect the results. A study that reports the method used to determine the minimal sample size has higher quality.
5. Were the outcome measures reliable and valid?	MCID should not be established for an outcome measure without established reliability and validity. Likewise, the gold standard must, of course, have established reliability and validity. Finally, even with established reliability and validity, an MCID study must demonstrate that reliable methods were used within the study to collect the outcome of interest and gold standard.
6. Were raters blinded to previous participant scores?	To avoid bias, raters should not have knowledge of previously collected scores on either the outcome of interest or the gold standard.
7. Was the follow-up rate sufficient?	Follow-up with participants to assess change over time is essential to MCID study results. As a rule of thumb, follow-up should exceed 80% at minimum.

Perhaps most useful of this category of psychometric properties, studies of MCID can help us assess whether therapy is resulting in meaningful change for our patients. MCID values can be used to inform patient goals and to substantiate the value of your interventions to all stakeholders — patients, caregivers, payers, your supervisors, and even yourself.

DIGGING DEEPER 10.1

Derivation of MCID

The receiver operator characteristic (ROC) curve (for review see Chapter 5) is a method of visually analyzing data used to derive MCID. To derive MCID, researchers need to determine what change score for an outcome measure best represents the minimal amount of change likely to be meaningful to patients. The ROC curve (Fig. 10.5) is used to plot the sensitivity and specificity of different potential change scores for detecting patients who experienced a meaningful change.

Consider the following hypothetical study:

Purpose: To determine the MCID for 10-cm Visual Analog Pain Scale among patients with acute total knee arthroscopy

Population: 100 persons within 3 days of total knee arthroplasty

Intervention: Ice pack for 20 minutes immediately following therapy

Outcome of Interest: All patients rated their pain on a 10-cm Visual Analog Pain Scale directly after therapy and 20 minutes later

Gold Standard: Directly after receiving a post-therapy ice pack, patients were asked to rate their change in pain from post-therapy to post–ice pack on a scale with a range from -7 (much worse) to +7 (much better).

- Responses of +7 to +3 are considered to represent a meaningful improvement.
- Reponses from +2 to -2 are considered to represent no meaningful change.
- Responses from -3 to -7 are considered to represent meaningful decline.

Results:

Visual Analog Pain Scale

Post-therapy mean (standard deviation)	7.3 cm (1.9)
Post-ice pack mean (standard deviation)	5.8 cm (1.9)
Mean change	-1.5 cm
Range of change	-3 to +3

Gold Standard	Number of Participants
Meaningful improvement (+3 to +7)	58
No meaningful change (-2 to +2)	41
Meaningful decline (-7 to -3)	1

Using the data provided, an ROC curve can be used to plot the sensitivity and specificity of Visual Analog Pain Scale change scores for identifying the 58 participants who experienced a meaningful improvement according to the gold standard (Fig. 10.5). The point closest to the upper left corner of the graph represents the change score that optimizes sensitivity and specificity.

Table 10.10 illustrates a 2x2 table comparing the meaningful change as defined by the gold standard and the optimally sensitive and specific cutoff point for the Visual Analog Pain Scale of 2.1, defined as the MCID. The -2.1-cm change score is 81% (47/58) sensitive and 83% (34/42) specific for identifying the 58 individuals who reported a meaningful improvement according to the gold standard measure. Hence a 2.1-cm change on the Visual Analog Pain Scale (in this hypothetical example) would be considered the MCID for *improvement* in pain.

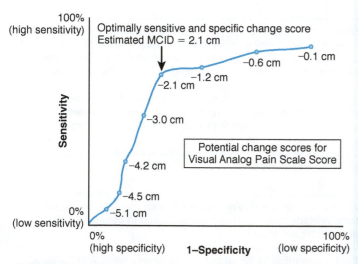

FIGURE 10.5 ROC curve for hypothetical study to determine the minimal clinically important difference for a Visual Analog Pain Scale among individuals with acute total knee arthroplasty. Sensitivity and specificity for identifying the 58 study participants who considered their pain to be meaningfully improved are plotted for 8 potential change scores. A change score of -2.1 has the highest combination of sensitivity and specificity, representing the estimated MCID.

DIGGING DEEPER 10.1 — cont'd

TABLE 10.10 2×2 Table for Hypothetical MCID Analysis

GOLD STANDARD			
Change: 10-cm Visual Analog Scale	Meaningful Improvement (+7 to +3)	No Meaningful Change (+2 to -2)	Meaningful Decline (-3 to -7)
≥−2.1 cm (meets or exceeds MCID)	47	7	0
<−2.1 cm (does not meet MCID)	11	34	1
Total	58	41	1

SUMMARY

Outcome measures allow physical therapists to measure and analyze the change that patients experience during the course of care. Outcome measures are also the primary tool used in research studies to quantify change in participants over time. Therefore, the ability to accurately appraise the quality of an outcome measure is a fundamental skill for evidence based therapists. Psychometric properties are used to describe the quality of an outcome measure. In this chapter we described the most common study types used to assess psychometric properties of outcome measures. Reliability studies assess the consistency of an outcome measure and include internal consistency and test-retest, intra-rater, and inter-rater reliability. Validity studies provide us with insight into whether an outcome measure actually measures what it is intended to measure. Validity studies can be divided into content, criterion, and context validity. Finally, an outcome measure can only be applied in practice if we understand how to interpret its clinical meaningfulness. Studies of clinical meaningfulness inform us about the presence of a floor or ceiling effect, the likelihood that an outcome measure will change when a patient experiences change (responsiveness), what change on a measure represents true change (MDC), and the amount of change that would be considered meaningful to a patient (MCID).

Throughout the chapter and the appendix, we provide key questions to ask when appraising the applicability and quality of studies that determine an outcome measure's reliability, validity, and/or clinical meaningfulness. By answering these questions, you will be able to determine whether the study is of sufficient quality to guide your use of a specific outcome measure.

REVIEW QUESTIONS

1. You are preparing your hospital-based outpatient clinic to provide cardiopulmonary rehabilitation services, and you want to select standard outcome measures to collect from each patient. What are the two main types of outcome measures to consider?

2. What are the three main categories of psychometric properties that should be considered for an outcome measure? Locate information about these properties for the 10-meter Walk Test (measure of walking speed).

3. Why is it important to consider the participant sample and the therapists studied when assessing the applicability of a study about outcome measure reliability?

4. What would be the problem with a test-retest reliability study that assessed patients' performance on a measure of cardiovascular performance at the beginning and end of their hospital stay?

5. What is the clinical impact of the inter-rater and intra-rater reliability for an outcome measure?

6. State the difference between content validity and criterion validity. What are three important questions to ask when assessing the quality of each type of study?

7. What is the difference between minimal detectable change and minimally clinically important difference? How would you use each psychometric property in clinical practice?

8. Find a measure of minimal clinically important difference, and use Table 10.9 to assess its quality. Is the study of high enough quality to guide clinical practice?

9. How would you determine if an outcome measure has a floor or ceiling effect in a population that you treat in clinical practice?

ANSWERS TO SELF-TESTS

■ SELF-TEST 10.1

Ambulatory Adults	Ambulatory Children	Adults Using Wheelchairs
1. Sitting while driving	1. Sitting at school	1. Sitting in chair while stationary
2. Lifting	2. Play that includes running	2. Propelling on level surfaces
3. Sleeping	3. Play that includes climbing	3. Propelling uphill or up curbs
4. Walking	4. Carrying a back-pack	4. Transfers
5. Household/yard chores	5. School sports	5. Sleeping

It would be difficult to develop one outcome measure with content validity for all three populations given the diversity of the lists for each population. The two adult populations (ambulatory and wheelchair user) could be combined if walking and propelling were considered the same activity, but this could diminish the validity for each individual group.

■ SELF-TEST 10.2

Abstract 1 describes a study that measures convergent validity. The authors compare the convergent validity between the 12-Item Short-Form Health Survey, version 2 (SF-12v2), with the 36-Item Short-Form Health Survey, version 2 (SF-36v2), in patients with spinal disorders.

Abstract 2 describes a study that measured construct validity. The authors assessed convergence of the HIV-Related Fatigue Scale with other measures of HIV fatigue.

REFERENCES

1. Fritz JM, Irrgang JJ. A comparison of a modified Oswestry Low Back Pain Disability Questionnaire and the Quebec Back Pain Disability Scale. *Phys Ther*. 2001;81:776–788.
2. Berg KO, Wood-Dauphinee SL, Williams JI, et al. Measuring balance in the elderly: validation of an instrument. *Can J Public Health*. 1992;83(suppl 2):7–11.
3. *International Classification of Functioning, Disability and Health: ICF*. Geneva, Switzerland: World Health Organization; 2001.
4. Vernon H, Mior S. The Neck Disability Index: a study of reliability and validity. *J Manipulative Physiol Ther*. 1991;14:409–415.
5. Karanicolas PJ, Bhandari M, Kreder H, et al. Evaluating agreement: conducting a reliability study. *J Bone Joint Surg Am*. 2009;91(suppl 3): 99–106.
6. Streiner DL, Norman GR. *Health Measurement Scales: A Practical Guide to Their Development and Use*. 4th ed. New York, NY: Oxford University Press; 2008.
7. Berg K, Wood-Dauphinee S, Williams JI. The balance scale: reliability assessment with elderly residents and patients with an acute stroke. *Scand J Rehabil Med*. 1995;27:27–36.
8. Yesavage JA, Brink TL, Rose TL, et al. Development and validation of a geriatric depression screening scale: a preliminary report. *J Psychiatr Res*. 1982;17:37–49.
9. McDowell I. *Measuring Health : A Guide to Rating Scales and Questionnaires*. 3rd ed. New York, NY: Oxford University Press; 2006.
10. Walters SJ. *Quality of Life Outcomes in Clinical Trials and Health-Care Evaluation: A Practical Guide to Analysis and Interpretation*. Hoboken, NJ: John Wiley & Sons; 2009.
11. Portney LG, Watkins MP. *Foundations of Clinical Research: Applications to Practice*. 3rd ed. Upper Saddle River, NJ: Pearson/Prentice Hall; 2009.
12. Whitney S, Wrisley D, Furman J. Concurrent validity of the Berg Balance Scale and the Dynamic Gait Index in people with vestibular dysfunction. *Physiother Res Int*. 2003;8:178–186.
13. George SZ, Valencia C, Zeppieri G Jr., et al. Development of a self-report measure of fearful activities for patients with low back pain: the fear of daily activities questionnaire. *Phys Ther*. 2009;89:969–979.
14. Fairbank JC, Pynsent PB. The Oswestry Disability Index. *Spine*. 2000;25:2940–2952; discussion.
15. Jensen TT, Asmussen K, Berg-Hansen EM, et al. First-time operation for lumbar disc herniation with or without free fat transplantation. Prospective triple-blind randomized study with reference to clinical factors and enhanced computed tomographic scan 1 year after operation. *Spine*. 1996;21:1072–1076.
16. Deyo RA, Battie M, Beurskens AJ, et al. Outcome measures for low back pain research. A proposal for standardized use. *Spine*. 1998;23:2003–2013.
17. Haley SM, Fragala-Pinkham MA. Interpreting change scores of tests and measures used in physical therapy. *Phys Ther*. 2006;86:735–743.
18. Steffen TM, Hacker TA, Mollinger L. Age- and gender-related test performance in community-dwelling elderly people: Six-Minute Walk Test, Berg Balance Scale, Timed Up & Go Test, and gait speeds. *Phys Ther*. 2002;82:128–137.
19. Ries JD, Echternach JL, Nof L, et al. Test-retest reliability and minimal detectable change scores for the timed "Up & Go" Test, the Six-Minute Walk Test, and gait speed in people with Alzheimer disease. *Phys Ther*. 2009;89:569–579.
20. Steffen T, Seney M. Test-retest reliability and minimal detectable change on balance and ambulation tests, the 36-item short-form health survey, and the unified Parkinson disease rating scale in people with parkinsonism. *Phys Ther*. 2008;88:733–746.
21. Brooks D, Solway S, Weinacht K, et al. Comparison between an indoor and an outdoor 6-minute walk test among individuals with chronic obstructive pulmonary disease. *Arch Phys Med Rehabil*. 2003;84:873–876.
22. Jaeschke R, Singer J, Guyatt GH. Measurement of health status. Ascertaining the minimal clinically important difference. *Control Clin Trials*. 1989;10:407.
23. Crosby R, Kolotkin R, Williams G. Defining clinically meaningful change in health-related quality of life. *J Clin Epidemiol*. 2003;56: 395–407.
24. Redelmeier D, Guyatt G, Goldstein R. Assessing the minimal important difference in symptoms: a comparison of two techniques. *J Clin Epidemiol*. 1996;49:1215–1219.
25. Beaton DE, Bombardier C, Katz JN, et al. Looking for important change/differences in studies of responsiveness. *J Rheumatol*. 2001;28:400–405.
26. Folstein MF, Folstein SE, McHugh PR. "Mini-mental state." A practical method for grading the cognitive state of patients for the clinician. *J Psychiatr Res*. 1975;12:189–198.
27. Powell LE, Myers AM. The Activities-Specific Balance Confidence (ABC) Scale. *J Gerontol A Biol Sci Med Sci*. 1995;50A:M28–34.
28. Tilson JK, Sullivan KJ, Cen SY, et al. Meaningful gait speed improvement during the first 60 days poststroke: minimal clinically important difference. *Phys Ther*. 2010;90:196–208.
29. Feldman AB, Haley SM, Coryell J. Concurrent and construct validity of the Pediatric Evaluation of Disability Inventory. *Phys Ther*. 1990;70:602–610.

11 Communicating Evidence for Best Practice

PRE-TEST

1. What is health literacy?

2. Who are the decision makers in physical therapy?

3. What is knowledge translation?

CHAPTER-AT-A-GLANCE

This chapter will help you understand the following:

- Integration of critically appraised research evidence with clinical expertise and the patient's values and circumstances

- Health literacy

- Communication with decision makers for physical therapy

- Profile for evidence storage and communication

- Communicating with critically appraised topics (CATs)

■ Introduction

Locating and appraising evidence is only a relevant process if it is integrated into your practice and it is successfully communicated to others (Fig. 11.1). Throughout this book we use examples of how to integrate best evidence into your physical therapy practice. A part of the integration process is to communicate the evidence for best practice to other people who are making decisions regarding physical therapy. These decision makers include patients, families, other professionals, managers, insurance companies, and makers of social policy. Each of these people or groups has a different set of questions, uses evidence for different purposes, and has different abilities to understand and effectively use what we communicate.

■ Integration of Research, Clinical Expertise, and the Patients' Values and Circumstances

Health Literacy

"Health literacy" can be defined as our ability to understand the factors and contexts that relate to our health, both in terms of prevention and how to manage our health conditions. Health education is aimed at improving health literacy. Effective health education requires an understanding of the social, educational, and economic realities of people's lives.[1]

One of our goals as physical therapists is to improve the health literacy of all health-care decision makers involved with physical therapy, beginning with our patients. To effectively communicate with our patients and their families, we must understand their comprehension of what we are saying, their ability to read materials that we give them, and their understanding of the value of our recommendations to them in the context of their lives. Effective communication requires careful listening

to our patients and incorporating time within the physical therapy sessions to determine the success of our communications. We may tell our patients about a home exercise program; we may write instructions for the program, and we may verbally stress the importance of our recommendations for their recovery. However, effective communication requires that we listen to our patient describe their home program; tell us which is better, written instructions or pictures; and tell us the importance of our recommendations in their everyday lives. Understanding a patient's reading level ensures that any written instructions are appropriate. A patient may not be able to read or may have a limited ability to do so, which may be embarrassing to the patient and so must be probed for carefully. However, knowing a patient's reading and comprehension levels is critical to effective physical therapy management.

The Harvard School of Public Health, Health Literacy Studies Web site (www.hsph.harvard.edu/healthliteracy) has excellent resources that support health literacy at both the individual and societal levels. Recommendations include the use of simple and direct language in terms that are relevant to the patient and the patient's goals. Brevity of communication is critical; there should be enough detail provided for clarity but not so much that the patient is overwhelmed. Repeating and clarifying specific and concrete actions that are planned and then checking for clarity will support good communication.

Communication With Decision Makers for Physical Therapy

Patients and Families

Patients and families are collaborators with us in making decisions regarding their care. They often rely on us to be informed about current research and recommendations for best practice. They arrive in physical therapy with knowledge they have gathered from a variety of sources. Together you can discuss the quality of evidence, including the quality of Web sites that each of you consult, the quality and applicability of published literature, and claims of therapeutic success encountered through the media or through friends and colleagues.

Communication requires practice, just as any skill does. Practicing communication of physical therapy information with people who are not familiar with physical therapy can help you to clarify your meaning and answer questions about care. When you communicate your interpretations of evidence, use simple, clear descriptions that address your patient's questions. Distinguish whether your evidence is from published research or the result of clinical experience. Your interpretations are always specific to your individual patient and thus are shaped by your patient's goals and personal context. For example, your patient may want to know how physical therapy

Step **1**	Identify the need for information and develop a focused and searchable **clinical question**.
Step **2**	Conduct a **search** to find the best possible research evidence to answer your question.
Step **3**	Critically **appraise** the research evidence for applicability and quality: **Outcome Measures**.
Step **4**	**Integrate** the critically appraised research evidence with clinical expertise and the patient's values and circumstances.
Step **5**	**Evaluate** the effectiveness and efficacy of your efforts in Steps 1–4 and identify ways to improve them in the future.

FIGURE 11.1 Step 4 in the EBP process is the integration of research evidence; clinical expertise; and patient's values, goals, and expectations.

will relieve his neck pain. You may have knowledge of the evidence on exercise for best postural alignment and the effects that physical therapy interventions can have on neck strength and range of motion for patients with neck pain. However, your patient cares about pain, and you must communicate how improving strength and range of motion with regular exercise will result in reduced pain.

Listening to patients and focusing on their goals will keep the lines of communication open and the shared information relevant. Asking patients to clarify their goals with specific examples supports good communication. For example, a patient may ask if she can return to work. Exploring the requirements of returning to work may assist the patient in self-identifying the necessary movements needed at work and help you to make a set of priorities toward this goal. Asking patients to summarize their understanding of our recommendations also gives clear insight into their understanding and attitude toward physical therapy.

You may have spent long hours searching and appraising the best possible evidence for your practice, but your patient wants to know that you are working toward goals that are relevant to her, that you understand how to achieve these goals, and that you have the evidence for your recommended plan. Useful phrases in working with your patient include the following:

- "The research and my clinical experience suggest that . . ."
- "There is not a lot of research on the best treatment, but my review of it coupled with my experience and your specific goal of . . . suggests that . . . might be our best course of action."
- "Yes, there is considerable research on physical therapy for your goal. Because you would like to review the research, I have some suggested Web sites or summaries that might be helpful. Let's discuss this again at your next visit, but here is my suggestion today: . . ."
- "I have not been able to locate published research evidence on . . . , but I have consulted with colleagues and with my own experience and theirs and I would suggest . . ."

Consumers of Your Practice

Creating a reputation as an evidence based practitioner can enhance referrals to you and your practice from physicians, colleagues, and members of your community. Summarizing evidence in the form of a newsletter or Web site on topics that you commonly treat can enhance your practice. Again, communicating in writing with decision makers is a skill that requires practice.

Managers, Funders, and Policy Makers

Managers want to develop and maintain programs that offer the highest quality physical therapy. Managers, funders, and policy makers are in positions to make important decisions for physical therapy practice. Approaching these decision makers requires that you know the research and clinical expertise that is used to serve your patients. "Knowledge translation" (KT) is a term used to describe the various methods for translating research evidence to practice. Evidence is developing that knowledge brokers (KBs) are effective in supporting evidence based practice (EBP).[2] A KB is a local champion of the change that is supported by evidence and that has been identified as a goal for practice. For example, a research team using KBs in Canada was successful in increasing awareness of and utilization across multiple clinics of the Gross Motor Classification System[3] for children with cerebral palsy (CP). This formed the basis of a system that could support intervention for specific groups of children with CP.

Decision makers are also concerned about cost of care and maintaining programs that are the most cost effective. As you develop your skills as an evidence based practitioner, you will become increasingly aware of the power of speaking from evidence when approaching decision makers in physical therapy. There are excellent examples in the literature of the power to change physical therapy through use of the evidence.[4,5]

■ Summarizing and Storing Research Evidence for Communication

There are many methods for summarizing and communicating evidence for practice. As suggested in Chapter 12, developing a technology profile assists you in becoming and remaining an efficient evidence based physical therapist. The profile should serve your information gathering and also link your profile to your personal system for summarizing and storing evidence for practice. One commonly used method for communicating research results is the critically appraised topic (CAT). A CAT is a summary that can be written in many forms and stored for your use as needed. The Centre for Evidence-Based Medicine (CEBM) in Oxford, United Kingdom, provides a method for writing CATs. The CAT maker can be found at www.cebm.net/; the site includes multiple examples of CATs. In this chapter, we provide details for one method of writing CATs. CATs can be used in journal clubs, and they are now being published at multiple Web sites and professional journals (e.g., *Pediatric Physical Therapy*).

The Critically Appraised Topic

The CAT has become an effective and efficient way to communicate and store the critique of a research study and its clinical application. You have already learned many of the necessary skills to complete a CAT, including:

- Writing clinical questions
- Extracting and recording the design of a study
- Appraising the quality and applicability of research

CATs are typically limited to a one-page or even a one-paragraph summary of the relevant information for making clinical decisions regarding the results of a published research study. Figure 11.2 is an example of a CAT form and contains explanations of the specific sections.

First, a clinical question is determined and an appropriate research study is identified. Next, the study quality is appraised. Most CAT forms include both a summary of the study design and a summary of the appraisal (design strengths and threats). The clinical bottom line is completed *after* you have

appraised the quality of the study. Before determining the clinical bottom line you should ask the following questions: What are the relevant outcomes from this study? Was the research conducted with sufficient rigor for the outcomes to be accepted? These questions are answered through completion of the CAT, which requires your appraisal of the study. Figure 11.3 includes an example of a CAT completed for an intervention study.

CAT Form and Examples

Web Resources for CATs

Table 11.1 includes two Web sites that offer support for creating CATs, CATs completed by others for reference, and additional materials on EBP. Other Web sites may contain CATs on specific topics.

Other Examples of Summaries of Evidence

The following are a few of the many methods for summarizing and communicating evidence for you and for others.

The CanChild Centre for Disabilities Research

The CanChild Centre for Disabilities Research Web site (www.canchild.ca/en/canchildresources/keepingcurrent.asp) hosts resources for children, families, and professionals. The organization maintains Keeping Current, which includes summaries of research on relevant topics in pediatric rehabilitation.

The BestBETs Web Site

The BestBETs (Best Evidence Topics) Web site (www.bestbets.org/) was designed by the Emergency Department of Manchester Royal Infirmary, UK, for emergency room physicians, but some of the topics are relevant to physical therapy. Over the years the Web site has expanded and now includes other professions such as physical therapy. BETs are different in form and content from a CAT. BETs are written using multiple research studies with a summary of results and applications. Multiple CATs can also be written on one topic with a summary paragraph included.

At the BestBETs Web site, click on Databases. Listed are appraisals of individual research articles and summaries of research on a topic or BETs. An example of a BET is included in Digging Deeper 11.1. The table is a useful format in which to record information for easy access and communication of results.

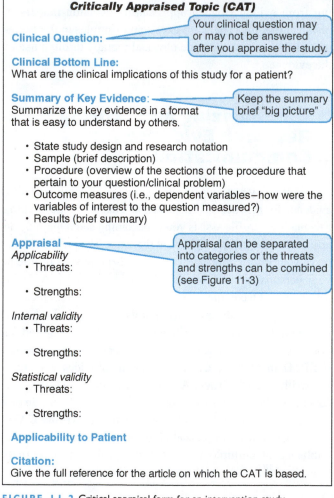

FIGURE 11.2 Critical appraisal form for an intervention study.

Critically Appraised Topic (CAT)

Clinical Question: What is the most effective physical therapy treatment for reduction of pain and increased function for a young female with plantar fasciitis?

Clinical Bottom Lines:
A plantar fascia (PF) stretching program combined with anti-inflammatory medication and insoles is an alternative treatment option to Achilles tendon (AT) stretching for patients with chronic plantar fasciitis to improve function and reduce pain. Pain subscale scores following PF on the Foot Function Index indicated less pain than scores following AT. Patient satisfaction and activity were increased for the PF group.

Summary of Key Evidence:
   A prospective randomized study ROXO
                                    OXO
- Subjects - 82 of 101 patients were randomized into the two treatment groups; mean age 46 ± 7.5 years; 58 females and 24 males.
- Procedure - Both groups received prefabricated soft insoles and a three-week course of anti-inflammatory medication; subjects viewed video on plantar fasciitis and received instructions for a home program of either PF or AT. Measurements at baseline and after 8 weeks of treatment.
- Outcome measures - The Foot Function Index scale for scaling pain and a questionnaire related to activity level and function.
- Results - The pain subscale scores of the Foot Function Index showed significantly better results for the patients in the PF group with respect to item 1 (worst pain; p = 0.02) and item 2 (first steps in the morning; p = 0.006). There were significant differences with respect to pain, activity limitations, and patient satisfaction, with greater improvement seen in the PF group.

Appraisal
Applicability
- Threats: 1) More women than men, hard to generalize to men. 2) Inclusion/exclusion criteria narrow down applicability. 3) Narrow age range, 46 ± 7.5 years.
- Strengths: 1) Noncontrolled environment for medication, activity level, and resistant to prior treatments – closer to reality. 2) Applicable at home and every clinic. 3) Narrow age and gender helps with making clinical decisions.

Quality
- Threats: 1) Groups not similar in duration of symptoms at baseline. 2) Medication not controlled. 3) Applicability of the stretching programs not controlled. 4) Other activities of the patients not controlled. 5) Uneven drop-out for both groups. 6) Usage of logs not mentioned for activities control.
- Strengths: 1) Randomization. 2) Drop-outs reported. 3) Inclusion/exclusion criteria to narrow down clinical differences. 4) Groups statistically similar at baseline in all characteristics other than duration of symptoms. 5) Different analyzing researchers for baseline and outcomes. 6) Follow-up visits. 7) Instructions for log keeping.

Statistical Quality
- Threats: 1) No SD for description of characteristics at baseline. 2) No analysis results for the 3 normal assumptions. 3) A violation of using an ordinal variable of duration of symptoms as a continuous. 4) Dichotomizing the response data. 5) Analyzing for specific items in the questionnaire with no validation for it.
- Strengths: 1) Statistical analysis of characteristics at baseline. 2) A multiple regression to adjust differences between groups. 3) Using the Fisher exact test for nonparametric. 4) Logistic regression was used to evaluate and control for covariates.

From: DiGiovanni BF, Nawoczenski DA, Lintal ME et al.: Tissue-specific plantar fascia-stretching exercise enhances outcomes in patients with chronic heel pain. A prospective, randomized study. *J Bone Joint Surg Am.* 2003; 85-A(7):1270-1277.

FIGURE 11.3 Example CAT for an intervention study.

TABLE 11.1 **CAT Web Sites**

WEB SITE	SPONSORING ORGANIZATION	CONTENT
EBM Resource Center Web Page www.ebmny.org/	The New York Academy of Medicine in partnership with the Evidence-Based Medicine Committee of the American College of Physicians, New York chapter, has received a grant from the National Institutes of Health to develop an evidence based medicine resource center.	The Web page contains references, bibliographies, tutorials, glossaries, and online databases to guide those embarking on teaching and practicing evidence based medicine. It offers practice tools to support critical analysis of the literature and MEDLINE searching as well as links to other sites that help enable evidence based medical care.
Centre for Evidence-Based Medicine CATmaker www.cebm.net/index. aspx?o=1216	The Centre for Evidence-Based Medicine (CEBM) was established in Oxford, UK, as the first of several UK centers having the aim of promoting evidence based health care. The CEBM provides free support and resources to doctors, clinicians, teachers, and others interested in learning more about EBP.	CATmaker is a software tool that helps you create Critically Appraised Topics (CATs) for the key articles you encounter about therapy, diagnosis, prognosis, etiology/harm, and systematic reviews of therapy. The site includes a form you may download to assist you in the CAT process.

DIGGING DEEPER 11.1 EXAMPLE COMMUNICATION

Beginning BestBETs

"Physiotherapy in acute lateral ligament sprains of the ankle"

- Report By: Jonathan Shaw—*SpR in Emergency Medicine*
- Search checked by Simon Clarke—*Consultant in Emergency Medicine and Health*

Protection

- Institution: Wythenshawe Hospital, Manchester
- Date Submitted: 15th January 2001
- Last Modified: 18th February 2005
- Status: Yellow dot (Internal BestBET edit)

In [patients with an ankle sprain] is [physiotherapy a useful adjunct to simple RICE instructions] at [speeding time to recovery]?

Clinical scenario

A 20-year-old man attends the emergency department, having sustained an inversion injury slipping off a curb. Clinical examination by an emergency nurse practitioner in the minor injuries unit reveals tenderness to the lateral malleolus, and you suspect an anterior talofibular ligament sprain. You prescribe a double-tubigrip bandage and advise him to follow rest, ice, compression, and elevation (RICE) instructions. You wonder whether it is worthwhile referring him to the physiotherapist in addition to this, to speed up his return to normal activity.

Search strategy

Medline 1966-week 3/09/04 using the OVID interface.

[exp ankle injuries OR (ankle.mp AND {exp soft tissue injuries OR exp "sprains and strains"})] AND [exp Physical Therapy Techniques OR physiotherapy.mp OR manipulation.mp] AND [controlled clinical trial.pt OR randomized controlled trial.pt OR review, academic.pt] LIMIT to human AND English.

Search outcome

Altogether 38 papers were found, of which 32 were irrelevant to the study question. An additional paper was found via reference checking. The remaining 6 papers and one systematic review are shown in the table here.

Relevant paper(s)

Author, Date, and Country	Patient Group	Study Type (level of evidence)	Outcomes	Key Results	Study Weaknesses
Pasila et al 1978 Finland	300 patients randomized to either Diapulse, Curapulse, or placebo therapy sessions	RCT	Strength measurements, range of movement; swelling	No significant differences found	Power settings of diathermy lower than previous studies
Wester et al 1996 Denmark	48 patients randomized to RICE alone or RICE + wobble board training	RCT	Swelling, reliance on support, activity Subjective opinion	No significant differences found Fewer recurrent sprains on treatment group ($p < 0.05$)	22% dropout rate No data on use of NSAIDs affecting outcome
Karlsson et al 1996 Sweden	86 patients <24 hours injury randomized to either compression pads and mobilization training or compression bandage and crutches	RCT	Validated orthopedic scoring scale for instability, pain, swelling, stiffness, activities	No significant differences found	Only difference between groups was more aggressive treatment in the first week

DIGGING DEEPER 11.1 EXAMPLE COMMUNICATION — cont'd

Author, Date, and Country	Patient Group	Study Type (level of evidence)	Outcomes	Key Results	Study Weaknesses
Holme et al 1999 Denmark	92 patients 5 days post-injury randomized to either RICE and exercise sheet or additional supervised 1 hour twice weekly physiotherapy sessions	Randomised controlled trial (RCT)	Position sense Isometric testing Postural control Patient interview	No significant differences found Reduced incidence of re-injury (7% vs. 29%, n = 65) in following 12 months	Questionable whether groups were comparable Significantly more positive anterior drawer signs in the experiment group
Green et al 2001 Australia	41 patients within 72 hours of injury randomized to RICE or RICE + passive manipulation every 2/7 for 2/52	RCT	Angle of dorsiflexion that produced pain; gait characteristics Return to work	No significant differences found 1.5 days quicker to return to normal walking. 0.7 days quicker to return to running. 1.2 days quicker to return to sport	Multiple assessors for goniometry Small sample size sports tape also applied Clinical relevance of results?
Van Der Windt 2001 Netherlands	Total of 572 patients (5 trials) — placebo or "sham ultrasound"	Systematic Review	General improvement Pain, swelling, functional disability, range of motion	No significant differences found for any outcome measure at 7 to 14 days of follow-up. Pooled relative risk for general improvement was 1.04 (CI 0.92 to 1.17)	Four of the trials were "of modest methodological quality"
Wilson DH, 1972, UK	40 patients all within 36 hours of acute injury, randomized to either Diapulse or placebo with exercise advice	RCT	Swelling, pain, and disability	Significant improvements in pain and disability noted, but not swelling	Small numbers (20 to each arm) Randomization not clear Outcome measures not taken beyond 3 days post-injury

Comment(s)

A number of different techniques are described, all of which purport to be of benefit in therapy for acute ankle sprains. These include passive manipulation, ultrasound, short-wave diathermy, and wobble-board training, among other exercise regimes. There does appear to be a paucity of evidence concerning the effectiveness of any of these methods at the present time. In addition, there is no clear demarcation concerning their effectiveness according to the three grades of injury that help to classify muscle and ligament damage equivalent to any loss of function, strength, fiber damage, and instability of the affected joint.

Clinical bottom line

Based on the current best evidence, home mobilisation facilitated by simple written instructions is suitable for the management of ankle sprains, and active physiotherapy offers no additional benefit.

Continued

DIGGING DEEPER 11.1 EXAMPLE COMMUNICATION — cont'd

References

1. Pasila M, Visuri T, Sundholm A. Pulsating shortwave diathermy: value in treatment of recent ankle and foot sprains. *Arch Phys Med Rehabil.* 1978;59(8):383-386.
2. Wester JU, Jespersen SM, Nielsen KD, et al. Wobble board training after partial sprains of the lateral ligaments of the ankle: a prospective randomised study. *J Orthop Sports Phys Ther.* 1996;23(5):332-336.
3. Karlsson J, Eriksson BI, Sward L. Early functional treatment for acute ligament injuries of the ankle joint. *Scand J Med Sci Sports.* 1996;6(6):341-345.
4. Holme E, Magnusson SP, Becher K, et al. The effect of supervised rehabilitation on strength, postural sway, position sense and re-injury risk after acute ankle ligament sprain. *Scand J Med Sci Sports.* 1996;9(2):104-109.
5. Green T, Refshauge K, Crosbie J, et al. A randomised control trial of a passive accessor joint mobilisation on acute ankle inversion sprains. *Phys Ther.* 2001;81(4):984-993.
6. Van Der Windt DA, Van Der Heijden GJ, Van Den Berg SG, et al. Ultrasound therapy for acute ankle sprains [Cochrane Review]. *Cochrane Libr 4.* Oxford: Update Software.
7. Wilson DH. Treatment of soft-tissue injuries by pulsed electrical energy. *BMJ.* 1972;2(808):269-270.

SUMMARY

Integration of research, clinical expertise, and the patient's values and circumstances is the goal of an evidence based physical therapy practitioner. Communicating evidence to patients, families, colleagues, and all stakeholders for physical therapy is a crucial skill for evidence based physical therapy practice. Understanding the health literacy of our patients is crucial to best practice. Educating our patients to improve their health literacy involves an understanding of their communication and comprehension abilities and requires time for listening during therapy sessions. Both a technology profile and a method of storing and retrieving appraised research evidence will increase the efficiency and effectiveness of physical therapy practice.

REVIEW QUESTIONS

1. State three ways to improve health education.

2. How can CATs be useful to your practice?

REFERENCES

1. Nutbeam D. Health literacy as a public health goal: a challenge for contemporary health education and communication strategies into the 21st century. *Health Promotion International.* 2000;15:259-267.
2. Knowledge brokers: a model to support evidence-based changes in practice. Teleconference summary: McMaster University, Centre for Childhood Disability Research, 2010. http://canchild.ca/en/resources/Participant_InBrief_Apr20_10.pdf. Accessed September 7, 2010.
3. Palisano R, Rosenbaum P, Walter S, Russell D, Wood E, Galuppi B. Gross Motor Function Classification System for cerebral palsy. *Dev Med Child Neurol.* 1997;39:214-223.
4. Fuhrmans V. Withdrawal treatment: a novel plan helps hospital wean itself off pricey tests—it cajoles big insurer to pay a little more for cheaper therapies. *Wall Street Journal.* January 12, 2007:A1.
5. Korthals-de Bos IB, Hoving JL, van Tulder MW, et al. Cost effectiveness of physiotherapy, manual therapy, and general practitioner care for neck pain: economic evaluation alongside a randomised controlled trial. *BMJ.* 2003;326:911.

12 Technology and Evidence Based Practice in the Real World

PRE-TEST

1. What technology resources can improve your EBP efficiency?

2. What push technology do you use to stay current with research evidence?

3. How do you combine push and pull technology resources?

4. How do you organize the articles you read for easy access?

CHAPTER-AT-A-GLANCE

This chapter will help you understand the following:

- How to evaluate and improve your EBP efforts

- How technology can support successful EBP

- The value and difference between push and pull technology

- How to develop your EBP technology profile

- Reference management systems that support EBP

Special Acknowledgment

The authors want to acknowledge and give special thanks to Pamela Corley, MLS, our medical librarian (Norris Medical Library, University of Southern California), who was integral to the accuracy and currency of this chapter and is a great supporter of EBP.

■ Introduction

Becoming an evidence based practitioner is an evolving process as you continue to expand and deepen your expertise. Part of this expertise includes the use and mastery of technology and management of the information that informs your practice (Fig. 12.1).

The History of Technology and Evidence Based Practice

One purpose of this chapter is to highlight the importance of technology for efficient evidence based practice (EBP) in the clinic. Clinicians consistently report "lack of time" as the greatest barrier to EBP.[1,2] Information technology was instrumental in the emergence of EBP, it is essential for EBP today, and it will make EBP easier and faster for you in the future. In this chapter, we briefly explore historical ties between technology and EBP, identify two main categories of technology (push and pull), and propose that every clinician develop an EBP technology profile. The recommended profile includes push and pull technology and a reference management system to make EBP more efficient and practical.

Evaluating and Improving Your EBP Efforts

The development of EBP has occurred in concert with the development of electronic databases that allow clinicians to efficiently access research evidence. In the late 1990s Sackett and Straus[3] described the use of an evidence cart on hospital ward rounds to facilitate access to research evidence within seconds of indentifying a clinical question. The cart consisted of a notebook computer with a CD-ROM drive; a computer projector with a collapsing projection screen; compact discs of MEDLINE, two reference books, and the Cochrane Library; several textbooks, and hard and electronic copies of critically appraised topics (CATs) created by the medical team. After one

attempt to push the cumbersome cart from room to room (as intended), it was parked in a team meeting room. Despite its lack of mobility, the cart enhanced residents' EBP activity because it increased the accessibility of research evidence.

Resources for EBP increased as the Internet and computing power developed. PubMed was launched by the U.S. National Library of Medicine in 1996, allowing the public to use the Internet to access the MEDLINE database.[4] By 2006, searches on PubMed grew to over 3 million per day. By the mid-2000s clinicians could download software applications to their Internet-enabled phones to search for research evidence. In less than 10 years, the portability of research databases progressed from a cart that was too wieldy to push through a hospital ward to a phone that fits in a pocket. As search technology continues to improve, the way we search for research evidence will change as well. Clinicians need to be ready adopters of new information technology as it emerges to support EBP. In the next section we provide a framework to organize and update your technology profile.

Developing Your Technology Profile

A technology profile is a select combination of technology resources used to support EBP. By explicitly developing and updating your technology profile, you may reduce the likelihood of becoming overwhelmed by the number of resources available or of missing new technologies that would be helpful. We propose that your profile consist of a balance of push and pull technologies and one reference management system.

Components of an EBP Technology Profile

Push and Pull Information Technology

In Chapter 2, we focused on strategies to find research evidence to answer a searchable clinical question. You learned the difference between a database (e.g., MEDLINE) and a search engine (e.g., PubMed) and explored skills required for efficiently identifying high-quality and applicable articles from among millions of research articles. The PubMed search engine is an example of pull technology. We use **pull technology** to retrieve information for a specific need on demand. Although the five steps for EBP emphasize using pull technology to search for research evidence in response to a clinical question, we propose that the addition of push technology is important to support your daily practice.

Push technology allows us to request that information be sent to us as soon as it is available. For example, if you commonly treat patients with nonspecific low back pain, by using appropriate push technology you are alerted to important studies when they are published. The alerts might also prompt you to use pull technology the next time you see a patient with

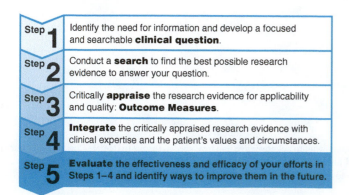

Step 1	Identify the need for information and develop a focused and searchable **clinical question**.
Step 2	Conduct a **search** to find the best possible research evidence to answer your question.
Step 3	Critically **appraise** the research evidence for applicability and quality: **Outcome Measures**.
Step 4	**Integrate** the critically appraised research evidence with clinical expertise and the patient's values and circumstances.
Step 5	**Evaluate** the effectiveness and efficacy of your efforts in Steps 1–4 and identify ways to improve them in the future.

FIGURE 12.1 Step 5 in the EBP process is evaluating the effectiveness and efficacy of your efforts in steps 1 to 4 and making a plan for improvement.

nonspecific low back pain. Examples of push technology include e-mails sent to you from previously established searches, podcasts, and Really Simple Syndication (RSS) feeds.

My NCBI[5] provides a mechanism for pushing new results to you from previously conducted PubMed searches. When signed into a freely available PubMed My NCBI account, you have the option to save searches and have new results automatically compiled and e-mailed to you (see Digging Deeper 12.1 for details on My NCBI).

Podcasts are episodically released digital media files (either audio or video) for automatic download to your computer or portable media player. This new form of media is generally free of charge and provides an alternative to reading new editions of your favorite journals each month. Many journals and professional associations, particularly in physical therapy, provide podcasts with each edition.[6–8]

Many research journals and other professional associations provide RSS feeds. The icon for an RSS feed in most Internet browsers is an orange square (Fig. 12.2). By clicking this icon you can request to have information updates (e.g., journal table of contents each month) sent to an RSS feed reader, which provides a user interface to read and organize the feeds.[9]

You can benefit from push technology for EBP by being selective and strategic about the information you request for push and how it is delivered. For example, iTunes is a proprietary tool that allows users to select from among a vast database of available podcasts. When using iTunes, or another podcast distribution service, it is important to (1) be selective about your subscriptions to podcasts and (2) ensure that the podcasts are sent to an easily accessible location. These principles can be applied to all push technologies. Too much push information can be overwhelming and poorly organized push information can be inefficient.

Reference Management Systems

Active and productive searching for research literature rapidly results in a large library of evidence. Managing research articles has been identified as a barrier to therapists engaging in EBP activities.[1] Numerous software and Web-based systems exist to help clinicians and scientists manage their journal articles. EndNote (www.endnote.com) and Reference

Manager (www.refman.com) are two commonly used reference management systems. Most systems allow users to easily create and search their reference lists and create bibliographies of subsets of references. For example, a reference from PubMed can be automatically downloaded into your reference system and includes the abstract, keywords, and links back to the original article. More sophisticated systems allow the user to append Portable Document Format files (PDFs) of articles and appraisal notes to the citation for easy access. You can access all of your references that relate to specific keywords and rapidly access evidence on a topic.

A developed reference management library allows you to quickly access your articles for reference. In addition, when you write professional documents, a reference management system allows you to easily find and accurately cite your references with just a few clicks. The cost for these systems ranges from free to hundreds of dollars for a user's license. Most universities provide students with access to one or more reference management systems.

Selecting Technologies for Your Profile

Technology resources support EBP efficiency; however, without careful attention to selecting your profile, the challenge of learning to use these resources may outweigh the benefits. Learning to use a focused set of information resources ensures that you have sufficient resources while allowing you to avoid the potential to feel overwhelmed by the many available tools.

Explore currently available resources before selecting your professional technology profile. Medical librarians are experts on this topic. We recommend that you meet with a librarian on a regular basis to explore the push, pull, and reference management systems available to you. Student should identify resources that continue to be available beyond graduation. Clarify with your librarian the costs of the technology for non-students.

Table 12.1 includes examples of established resources for each type of technology for your profile. Over time we can expect to see tools (such as PubMed and My NCBI) that combine push, pull, and reference management components for convenience. By their nature, new technology tools for EBP are constantly emerging. In the near future, we may see electronic medical records that are linked to specific research evidence databases so that you can access research evidence from the same interface used to document patient care. For example, the National Library of Medicine has developed MedlinePlus Connect[10] which links MedlinePlus[11] (see Chapter 2) to electronic health records to provide clinicians and patients with high-quality research evidence customized to a specific patient's health conditions.

Depending on your preferences for technology, you may be more drawn to established or emerging technologies or a

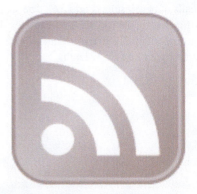

FIGURE 12.2 Icon for RSS for most Internet browsers.

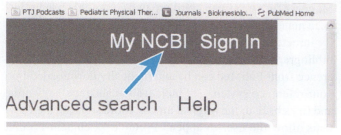

FIGURE 12.3 Screen shot from PubMed highlighting My NCBI sign-in page.

balance between the two. We recommend that clinicians choose one to three favorite resources each from the push and pull categories and one reference management system. Table 12.2 illustrates a sample professional technology profile for a clinician in 2011. Medical librarians are a fundamental resource for learning how to use technology to improve our access to medical information. Identify a medical librarian who, over the course of your professional career, can guide you through selecting and learning to use new EBP technology resources. To identify this person, start at your closest university medical library. The National Network of Libraries of Medicine (NN/LM) Web site (http://nnlm.gov) provides a directory of specially designated NN/LM resource libraries for your reference.

 DIGGING DEEPER 12.1

My NCBI

My NCBI, mentioned briefly in this chapter and in Chapter 2, is provided by the National Center for Biotechnology Information (NCBI) of the U.S. National Library of Medicine.[5] This service is linked to the PubMed search engine and allows registered users to save information, sign up for push services, and customize their PubMed search interface. In this section, we highlight several elements of My NCBI and we encourage you to explore them. Although the exact look of My NCBI will change over time, we anticipate that the general concepts of how to use the service will remain relatively constant. Therefore, we have included screen shots to facilitate your learning.

Register for My NCBI Registration for My NCBI is free of charge. A link to registration can be found on the top right margin of most PubMed pages (Fig. 12.3). Complete your registration by following the instructions in the confirmation e-mail that you will receive; this establishes the e-mail account to receive your *requested* push e-mails. Sign in to My NCBI to gain access to the services that follow.

Customize your PubMed search filters Use the Search Filters tab on the My NCBI home page to customize filters that appear for each of your PubMed searches. The screen shots in Figure 12.4 illustrate that you have options to sort (or filter) your search results into categories, such as Clinical Trial, English and Humans, Items with Abstracts, or Published in the Last 5 Years, with a single click. (For those searching PubMed through a university library, the Free Full Text filter is *not* recommended. Using this filter will exclude citations

with full text available through your library's subscription packages.)

Save collections of article citations My NCBI allows you to save collections of article citations. The *clipboard* is useful for temporarily setting aside citations (within a search session) and does not require that you be signed into My NCBI. *Collections* are stored in your My NCBI account and can be kept for an unlimited period of time. To send citations to a collection, check the box to the left of the citations and select, Send to: and Collections (Fig. 12.5). Access collections by clicking on Collections under My Saved Data on your My NCBI page. To share a collection with a colleague, click the Manage button next to your list of collections. You will see the option to make a collection public. If you make a collection public, My NCBI provides you with a Web site URL to distribute.

Save searches and updates e-mailed to you The Save Search option allows My NCBI users to save a search strategy. With the search strategy saved, you have the option to re-run the search manually or request that My NCBI re-run the search and e-mail you newly published results at selected intervals. When you are signed in to My NCBI and complete a search, you see the option to Save Search above the search box. Simply click this option and answer the questions, which will include the option to set up automatic e-mails of new results (Fig. 12.6). The settings for automatic notifications of any search can be modified on your My NCBI page under Saved Searches, Manage, and then click on Settings to the right of a saved search.

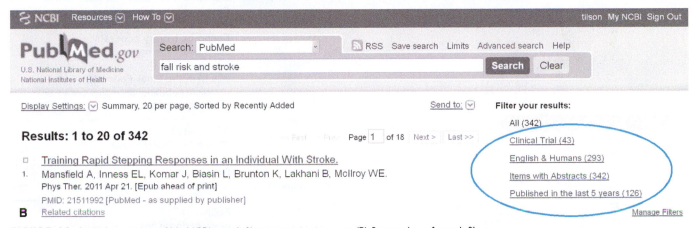

FIGURE 12.4 (A) Screen shot of My NCBI search filter customization page. (B) Screen shot of search filters for a PubMed search.

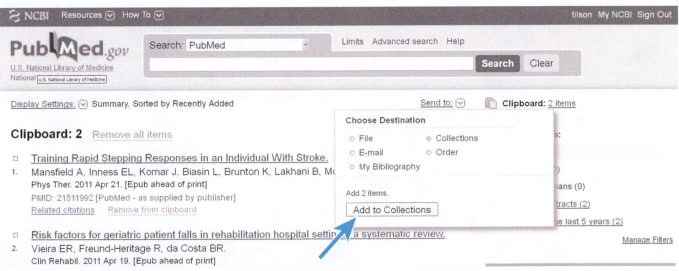

FIGURE 12.5 Screen shot of saving articles to collections on a My NCBI account.

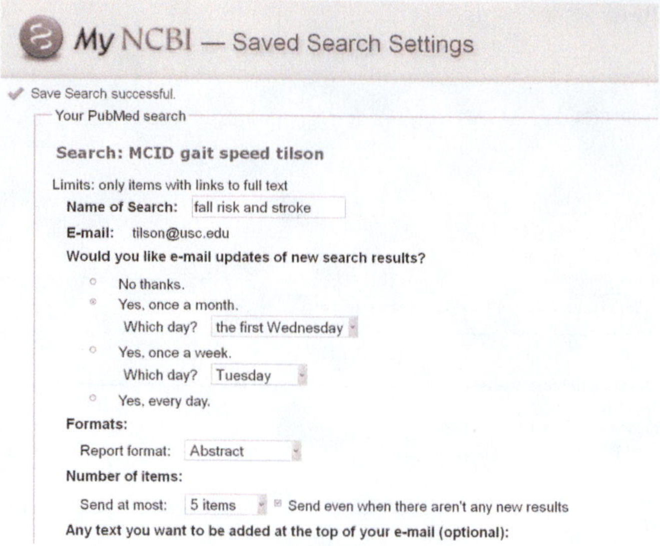

My NCBI — Saved Search Settings

Save Search successful.

Your PubMed search

Search: MCID gait speed tilson

Limits: only items with links to full text

Name of Search: fall risk and stroke

E-mail: tilson@usc.edu

Would you like e-mail updates of new search results?

- No thanks.
- Yes, once a month.
  Which day? the first Wednesday
- Yes, once a week.
  Which day? Tuesday
- Yes, every day.

Formats:

Report format: Abstract

Number of items:

Send at most: 5 items ☑ Send even when there aren't any new results

Any text you want to be added at the top of your e-mail (optional):

FIGURE 12.6 Setting up automatic e-mails for a search.

TABLE 12.1 **Push and Pull Technology Resources in 2010**

EXAMPLES OF ESTABLISHED TECHNOLOGIES	
Pull	PubMed*† www.pubmed.gov
	TRIP database† www.tripdatabase.com
	PEDro database www.pedro.org.au
	Essential Evidence Plus*‡ www.essentialevidenceplus.com
Push	My NCBI*—automatic e-mails of saved searches www.ncbi.nlm.nih.gov/sites/myncbi/, www.pubmed.gov
	Journal-produced podcasts* (abstracts, discussions, bottom-line summaries). Check your favorite journal.
	Cochrane Library podcasts* www.cochrane.org/podcasts
	POEM of the Week Podcast* www.essentialevidenceplus.com/subscribe/netcast.cfm
	RSS feed of highlighted articles from the *British Medical Journal*
Reference management	RefWorks‡ www.refworks.com
	EndNote‡ www.endnote.com
	Bookends‡ www.sonnysoftware.com
	Reference Manager‡ www.refman.com

*Technologies that have components designed for use with handheld devices as of 2010.

† Facilitates access to full text.

‡ Paid subscription required. The subscriptions, however, are often covered by medical libraries for students and others with library membership.

TABLE 12.2 **Sample Professional Technology Profile for a Physical Therapist in 2012**

TECHNOLOGY CATEGORY	CLINICIAN'S TECHNOLOGY PROFILE	
Pull	Primary	PubMed—clinical queries
	Secondary	TRIP database
Push	Disease specific	My NCBI—three monthly autosearches for most common diagnoses seen in practice are sent by e-mail
	Discipline specific	*Physical Therapy* journal podcast via iTunes
Reference manager		EndNote*

*License fee required, often provided through university libraries.

■ SELF-TEST 12.1

Make an appointment with your medical librarian to complete Table 12.3. After testing resources, highlight those to include in your profile. We recommend a conservative approach to adding new technologies to your profile. Too many options may reduce your efficiency. Your librarian can help you become familiar with new tools and learn to improve your use of familiar tools. In addition, many technologies provide online tutorials that facilitate learning. Finally, commit to a date on which you will revisit the librarian to fine-tune your skills and learn about emerging technologies.

TABLE 12.3 **Develop Your Information Technology Profile**

TECHNOLOGY	TYPE (PUSH, PULL, REFERENCE MANAGEMENT)	COST	USER FRIENDLY?	PORTABLE?	ACCESSES OR MANAGES FULL TEXT?	ADD TO PROFILE?

Date to revisit:

SUMMARY

Technology tools are essential to efficient EBP. Establishing a personal profile of technologies that provide pull, push, and reference management resources provides you with the fundamental technology resources needed to support EBP. Pull technologies are most commonly used and include search engines such as PubMed, PEDro, and the TRIP database. Push technologies have emerged since the mid-2000s and allow clinicians to select information that is sent to the user as it becomes available. Reference management systems provide clinicians with efficient means to organize and access research articles collected over time. Medical librarians are experts in established and emerging information technology for health-care professionals. We recommend working with your librarian to establish your technology profile and become proficient with it.

REVIEW QUESTIONS

1. What is the difference between push and pull technologies?

2. Would push or pull technology be most useful when you have a clinical question about the sensitivity and specificity of a certain diagnostic test?

3. Would push or pull technology be most useful for keeping you up to date about new diagnostic tests emerging for a particular patient population?

4. Use PubMed to conduct a search on a topic of interest. Use My NCBI to save your search, set up automatic e-mails from your search, and save a collection of articles.

5. Outline your current technology profile. What technologies do you already use? What are their strengths and weaknesses? Categorize them as push, pull (or both), or as a reference management system.

6. Make an appointment with a medical librarian to develop and/or review your EBP technology profile. Be sure to schedule a follow-up appointment to ask questions that emerge as you learn to use new technology.

7. If you had unlimited resources to build a new EBP technology tool, what would it do?

REFERENCES

1. Salbach NM, Jaglal SB, Korner-Bitensky N, et al. Practitioner and organizational barriers to evidence-based practice of physical therapists for people with stroke. *Phys Ther.* 2007;87:1284–1303; discussion at 1304–1286.
2. Jette DU, Bacon K, Batty C, et al. Evidence-based practice: beliefs, attitudes, knowledge, and behaviors of physical therapists. *Phys Ther.* 2003;83:786–805.
3. Sackett DL, Straus SE; Firm ANDM. Finding and applying evidence during clinical rounds—the "evidence cart." *JAMA.* 1998;280: 1336–1338.
4. NLM Training: PubMed: National Library of Medicine; 2010.
5. My NCBI. www.ncbi.nlm.nih.gov/sites/myncbi/.
6. Physical Therapy Journal. Podcast Central. http://ptjournal.apta.org/misc/podcasts.dtl. Accessed August 13, 2010, 2010.
7. Journal of Neurologic Physical Therapy—JNPT. Podcast. http://journals.lww.com/jnpt/Pages/podcastepisodes.aspx?podcastid=1. Accessed August 13, 2010, 2010.
8. Pediatric Physical Therapy. Podcasts. http://journals.lww.com/pedpt/Pages/podcastepisodes.aspx?podcastid=1. Accessed August 13, 2010, 2010.
9. Wikipedia. RSS. http://en.wikipedia.org/wiki/RSS. Accessed December 22, 2010.
10. Medline Plus Connect. www.nlm.nih.gov/medlineplus/connect/overview.html. Accessed December 22, 2010.
11. MedlinePlus. http://medlineplus.gov. Accessed October 24, 2008.

Key Question Tables

TABLE 3.3 **Key Questions to Determine an Intervention Research Study's *Applicability* and *Quality***

QUESTION	YES/NO	WHERE TO FIND THE INFORMATION	COMMENTS AND WHAT TO LOOK FOR
1. Is the study's purpose relevant to my clinical question?	__ Yes __ No	Introduction (usually at the end)	The study should clearly describe its purpose and/or hypothesis. Ideally, the stated purpose will contribute to answering your clinical question.
2. Is the study population (sample) sufficiently similar to my patient to justify the expectation that my patient would respond similarly to the population?	__ Yes __ No	Results section	The study should provide descriptive statistics about pertinent study population demographics. Ideally, the study population would be relatively similar to your patient with regard to age, gender, problem severity, problem duration, co-morbidities, and other socio-demographic and medical conditions likely to affect the results of the study.
3. Are the inclusion and exclusion criteria clearly defined and would my patient qualify for the study?	__ Yes __ No	Methods section	The study should provide a list of inclusion and exclusion criteria. Ideally, your patient would have characteristics that meet the eligibility criteria or at least be similar enough to the subjects. Remember, you will not find "the perfect study"!
4. Are the intervention and comparison/control groups receiving a realistic intervention?	__ Yes __ No	Methods (some post-study analysis about the intervention may be found in the Results)	The study should clearly describe the treatment regimen provided to all groups. Ideally, the intervention can be reproduced in your clinical setting and the comparison/control is a realistic contrasting option or well-designed placebo. Consider the quality of the dose, duration, delivery method, setting, and qualifications of the therapists delivering the intervention. Could you implement this treatment in your setting?
5. Are the outcome measures relevant to the clinical question and were they conducted in a clinically realistic manner?	___ Yes ___ No	Methods	The study should describe the outcome measures used and the methods used to ensure their reliability and quality. Ideally, the outcome measures should relate to the clinical question and should include measures of quality of life, activity, and body structure and function. For diagnostic studies, it is important that the investigated measure is realistic for clinical use.

Continued

TABLE 3.3 **Key Questions to Determine an Intervention Research Study's *Applicability* and *Quality*—cont'd**

QUESTION	YES/NO	WHERE TO FIND THE INFORMATION	COMMENTS AND WHAT TO LOOK FOR
6. Were participants randomly assigned to intervention groups?	__ Yes __ No	Methods	The study should describe how participants were assigned to groups. **Randomization** is a robust method for reducing **bias.** Computerized randomization in which the order of group assignment is concealed from investigators is the strongest method.
7. Is the sampling procedure (recruitment strategy) likely to minimize bias?	__ Yes __ No	Methods	The study should describe how and from where participants were recruited. **Consecutive recruitment,** in which any participant who meets eligibility criteria is invited to join the study, is the strongest design. Studies in which the authors handpick participants may demonstrate the best effects of a specific treatment, but they will lack applicability across patient types.
8. Are all participants who entered the study accounted for?	__ Yes __ No		The study should describe how many participants were initially allocated to each group and how many completed the study. Ideally, >80% of participants complete the study and the reason for any participants not completing is provided.
9. Was a comparison made between groups with preservation of original group assignments?	__ Yes __ No	Methods will describe the planned analysis. Results will report findings.	The study should make comparisons between groups (not just a comparison of each group to itself). Ideally, an **intention-to-treat analysis** is conducted to compare groups' participants according to their original group assignment.
10. Was blinding/masking optimized in the study design? (evaluators, participants, therapists)	__ Yes __ No	Methods	The study should describe how/if **blinding** was used to reduce bias by concealing group assignment. Most physical therapy–related studies cannot blind therapists or participants due to the physical nature of interventions. Bias can be reduced, however, by blinding the evaluators (who conduct the outcome measures).
11. Aside from the allocated treatment, were groups treated equally?	__ Yes __ No	Methods will describe the treatment plan. Results may report adherence to plan.	The study should describe how **equivalency,** other than the intended intervention, is maintained between groups. Ideally, all participants will have exactly the same experience in the study except for the difference between interventions.

TABLE 4.5 **Key Questions to Interpret the Results and Determine the Clinical Bottom Line for an Intervention Research Study**

QUESTIONS	YES/NO	WHERE TO FIND INFORMATION	COMMENTS AND WHAT TO LOOK FOR
1. Were the groups similar at baseline?	__ Yes __ No	Results (occasionally listed in Methods)	The study should provide information about the **baseline characteristics** of participants. Ideally, the randomization process should result in equivalent baseline characteristics between groups. The authors should present a statistical method to account for baseline differences.

TABLE 4.5   **Key Questions to Interpret the Results and Determine the Clinical Bottom Line for an Intervention Research Study—cont'd**

QUESTIONS	YES/NO	WHERE TO FIND INFORMATION	COMMENTS AND WHAT TO LOOK FOR
2. Were outcome measures reliable and valid?	__ Yes __ No	Methods will describe the outcome measures used. Results may report evaluators' inter- and/or intra-rater reliability.	The study should describe how **reliability** and **validity** of **outcome measures** were established. The study may refer to previous studies. Ideally, the study will also provide an analysis of rater reliability for the study. Reliability is often reported with a Kappa or intra-class correlation coefficient score—values >0.80 are generally considered to represent high reliability (Table 4.1).
3. Were CIs reported?	__ Yes __ No	Results	The study should report a **95% CI** for the reported results. The size of the CI helps the clinician understand the precision of reported findings.
4. Were descriptive and inferential statistics applied to the results?	__ Yes __ No	Methods and Results	Descriptive statistics will be used to describe the study subjects and to report the results. Were the groups tested with inferential statistics at baseline? Were groups equivalent on important characteristics before treatment began?
5. Was there a treatment effect? If so, was it clinically relevant?	__ Yes __ No	Results	The study should report whether or not there was a **statistically significant difference** between groups and if so, the magnitude of the difference (effect sizes). Ideally, the study will report whether or not any differences are **clinically meaningful.**

TABLE 5.7   **Key Questions for Appraising Studies of Diagnosis***

QUESTION	YES/NO	WHERE TO FIND THE INFORMATION	COMMENTS AND WHAT TO LOOK FOR
1. Is the entire spectrum of patients represented in the study sample? Is my patient represented in this spectrum of patients?	__ Yes __ No	Methods	The study should report specific details about how the sample of participants was selected. It is important that participants are at a similar stage in the event of interest (or recovery process) prior to starting the study. Finally, it is important that all participants are measured at study outset on the primary outcome that will be used to detect change in status.
2. Was there an independent, blind comparison with a reference (gold) standard of diagnosis?	__ Yes __ No	Methods	Development of a valid and reliable diagnostic measure requires the use of two tests, the index test and the gold standard test for each subject.
3. Were the diagnostic tests performed by one or more reliable examiners who were masked to results of the reference test?	__ Yes __ No	Methods	Because all outcome measures are subject to bias, when possible, it is ideal for evaluators to be blinded to the primary hypothesis and previous data collected by a given participant.
4. Did all subjects receive both tests (index and gold standard tests) regardless of test outcomes?	__ Yes __ No	Methods	Even if the gold standard test is completed first and indicates the best diagnosis in current practice, the comparison test must be completed for each subject.
5. Was the diagnostic test interpreted independently of all clinical information?	__ Yes __ No	Methods	The person interpreting the test should not know the results of the other test, or other clinical information regarding the subject.
6. Were clinically useful statistics included in the analysis and interpreted for clinical application?	__ Yes __ No	Methods and Results	Have the authors formed their statistical statement in a way that has application to patients?

Continued

TABLE 5.7 **Key Questions for Appraising Studies of Diagnosis*—cont'd**

QUESTION	YES/NO	WHERE TO FIND THE INFORMATION	COMMENTS AND WHAT TO LOOK FOR
7. Is the test accurate and clinically relevant to physical therapy practice?	__ Yes __ No	Methods, Results, and Discussion	Accuracy is estimated by comparison to the gold standard. Does the test affect practice?
8. Will the resulting post-test probabilities affect my management and help my patient?	__ Yes __ No	Results and Discussion	This requires an estimate of pre-test probabilities. If the probability estimates do not change, then the test is not clinically useful.

*The key questions were adapted from previous literature and applied to physical therapy.
From: Sackett DL, Straus SE, Richardson WS, Rosenberg W, Haynes RB. *Evidence-Based Medicine.* 2nd ed.
New York, NY: Churchill Livingstone; 2000; and Straus SE, Richardson WS, Glaszious P, Haynes RB. *Evidence Based Medicine.* 3rd ed. Philadelphia, PA: Elsevier; 2003, and applied to physical therapy.

TABLE 6.3 **Key Questions for Appraising Studies of Prognosis**

QUESTION	YES/NO	WHERE TO FIND THE INFORMATION	COMMENTS AND WHAT TO LOOK FOR
1. Is there a defined, representative sample of patients assembled at a common point that is relevant to the study question?	__ Yes __ No	Methods and Results	The study should report specific details about how the sample of participants was assembled. It is important that participants are at a similar stage in the event of interest (or recovery process) prior to starting the study. Finally, it is important that all participants are measured at study outset on the primary outcome that will be used to detect change in status.
2. Were end points and outcome measures clearly defined?	__ Yes __ No	Methods	The study should describe specific details about how participants' change in status will be measured. Ideally, a standardized outcome measure will be used to determine change in status.
3. Are the factors associated with the outcome well justified in terms of the potential for their contribution to prediction of the outcome?			The factors chosen for association to the outcomes should be justified from previous literature combined with the logic of clinical reasoning in associating the factors with the outcome.
4. Were evaluators blinded to reduce bias?	__ Yes __ No	Methods	Because all outcome measures are subject to bias, when possible, it is ideal for evaluators to be blinded to the primary hypothesis and previous data collected by a given participant.
5. Was the study time frame long enough to capture the outcomes of interest?	__ Yes __ No	Methods and Results	The study should report the anticipated follow-up time in the methods and the actual follow-up time in the results. Ideally, the follow-up time will be sufficient to ensure that the outcome of interest has sufficient time to develop in study participants.
6. Was the monitoring process appropriate?	__ Yes __ No	Methods	The study should report how information was collected over the length of the study. Ideally, the monitoring process results in valid and reliable data and does not cause participants to be substantially different from the general population.
7. Were all participants followed to the end of the study?	__ Yes __ No	Methods and Results	The greater the percentage of participants who have complete a study, the better. Ideally, >80% of participants will have follow-up data and the reason for those without follow-up data will be reported.

TABLE 6.3 **Key Questions for Appraising Studies of Prognosis—cont'd**

QUESTION	YES/NO	WHERE TO FIND THE INFORMATION	COMMENTS AND WHAT TO LOOK FOR
8. What statistics were used to determine the prognostic statements? Were the statistics appropriate?	__ Yes __ No	Methods and Results	The statistical analysis should be clearly described and a rationale given for the chosen methods.
9. Were clinically useful statistics included in the analysis?	__ Yes __ No	Methods and Results	Have the authors formed their statistical statement in a way that has an application to your patient?
10. Will this prognostic research make a difference for my recommendations to my patient?	__ Yes __ No	Discussion and Conclusions	How will your recommendations or management of your patient change based on this study?

TABLE 7.6 **Key Questions for Appraising Systematic Reviews**

QUESTION	YES/NO	EXPLAIN
1. Is the study's purpose relevant to my clinical question?	__ Yes __ No	
2. Are the inclusion and exclusion criteria clearly defined and are studies that would answer my clinical question likely to be included?	__ Yes __ No	
3. Are the types of interventions investigated relevant to my clinical question?	__ Yes __ No	
4. Are the outcome measures relevant to my clinical question and are they conducted in a clinically realist manner?	__ Yes __ No	
5. Is the study population (sample) sufficiently similar to my patient to justify expectation that my patient would respond similarly to the population?	__ Yes __ No	
6. Was the literature search comprehensive?	__ Yes __ No	
7. Was an objective, reproducible, and reliable method used to judge the quality of the studies in the systematic review?	__ Yes __ No	
8. Was a standardized method used to extract data from studies included in the systematic review?	__ Yes __ No	
9. Was clinical heterogeneity assessed to determine whether a meta-analysis was justified?	__ Yes __ No	
10. If a meta-analysis was conducted, was statistical heterogeneity assessed?	__ Yes __ No	
11. What methods were used to report the results of the systematic review?		
12. How does the systematic review inform clinical practice related to my clinical question?		

TABLE 8.6 **Key Questions for Appraising Clinical Practice Guidelines**

DOMAIN	STATEMENT	YES/NO
	Part A: Applicability	
Scope and purpose	1. The overall objective(s) of the guideline is (are) specifically described and addresses my clinical question.	
	2. The clinical question(s) addressed by the guideline is(are) specifically described and addresses my clinical question.	
	3. The patients to whom the guideline is meant to apply are specifically described and match my clinical question.	
	Part B: Quality **Part C: Interpreting Results**	
Stakeholder involvement	4. The guideline development group includes individuals from all the relevant professional groups.	
	5. The patients' views and preferences have been sought.	
	6. Target users of the guideline are clearly defined.	
Rigor of development	7. Systematic methods were used to search for evidence	
	8. The criteria for selecting the evidence are clearly described.	
	9. The strengths and limitations of the body of evidence are clearly described.	
	10. The methods used for formulating the recommendations are clearly described.	
	11. The health benefits, side effects, and risks have been considered in formulating the recommendations.	
	12. There is an explicit link between the recommendations and the supporting evidence.	
	13. The guideline has been externally reviewed by experts prior to its publication.	
	14. A procedure for updating the guideline is provided.	
Editorial independence	15. The views of the funding body have not influenced the content of the guideline.	
	16. Competing interests of guideline development members have been recorded and addressed.	
	Part D: Clinical Bottom Line	
Clarity of presentation	17. The recommendations are specific and unambiguous.	
	18. The different options for management of the condition are clearly presented.	
	19. Key recommendations are easily identifiable.	
Attention to implementation	20. The guideline describes facilitators and barriers to its application.	
	21. The guideline provides advice and/or tools on how the recommendations can be put into practice.	
	22. The potential cost implications of applying the recommendations have been considered.	
	23. The guideline presents key review criteria for monitoring and/or audit purposes.	

Modified from: AGREE Next Steps Consortium. *The AGREE II Instrument* [Electronic version]. http://www.agreetrust.org. Published 2009. Accessed Septermber 3, 2010.

TABLE 9.1   Key Questions to Determine an SSR Study's Applicability and Quality

	YES/NO
Question 1: Is the study's purpose relevant to my clinical question?	
Question 2: Is the study subject sufficiently similar to my patient to justify the expectation that my patient would respond similarly to the population?	
Question 3: Are the inclusion and exclusion criteria clearly defined and would my patient qualify for the study?	
Question 4: Are the outcome measures relevant to the clinical question and are they conducted in a clinically realistic manner?	
Question 5: Was blinding/masking optimized in the study design (evaluators)?	
Question 6: Is the intervention clinically realistic?	
Question 7: Are the outcome measures relevant to the clinical question and are they conducted in a clinically realistic manner?	
Question 8: Aside from the planned intervention, could other events have contributed to my patient's outcome?	
Question 9: Were both visual and statistical analyses applied to the data?	
Question 10: Were data trends in the baseline removed from the intervention data?	
Question 11: Were outcome measures clinically important and meaningful to my patient?	

TABLE 9.3   Key Questions for Appraisal of Qualitative Research

	YES	NO
1. Is the study's purpose relevant to my clinical question?		
2. Was a qualitative approach appropriate? Consider: Does the research seek to understand or illuminate the experiences and/or views of those taking part?		
3. Was the sampling strategy clearly defined and justified? Consider: • Has the method of sampling (subjects and setting) been adequately described? • Have the investigators studied the most useful or productive range of individuals and settings relevant to their question? • Have the characteristics of the subjects been defined? • Is it clear why some participants chose not to take part?		
4. What methods did the researcher use for collecting data? Consider: • Have appropriate data sources been studied? • Have the methods used for data collection been described in enough detail to allow the reader to determine the presence of any bias? • Was more than one method of data collection used (e.g., triangulation)? • Were the methods used reliable and independently verifiable (e.g., audiotape, videotape, field notes)? • Were observations taken in a range of circumstances (e.g., at different times)?		
5. What methods did the researcher use to analyze the data, and what quality control measures were implemented? Consider: • How were themes and concepts derived from the data? • Did more than one researcher perform the analysis, and what method was used to resolve differences of interpretation? • Were negative or discrepant results fully addressed, or just ignored?		

Continued

TABLE 9.3 **Key Questions for Appraisal of Qualitative Research—cont'd**

	YES	NO
6. What are the results, and do they address the research question? Are the results credible?		
7. What conclusions were drawn and are they justified by the results? In particular, have alternative explanations for the results been explored?		

Data from: Critical Appraisal Skills Programme (CASP), Public Health Resource Unit, Institute of Health Science, Oxford. Greenhalgh T. Papers that go beyond numbers (qualitative research). In: Dept. of General Practice, University of Glasgow. *How to Read a Paper. The Basics of Evidence Based Medicine.* London, England: BMJ Publishing Group; 1997.

TABLE 10.6 **Key Questions for Appraising Studies of Outcome Measure Reliability**

QUESTION	ANSWER	WHY IT MATTERS
1. Is the study's purpose relevant to my clinical question?	Yes____ No____	If the purpose of the study is not relevant to your question, it is unlikely to be applicable.
2. Are the inclusion and exclusion criteria clearly defined and would my patient qualify for the study?	Yes____ No____	Ideally, the study inclusion and exclusion criteria for both study participants (e.g., patients) and testers (e.g., therapists) should be similar to your clinical environment. If they are not, you need to take this into consideration when integrating the study findings into your practice.
3. Are the outcome measures relevant to my clinical question and are they conducted in a clinically realistic manner?	Yes____ No____	Consider if the outcome measure was applied in a clinically replicable manner. This includes consideration of the amount of training provided to testers.
4. Is the study population (sample) sufficiently similar to my patient and to my clinical setting to justify the expectation that I would experience similar results?	Yes____ No____	Beyond the inclusion and exclusion criteria (question 2), it is important to consider the similarity of the study participants and therapists to your clinical environment.
5. Consider the number of participants being rated and the number of raters. Does the study have sufficient sample size?	Yes____ No____	Sufficient sample size is required to reduce the chance for random error to affect the results. A study that reports the method used to determine the minimum sample size (i.e., sample size calculation) has higher quality.
6. Do participants have sufficient diversity to assess the full range of the outcome measure?	Yes____ No____	A study of reliability should include the full spectrum of people that the outcome measure was designed to test. For example, consider a measure designed to assess a child's ability to engage in elementary school activities. Study participants should include all ages of elementary school children and children with a full range of participation abilities.
7. Are study participants stable in the characteristic of interest?	Yes____ No____	If the participants in a reliability study change substantially in the characteristic of interest, the reliability result will not be accurate. For example, in the case of an outcome measure designed to assess urinary incontinence, it is important that the participants not change any medication regimen that could change the severity of their incontinence between study assessments. Such a change would produce erroneous results for a study of reliability.
8. Is there evidence that the outcome measure was conducted in a reasonably consistent manner between assessments?	Yes____ No____	If it is conducted differently between assessments, the reliability of the outcome measure will be inaccurate. Consider a questionnaire completed by patients regarding their satisfaction with therapy services. If the first assessment is conducted in a quiet, private room and the second assessment is conducted over the phone and without privacy, patients might be prone to give different answers. This scenario would give inaccurate estimates of the measure's test-retest reliability.

TABLE 10.6 **Key Questions for Appraising Studies of Outcome Measure Reliability—cont'd**

QUESTION	ANSWER	WHY IT MATTERS
9. Were raters blinded to previous participant scores?	Yes____ No____	Raters should not have knowledge of previously collected scores. For example, for a study of PT students' inter-rater reliability in taking manual blood pressure measurements, students must be blinded to the measures collected by other students. Lack of blinding is likely to produce inaccurate results.
10. Is the time between assessments appropriate?		If assessments are conducted within too short a time interval, the reliability may be inaccurate because raters (or participants) are influenced by the initial test. Consider a study of the intra-rater reliability of manual muscle testing. If assessments are taken with only a minute between tests, the raters are likely to remember the strength scores from one test to another and participants may have fatigue that causes a decrease in their strength. In this case, rater recall could *overestimate* intra-rater reliability and participant fatigue could *underestimate* intra-rater reliability, making the results difficult to interpret.

TABLE 10.8 **Key Questions for Appraising Quality of Studies of Outcome Measure Validity**

QUESTION	EXPLANATION
1. Is the study's purpose relevant to my clinical question?	If the purpose of the study is not relevant to your question, it is unlikely to be applicable.
2. Are the inclusion and exclusion criteria clearly defined and would my patient qualify for the study?	Ideally, the study inclusion and exclusion criteria for both study participants (e.g., patients) and testers (e.g., therapists) should be similar to your clinical environment. If not, you need to take this into consideration when integrating the study findings into your practice.
3. Are the outcome measures relevant to my clinical question and are they conducted in a clinically realistic manner?	Consider if the outcome measure was applied in a clinically replicable manner. This includes consideration of the amount of training provided to testers.
4. Is the study population (sample) sufficiently similar to my patient and to my clinical setting to justify the expectation that I would experience similar results?	Beyond the inclusion and exclusion criteria (question 2), it is important to consider the similarity of the actual participants enrolled in the study to your clinical environment.
CONTENT VALIDITY	
Content validity is the appraisal of a study that assesses face validity and involves assessment of the quality of the expert panel.	
5. Did the experts have diverse expertise to allow the outcome measure to be assessed from different perspectives?	The purpose of the expert panel is to ensure that the measure addresses all aspects of the characteristics of the construct. A diverse panel helps to ensure the panel's success.
6. Did the researchers systematically collect and respond to the experts' feedback?	Researchers should report their process for collection and analysis to ensure full transparency for the face validity process.
CRITERION AND CONSTRUCT VALIDITY	
Criterion validity establishes the validity of an outcome measure by comparing it to another, more established measure. **Construct validity** establishes the ability of an outcome measure to assess an abstract characteristic or concept.	
7. Have the authors made a satisfactory argument for the credibility of the gold standard or reference criterion measure?	The internal validity of the study is suspect if the gold standard or reference measures were not strong criteria for assessing the validity of the measure of interest.

Continued

TABLE 10.8 **Key Questions for Appraising Quality of Studies of Outcome Measure Validity—cont'd**

CRITERION AND CONSTRUCT VALIDITY	
8. Were raters blinded to the results of the outcome measure of interest and the criterion measure?	It is important to minimize the impact of the outcome measures on each other.
9. Did all participants complete the outcome measure of interest and the gold standard or reference criterion measure?	All participants should be have completed both measures. There is bias if only a subset of subjects had both measures.
10. Was the time between assessments appropriate?	The measures should be conducted either concurrently (concurrent, convergent, and discriminant validity) or with an intervening time period (predictive validity). This depends on the purpose of the study. In the former situation it is important that the assessments be done close together but not so close as to have one assessment affect the other. In the case of predictive validity, it is important for enough time to elapse for the characteristic the researchers are trying to predict (e.g., falls) to occur.
11. For known-groups construct validity studies: Are the groups established as being distinctly different on the characteristic of interest?	The groups must be known to be different. If not, the study validity is in question. The authors must provide evidence that they can establish the difference between groups prior to starting the study.

TABLE 10.9 **Key Questions for Appraising Quality of Studies of Outcome Measure Clinical Meaningfulness**

QUESTION	EXPLANATION
1. Is the study's purpose relevant to my clinical question?	If the purpose of the study is not relevant to your question, it is unlikely to be applicable.
2. Are the inclusion and exclusion criteria clearly defined and would my patient qualify for the study?	Ideally, the study inclusion and exclusion criteria for both study participants (e.g., patients) and testers (e.g., therapists) should be similar to your clinical environment. If not, you need to take this into consideration when integrating the study findings into your clinic.
3. Are the outcome measures relevant to my clinical question and are they conducted in a clinically realistic manner?	Consider if the outcome measure was applied in a clinically replicable manner. This includes consideration of the amount of training provided to testers.
4. Is the study population (sample) sufficiently similar to my patient and to my clinical setting to justify the expectation that I would experience similar results?	Beyond the inclusion and exclusion criteria (question 2), it is important to consider the similarity of the study participants and therapists to your clinical environment.
FLOOR AND CEILING EFFECTS	
Floor and ceiling effects reflect a lack of sufficient range in the measure to fully characterize a group of patients.	
5. Does the study sample represent individuals who are likely to score across the full range of the outcome measure of interest?	To determine if an outcome measure has a floor and/or ceiling effect, individuals who are likely to perform very poorly (to assess for presence of floor effect) and very well (to assess for presence of ceiling affect) are required.
MINIMAL DETECTABLE CHANGE (MDC)	
MDC is the minimum amount of change required on an outcome measure to exceed anticipated measurement error and variability. Use questions for assessing quality of studies of reliability.	

TABLE 10.9   **Key Questions for Appraising Quality of Studies of Outcome Measure Clinical Meaningfulness—cont'd**

MINIMAL CLINICALLY IMPORTANT DIFFERENCE (MCID)	

MCID represents the minimum amount of change on an outcome measure that patients perceive as beneficial and that would justify a change in care.

6. Is the sampling procedure (recruitment strategy) likely to minimize bias?	The study should describe how and from where participants were recruited. Consecutive recruitment, in which any participant that meets eligibility criteria is invited to join the study, is the strongest design. To understand what change is meaningful to patients as a whole, it is important to have a diverse and unbiased sample.
7. Were the participants recruited likely to experience change during the course of the study?	In the case of studies of MCID (unlike studies of reliability and MDC) it is important that participants are likely to experience change in the outcome of interest. If some participants do not experience meaningful change, then a useful result cannot be generated.
8. Were sufficient time and circumstance afforded for participants to experience a meaningful change?	A useful result cannot be generated without sufficient time for meaningful change to occur among participants.
9. Does the study have sufficient sample size?	Sufficient sample size is required to reduce the chance that random error will affect the results. A study that reports the method used to determine the minimal sample size has higher quality.
10. Were the outcome measures reliable and valid?	MCID should not be established for an outcome measure without established reliability and validity. Likewise, the gold standard must, of course, have established reliability and validity. Finally, even with established reliability and validity, an MCID study must demonstrate that reliable methods were used within the study to collect the outcome of interest and gold standard.
11. Were raters blinded to previous participant scores?	Raters should not have knowledge of previously collected scores on both the outcome of interest and the gold standard to avoid bias.
12. Was the follow-up rate sufficient?	Follow-up with participants to assess change over time is essential to MCID study results. As a rule of thumb, follow-up should exceed 80% at minimum.

From: Haley SM, Fragala-Pinkham MA. Interpreting change scores of tests and measures used in physical therapy. *Phys Ther.* 2006;86:735-743; and Jaeschke R, Singer J, Guyatt GH. Measurement of health status. Ascertaining the minimal clinically important difference. *Control Clin Trials.* 1989;10:407.

Glossary

Activity: An ICF term that describes actions such as walking, climbing stairs, or getting out of bed.

AGREE II: A published, open access tool for the appraisal of clinical practice guidelines; the product of the AGREE Collaboration (http://www.agreecollaboration.org), an international collaboration of researchers and policy makers.

Alpha Level: The agreed-on value for the probability of chance in explaining the results of a study; it is typically 5% (0.05).

Analysis of Covariance (ANCOVA): A parametric statistic used to compare means and to remove the contribution of a factor that is present during treatment that was not controlled in the experimental design.

Analysis of Variance (ANOVA): A parametric statistic used to compare results for more than two groups.

Applicability: The relevance of a sample or study to your patient or patient group.

Appraise: To critically evaluate a research study.

Autocorrelation: Positive correlation among data points from the same subject.

Background Questions: Questions that supply general information and are not specific to an individual patient.

Basic Science Research: Often involves non-human research and is fundamental to evidence based physical therapy; typically tests theory.

Beta Weight: A standardized value that gives a weight (amount of contribution) to each of the independent variables in a regression equation.

Bias: Attitudes or design features that shape the results of a study.

Blinding: Restricting knowledge of the purpose of a research study, participant group, or other factors that would influence the conducting of or results from a research study (masking).

Body Functions and Structures: An ICF term that describes variables at the level of bodily functions and specific structures.

Bonferroni Correction: A planned statistical test used to correct for conducting multiple statistical tests and the possibility of a type I error.

C Statistic: A statistic to determine the probability of chance; used with small data sets or data with serial dependency.

Case Control Studies: Studies conducted after an outcome of interest has occurred. The factors that contributed to the outcome are studied in a group that has the outcome (case group) and compared to a group that does not have the outcome of interest but is similar to the case group in other factors (control group).

Case Studies: A written case description completed retrospectively and detailing the characteristics of one case and the course of intervention for that case; not a controlled single case experimental study.

Ceiling Effects: Reflect a lack of sufficient range in a measure to fully characterize a group of patients.

Celeration Line: A "best fit" line through the data beginning in the first phase of a single-subject study and extending through each phase in the study; assumes a linear trend.

Chi-square (χ^2): A statistic used to analyze nominal (categorical) data; compares the observed frequency of a particular category to the expected frequency of the category.

Clinical Meaningfulness: Refers to an outcome measure's ability to provide the clinician and the patient with consequential information.

Clinical Practice Guidelines (CPGs): Systematically developed statements designed to facilitate evidence based decision making for the management of specific health conditions.

Clinical Prediction Rule: A set of clinical guidelines using patient criteria for applying a specific intervention or used for prognosis of a patient with a specific set of clinical criteria.

Clinical Research: Involves human subjects and answers questions about diagnosis, intervention, prevention, and prognosis in relation to disease or injury.

Clinically Relevant: Results that show change on a measure that has value to the patient in terms of his or her daily life (patient values).

Cochrane Collaboration, The: Founded by Archie Cochrane, a British medical researcher and epidemiologist; was formally launched in 1993. Consists of groups of expert clinicians and scientists that conduct and publish systematic reviews of health-care interventions.

Cochrane Library of Systematic Reviews: A database of systematic reviews conducted by Cochrane-approved reviewers.

Coefficient of Determination: The square of the correlation coefficient and is expressed in the literature as r^2. This expresses the percentage of variance that is shared by the two variables.

Cohen's *d*:   The most common form of effect size (computed as the difference between treatment means divided by the standard deviation of the control group).

Cohort Design: A study design in which an identified group is followed prospectively; the most common study design for the development of a diagnostic test.

Cohort Study: In a cohort study, a group of subjects who are likely to develop a certain condition or outcome is followed into the future (prospectively) for a sufficient length of time to observe whether they develop the condition.

Concurrent Validity: Established when researchers demonstrate that an outcome measure has a high correlation with a criterion measure taken at the same point in time.

Confidence Intervals: A range of values that includes the real (or true) statistic of interest; states the probability that the estimate of the true statistic is within the given range.

Consecutive Sample: Subjects are entered into a research study as they enter a clinic, hospital, physical therapy practice, etc.

Construct Validity: Establishes the ability of an outcome measure to assess an abstract characteristic or concept; the most complex form of validity to establish.

Content Validity: Establishes that an outcome measure includes all the characteristics that it purports to measure.

Continuous Variable: A variable on a ratio or interval scale.

Convergent Validity: Establishes that a new measure correlates with another measure thought to measure a similar characteristic or concept.

Correlation: A measure of the extent to which two variables are associated; a measure of how these variables change together.

Correlation Coefficient: The pattern of change or association of the two variables over different levels of the variables; represented as *r*.

Criterion Validity: Establishes the validity of an outcome measure by comparing it to another, more established measure.

Critically Appraised Topic (CAT):   A summary that can be written in many forms for communication of research results.

Cronbach Alpha: A statistic that measures the internal consistency of items in a scale or other measurement tool.

Crossover Design: A research study design in which all subjects receive all treatment given in random order.

Cross-sectional Studies: In cross-sectional studies data are collected at one time point. A group of people with an outcome of interest might all be measured during 1 week or over a longer period of time but at the time of the presenting problem.

Data: Measured variables.

Database: A compilation of research evidence resources, primary lists of peer-reviewed journal articles, designed to organize the large amount of research published every year.

Dependent Variable: The variable that is a measured outcome in a research study.

Descriptive Statistics: Statistics including mean, mode, median, standard deviation, and standard error that give an overall impression of the typical values for the group as well as the variability within and between the groups.

Detrend: The removal of trends that occur in the baseline period of a single-subject design research study from the intervention and post-intervention periods. Detrending should be completed before visual and statistical analyses.

Dichotomous Outcomes: Outcome with two categories, e.g., healthy or sick, admitted or not admitted, relapsed or not relapsed.

Discriminant Validity: Establishes that a measure does not correlate with a measure thought to assess a distinctly different characteristic or concept.

Effect Size: A statistical approach to evaluate the magnitude of the difference between treatment groups following treatments.

Effectiveness: Refers to the effect of a treatment under typical clinical conditions; speaks to what is likely to happen given a treatment is typically implemented; contrasts with *efficacy*.

Efficacy: Refers to the effect of treatment under highly controlled conditions; contrasts with *effectiveness*.

Epidemiological Research: Research into the causes and occurrences of aspects of health and disease.

Ethnology: A qualitative study design typically used to study questions of individuals or groups of people with common heritage.

Evidence Based Practice (EBP): A method of clinical decision making and practice that integrates the best available scientific research evidence with clinical expertise and a patient's unique values and circumstances.

Face Validity: Based on informal evaluation by experts that a measure appears to measure what it is intended to measure.

False Negative: A negative test result when a movement problem is present.

False Positive: A positive test result when a movement problem is absent.

Five Steps of the EBP Process: Step 1: Identify the need for information and develop a focused and searchable clinical question. Step 2: Conduct a search to find the best possible research evidence to answer your question. Step 3: Critically appraise the research evidence for applicability and quality. Step 4: Integrate the critically appraised research evidence with clinical expertise and the patient's values and circumstances. Step 5: Evaluate the effectiveness and efficacy of your efforts in steps 1–4 and identify ways to improve them in the future.

Floor Effects: Reflect a lack of sufficient range in the measure to fully characterize a group of patients.

Foreground Questions: Questions that are specific to a particular patient, condition, and clinical outcome of interest.

Forest Plots: A graphical representation of the results of studies included in a systematic review.

Gaussian Distribution: A distribution of data that is symmetrical, continuous, and bell shaped (normal distribution).

Gold Standard: A measure that is accepted as the most valid measure available; typically used for comparison when developing a new test or measure.

Gold Standard: The criterion test that is used to define the presence or absence of a movement problem.

Google Scholar: A search engine developed by the company Google; designed to search the Internet for journal articles.

GRADE: Grading of Recommendations Assessment, Development and Evaluation; used to describe the quality of literature on a clinical topic and communicate the strength of recommendations.

Grounded Theory: A qualitative study design typically used to construct or validate a theory.

Health Literacy: The ability to understand the factors and contexts that relate to our health, both in terms of disease prevention and management of our health conditions.

Hooked on Evidence: A physical therapy–specific database developed by the American Physical Therapy Association. This database is a grassroots project available to APTA members.

Independent Variable: The variable that is used to separate groups in a randomized clinical trial.

Inferential Statistics: Statistical tests that use the mathematics of probability to interpret the differences observed in research studies; helpful in making conclusions about the differences between groups. These statistics focus on the question, Is the outcome due to the intervention or could it be due to chance?

Intention to Treat: All subjects in a research study are analyzed in the groups to which they were initially assigned, even if they did not complete the study.

Intercept: The Y-intercept is the value of Y when the value of X is zero in a regression analysis.

Interclass Correlation Coefficient (ICC): One of several common statistical methods that can be used for making comparisons of test-retest, intra-rater, and inter-rater reliability; used when data are continuous.

Internal Consistency: Establishes the extent to which multiple items within an outcome measure reflect the same construct.

International Classification of Function (ICF): The International Classification of Functioning, Disability and Health (ICF); a classification of health and health-related domains developed by the World Health Organization (WHO).

Inter-Rater Reliability: Agreement of score between individuals completing the same measurement.

Interval: Variables that are measured precisely and share the properties of equal intervals as with ratio scales.

Intra-Rater Reliability: Agreement within an individual with repeat administrations of a measurement.

Kappa (κ): One of several common statistical methods that can be used for making comparisons of test-retest, intra-rater, and inter-rater reliability; used when data are nominal with more than two categories.

Key words: Important words from your searchable clinical question and/or synonyms of those words.

Knowledge Brokers (KB): A local champion of the change in practice that is supported by evidence and that has been identified as a goal for practice.

Knowledge Translation (KT): A term used to describe the various methods for translating research evidence into practice.

Known-Groups Validity: Establishes that an outcome measure produces different scores for groups with known differences on the characteristic being measured.

Language Bias: Results when important study results are excluded from a systematic review because of language.

Likelihood Ratio, Negative: The probability that a person with a negative diagnostic test result does not have the suspected problem.

Likelihood Ratio, Positive: The probability that a person with a positive diagnostic test result has the suspected problem.

Logistic Regression: Used when the outcome measure of interest is categorical, typically dichotomous (two categories).

Longitudinal: A study design that collects repeated data on the same individuals over a period of time.

Masking: Restricting knowledge of the purpose of a research study, participant group, or other factors that would influence the conducting of or results from a research study (blinding).

Mean: The arithmetic average—the mean of a set of observations is simply their sum, divided by the number of observations.

Measures of Association: Statistical tests that determine the similarity of change in variables or the values of two variables at one time point.

Measures of Central Tendency: Measures of the average or most typical; the most widely used statistical description of data.

Measures of Variability: Reflect the degree of spread or dispersion that characterizes a group of scores and the degree to which a set of scores differs from some measure of central tendency.

Median: The 50th percentile of a distribution—the point below which half of the observations fall.

MEDLINE: MEDLINE is a component of PubMed, an open access online database of biomedical journal citations and abstracts created by the U.S. National Library of Medicine.

Member Checking: A method to verify that the investigator has adequately represented the participant's contributions to the question under study.

MeSH Terms: Words that are designed to provide a common and consistent language across published articles.

Meta-analysis: A statistical method used to summarize outcomes across multiple primary studies as a part of a systematic review.

Minimal Clinically Important Difference (MCID): A measure of responsiveness that represents the minimum amount of change on an outcome measure that patients perceive as beneficial and would justify change in care.

Minimal Detectable Change (MDC): The minimum amount of change required on an outcome measure to exceed anticipated measurement error and variability.

Mode: The most frequently occurring observation—the most popular score of a class of scores.

Multiple Regression: A statistical test that determines a numerical prediction given multiple contributing variables.

My NCBI: National Center for Biotechnology Information (NCBI); provides a mechanism for pushing new research results from previously conducted PubMed searches.

Narrative Review: Author interpretation of research literature; typically without statistical analyses; commonly published in peer-reviewed research journals.

National Guidelines Clearinghouse: An open access resource for evidence based clinical practice guidelines.

Negative Correlation: A value of –1.0; as one variable increases, the other variable decreases.

Negative Likelihood Ratio: Expresses the numeric value of a negative test if the movement problem is present.

Negative Predictive Value: Proportion of people with a negative test who do not have the movement problem as defined by the gold standard.

Nominal: Variables that are in categories; nominal scales are also termed categorical, and there is no order of the categories in nominal scales.

Non-normally Distributed Data: A distribution of data that is not bell shaped (normal distribution).

Normal Distribution: The distribution of data based on repeated measures in a large sample of people.

Null Hypothesis: The hypothesis in a research study that groups are considered (in statistical terms) to be equal, i.e., there is no difference between groups.

Number Needed to Treat (NNT):   A ratio between the rate of the desired outcome in the experimental group and the rate of the desired outcome in the control or comparison group.

Odds Ratios: A commonly used expression of relative risk statistics.

Operational Definition: A specific definition that is used in a research study.

Ordinal: Variables that are in categories that are ordered; the ranking within the scale typically indicates most to least, but the distance between ranks is not uniform within the scale.

Outcome Measure: Any characteristic or quality measured to assess a patient's status; commonly collected at the beginning, middle, and end of a research study.

Ovid: An electronic access system allowing access to electronic databases such as MEDLINE.

p **Values:** An expression of the probability that the difference that has been identified is due to chance ($p =$)

Participation: An ICF term that includes work, school, and community involvement and participation restrictions describes problems at this level.

Pearson Product-Moment Coefficient of Correlation: A statistical test of the association of two variables; range from +1 to –1.

PEDro: The Physiotherapy Evidence Database (PEDro); a free, Web-based database of evidence relevant to physical therapy.

Performance-Based Measure: A type of outcome measure that measures patient action; requires the patient to perform a new set of tasks.

Phenomenology: A qualitative study design typically used to study experiences in life.

PICO: An acronym used to illustrate key components of a searchable clinical question about interventions: Patient (or Population) and clinical characteristics, Intervention, Comparison (referring to an alternative intervention), and Outcome.

Podcasts: Episodically released digital media files (either audio or video) for automatic download to your computer or portable media player; generally free of charge.

Positive Correlation: A value of +1.0; as one variable increases or decreases, the other variable varies in the same direction.

Positive Likelihood Ratio: Expresses the numerical value of a positive test if the movement problem is present.

Positive Predictive Value: Proportion of people with a positive test who have the movement problem as defined by the gold standard.

Post-Test Probability: The probability that a person has a movement problem after a diagnostic.

Power: A statistical term; the likelihood that the test will detect a difference between groups if there is a difference.

Predictive Validity: Established when researchers demonstrate that an outcome measure has a high correlation with a future criterion measure.

Predictor Variables: Independent variables used in regression analysis that are thought to relate to the predicted variable.

Pre-Test Probability: The probability that a person has a movement problem before diagnostic testing; estimated from prevalence of the problem; more often in PT estimated from history and patient symptoms.

Primary Studies: Original studies such as randomized clinical trials or cohort studies.

Prognostic Equation: An equation used in regression analysis that includes the independent variables thought to relate to the prediction of the dependent variable.

ProQuest: An electronic database library.

Prospective Studies: Research designs in which data are collected toward the future (opposite of retrospective design); typically used to study cause.

Psychometric Properties: The intrinsic properties of an outcome measure; include the concepts of reliability, validity, and clinical meaningfulness.

Publication Bias: The tendency for studies with positive results to be published more often than studies with nonsignificant results.

PubMed: An open-access, online database of biomedical journal citations and abstracts created by the U.S. National Library of Medicine.

Pull Technology: Used to retrieve electronic information for a specific need on demand.

Push Technology: Information is sent to an individual.

Qualitative Research: Focuses on questions of experience, culture, and social/emotional health. Study designs used in qualitative research facilitate understanding of the processes that are experienced by an individual, group of individuals, or an entire culture of people during everyday life.

Quality: Used to infer the validity of a research study.

Quality Assessment of Diagnostic Accuracy Studies (QUADAS):   A guide for the appraisal of applicability and quality of a diagnostic study.

Questionnaire: A type of outcome measure; requires that either a therapist interviews a patient or the patient independently answers questions.

Randomized Clinical Trial (RCT):   An experimental design in which treatments are compared. The RCT is considered one of the most valid designs to determine if a particular physical therapy treatment has a positive effect.

Randomized Controlled Trial (RCT):   An experimental design in which treatments are compared. The RCT is considered one of the most valid designs to determine whether a particular physical therapy treatment has a positive effect.

Range: The values between the highest and lowest scores in a distribution.

Ratio Level Variable: Variables that are ordered precisely and continuously; the measured intervals on the scale are equal.

Receiver Operating Characteristics Curve (ROC):   A graph of sensitivity and specificity values determined from various cut points on a study test; used to determine the best cut points for the test.

Reference Interval: The range of values from a sample group representing people without a specific movement problem; used to define the cut points for diagnostic tests.

Reference Intervals: A range of scores that captures individuals without a movement problem.

Reference Management Systems: Software databases for managing research and other literature.

Reference Standard: Used when a gold standard criterion does not exist for a given characteristic; less irrefutable than a gold standard, but considered a reasonable comparison for the outcome measure of interest.

Regression: A statistical analysis based on correlation statistics that relates independent variable(s) to a dependent variable with a prediction equation.

Relative Risk: A type of commonly used statistics in epidemiology for risk analysis in prognostic studies.

Reliability: The ability for people and instruments to produce consistent values over time.

Repeated Measures: A parametric statistic (Analysis of Variance) used to compare multiple measures from the same subjects. The multiple measures may be taken within a short or long period of time.

Research Notation: Helpful shorthand to diagram the design of an intervention study and highlight the "big picture" of the overall study.

Responsiveness: Reflects an outcome measure's ability to detect change over time.

Risk Ratio: A commonly used expression of relative risk statistics; computed as the incidence rate of one group compared to the incidence rate of another group.

Sample: Participants chosen for a study.

Scale of Measurement: Defines the type of data; all measurement tools have a specific scale that is used to describe the variable of interest.

Scientific Research: Empirical evidence acquired through systematic testing of a hypothesis.

Search Engine: The user interface that allows specific articles to be identified in a database.

Searchable Clinical Question: A question with a specific structure that makes it easier to search databases for the best available research evidence.

Secondary Research Studies: "Studies of studies" that summarize information from multiple, primary studies.

Selective Sample: A sample in a research study that is specifically selected, e.g., the test or treatment that might be effective for patients with specific characteristics.

Sensitivity: Expresses test accuracy in correctly identifying a problem as established by the gold standard.

Sensitivity: The proportion of people with the movement problem identified by the gold standard who test positive on the study test; the ability of a test to identify a movement problem when it is present.

Serial Dependency: Repeated measures on the same person, creating dependency in the data.

Simple Linear Regression: One variable (X) is used to predict the level of another variable (Y), with the assumption that the two variables have a linear relationship.

Single-Subject Design (SSD):   One participant is followed and treated repeatedly and intensely.

Slope: The angle of the regression line, indicating the rate of change of one variable in relation to another.

Slope of the Celeration Line: A part of visual interpretation of data; the direction and pitch of the slope convey the amount and rate of increase or decrease in the data; assumes a linear trend.

SnNout: Indicates that a negative test result from a highly sensitive test can assist in ruling out the diagnosis.

Spearman's Rho: One of several common statistical methods that can be used for making comparisons of test-retest, intra-rater, and inter-rater reliability; used to compare two ranked variables.

Specificity: Expresses the test's ability to correctly identify the absence of a problem as established by the gold standard.

Specificity: The proportion of people without a movement problem as identified by the gold standard who test negative on the study test; the ability of a test to identify that a movement problem is not present.

SpPin: Indicates that a positive test result from a highly specific test can assist you in ruling in the diagnosis.

Standard Deviation: The most commonly used measure of variability; the average amount that each of the individual scores varies from the mean of the set of scores.

Standards for Reporting of Diagnostic Accuracy (STARD):   Used to systematically report diagnostic study research for publication; not directly applicable to the appraisal process for individual diagnostic studies.

Statistical Heterogeneity: Also called a test of statistical homogeneity; assesses the likelihood that the variability between studies is due to chance.

Stratification: A sampling technique in which a subgroup of subjects is represented in percentage or absolute numbers in each treatment group.

Strength: A factor in a research study that is well controlled and contributes to the conclusion that the treatment was responsible for the change in the patients and not other uncontrolled factors.

Systematic Review: A special type of research study that includes a statistical analysis and summary of research on a specific topic; characterized as secondary research.

t-**Test:** A parametric statistic that is used to compare the means of two groups.

Technology Profile: A select combination of technology resources used to support EBP.

Test-retest reliability: Establishes the extent to which an outcome measure remains the same when no patient change has occurred.

Threat: A factor in a research study that is not controlled in a study and that might affect the results.

Translating Research Into Practice (TRIP):   A search engine that searches over 21 databases simultaneously.

Triangulation: The use of different perspectives to study the identified process.

TRIP Database: An electronic database for clinical research evidence.

True Negative: A negative test result when the movement problem is absent.

True Positive: A positive test result when the movement problem is present.

Two-Standard Deviation: A statistic used in single-subject research analysis; data must be normally distributed and not have a significant autocorrelation coefficient; means and standard deviations (SD) are computed in the baseline and extended into treatment phases; data are significant if two data points fall above or below the values extended from the baseline.

Type I Error: The false conclusion that there is a statistically significant difference when there is no difference.

Type II Error: The false conclusion that there is no statistically significant difference between groups when there truly is a difference.

Validity: The quality of a research study; also the extent to which an outcome measure is useful.

Variance: A measure of the variability in a sample. The standard deviation is the square root of the variance.

Index